Canine Lameness

Canine Lameness

Edited by

Felix Michael Duerr, Dr. med. vet., MS, DACVS-SA, DECVS, DACVSMR

Associate Professor, Small Animal Orthopedics
Department of Clinical Sciences
College of Veterinary Medicine and Biomedical Sciences
Colorado State University
Fort Collins, CO, USA

WILEY Blackwell

Registered Office
John Wiley & Sons, Inc., 111 River Street, Hoboken, NJ 07030, USA

Editorial Office
111 River Street, Hoboken, NJ 07030, USA

For details of our global editorial offices, customer services, and more information about Wiley products visit us at www.wiley.com.

Wiley also publishes its books in a variety of electronic formats and by print-on-demand. Some content that appears in standard print versions of this book may not be available in other formats.

Library of Congress Cataloging-in-Publication Data

Names: Michael Duerr, Felix, editor.
Title: Canine lameness / edited by Felix Michael Duerr, Dr. med. vet., MS,
    DACVS-SA, DECVS, DACVSMR, Associate Professor, Small Animal Orthopedics,
    Department of Clinical Sciences, College of Veterinary Medicine and
    Biomedical Sciences, Colorado State University, USA.
Description: Hoboken : Wiley-Blackwell, 2020. | Includes bibliographical
    references and index.
Identifiers: LCCN 2019045104 (print) | LCCN 2019045105 (ebook) | ISBN
    9781119474029 (paperback) | ISBN 9781119474036 (adobe pdf) | ISBN
    9781119474050 (epub)
Subjects: LCSH: Lameness in dogs.
Classification: LCC SF992.L36 C36 2020 (print) | LCC SF992.L36 (ebook) |
    DDC 636.7/089758–dc23
LC record available at https://lccn.loc.gov/2019045104
LC ebook record available at https://lccn.loc.gov/2019045105

Cover Design: Wiley
Cover Images: Courtesy of Felix Duerr

Set in 9.5/12.5pt STIX Two Text by SPi Global, Pondicherry, India

10 9 8 7 6 5 4 3 2 1

This book is dedicated to Alice, Banjo, Karla, Connor, Enno, Fine, Frankie, Harley, Keester, Kelsey, Kono, Kutya, Lefty, Tide, Tootle, and Zach, and their phenomenal people at the other end of the leash.

Contents

20 Hip Region *347*

Nina R. Kieves

List of Contributors

Lisa Bartner, DVM, MS, DACVIM (Neurology)
Assistant Professor
Neurology/Neurosurgery
Department of Clinical Sciences
College of Veterinary Medicine and
Biomedical Sciences
Colorado State University
Fort Collins, CO
USA

**Felix Michael Duerr, Dr. med. vet., MS,
DACVS-SA, DECVS, DACVSMR**
Associate Professor
Small Animal Orthopedics
Department of Clinical Sciences
College of Veterinary Medicine and
Biomedical Sciences
Colorado State University
Fort Collins, CO
USA

Sasha Foster, MSPT, CCRT
James L. Voss Veterinary Teaching Hospital
Colorado State University
Fort Collins, CO
USA

Adam Harris, DVM
Resident
Clinical Pathology
Department of Microbiology, Immunology,
and Pathology
College of Veterinary Medicine and
Biomedical Sciences
Colorado State University
Fort Collins, CO
USA

Kristina M. Kiefer, DVM, PhD, CCRP, DACVSMR
VetSSMART, LLC
Veterinary Surgery and
Sports Medicine Assistance,
Research and Tutelage
St. Paul, MN
USA

Nina R. Kieves, DVM, DACVS-SA, DACVSMR
Assistant Professor
Small Animal Orthopedic Surgery
Department of Veterinary
Clinical Sciences
The Ohio State University
Columbus, OH
USA

**Nicolaas E. Lambrechts, BVSc, MMedVet
(Surgery), DECVS, DACVSMR**
Associate Professor
Small Animal Orthopedics
Department of Clinical Sciences
College of Veterinary Medicine and
Biomedical Sciences
Colorado State University
Fort Collins, CO
USA

Kathleen Linn, DVM, MS, DACVS
Associate Professor
Small Animal Surgery
Department of Small Animal Clinical
Sciences
Western College of Veterinary Medicine
University of Saskatchewan
Saskatoon, Saskatchewan
Canada

Denis J. Marcellin-Little, DEDV, DACVS, DACVSMR (Charter)
Professor
Orthopedic Surgery
Department of Veterinary Surgical and
Radiological Sciences
School of Veterinary Medicine
University of California
Davis, CA
USA

Angela J. Marolf, DVM, DACVR
Associate Professor
Radiology
Department of Environmental and
Radiological Health Sciences
College of Veterinary Medicine and
Biomedical Sciences
Colorado State University
Fort Collins, CO
USA

Kelly Santangelo, DVM, PhD, DACVP
Associate Professor
Clinical Pathology
Department of Microbiology, Immunology,
and Pathology
College of Veterinary Medicine and
Biomedical Sciences
Colorado State University
Fort Collins, CO
USA

Bernard Séguin, DVM, MS, DACVS
ACVS Founding Fellow
Surgical Oncology
Associate Professor
Surgical Oncology
Department of Clinical Sciences
College of Veterinary Medicine and
Biomedical Sciences
Flint Animal Cancer Center
Colorado State University
Fort Collins, CO
USA

Bryan T. Torres, DVM, PhD, DACVS-SA, DACVSMR
Assistant Professor
Small Animal Orthopedic Surgery
Director of the Motion Analysis Laboratory
Department of Veterinary Medicine and
Surgery
College of Veterinary Medicine
University of Missouri
Columbia, MO
USA

Dirsko J.F. von Pfeil, Dr. med. vet., DVM, DACVS, DECVS, DACVSMR
Owner, Surgeon:
Small Animal Surgery Locum, PLLC
Dallas, TX
USA
Staff Surgeon:
Sirius Veterinary Orthopedic Center
Omaha, NE
USA

Rick Wall, DVM, DACVSMR
Animal Clinics of The Woodlands
The Woodlands, TX
USA
Center for Veterinary Pain Management and
Rehabilitation
The Woodlands, TX
USA

Jennifer Warnock, DVM, PhD, DACVS-SA
Carlson College of Veterinary Medicine
Oregon State University
Corvallis, OR
USA

Preface

Canine lameness is a common problem in clinical practice. While there is a plethora of equine literature illuminating causes of equine lameness, few such resources are available in the canine field. This is likely because of the greater emphasis on lameness in daily equine practice. However, with the recent surge of canine sports and pet owners placing increasingly more emphasis on maximizing their dogs' happiness and activity, the field of canine orthopedics is changing – thus, determining an accurate diagnosis and the prevention of orthopedic disease are playing a larger role in canine practice. The goal of this textbook, therefore, is to address this gap in the literature by providing a single resource of clinically relevant information for the veterinary health professional faced with canine lameness problems.

Within the orthopedic community, lameness is generally defined as an alteration of normal locomotion that may be due to pain (e.g. arthritis or fractures), mechanical dysfunction (e.g. muscle contractures), or neurologic conditions (e.g. spinal cord compression from disc disease; Renberg 2001; Baxter and Stashak 2011). However, within the neurologic community, lameness is more specifically defined as pain from compression of the nerve roots and meninges (Chapter 4; Dewey et al. 2016). This "neurogenic lameness" and monoparesis (i.e. lower motor neuron disease of a single limb) are the most common reason for confusion between orthopedic and neurologic disease. For the purpose of this book, the term lameness is applied in its broader meaning, unless specified otherwise (i.e. Chapters 4, 16, 21).

This book is divided into two sections. Section 1 focuses on lameness evaluation, describing the different types of exams (e.g. orthopedic and neurologic examination, etc.) that aid in localization of a problem causing gait abnormalities (Part I) and the recommendations regarding specific diagnostic procedures that aid in establishing a definitive diagnosis (Part II). Section 2 describes the most common reasons for lameness, organized by the anatomical regions of the distal limb (Part III), thoracic (Part IV), and pelvic (Part V) areas including the major joints and surrounding areas. For ease of identification these chapters are marked with colored tabs. This organization was chosen to provide a resource that mimics the hypothetical clinical scenario where the examiner first identifies an abnormality (e.g. pain or swelling) in a specific area and then develops a differential diagnosis list and diagnostic plan based on that finding. Thus, each region chapter focuses on musculoskeletal diseases of the specific area. The other two causes of lameness, namely oncologic and neurologic, are described in the individual Chapters 16, 17 and 21, 22 for the thoracic and pelvic limb, respectively.

The emphasis of this text is to provide the necessary resources to establish a diagnosis for dogs presenting with lameness, with a particular focus on physical exam and radiographic findings. While neurologic conditions are included, the scope of the book is limited to conditions that can be confused with lameness. For this reason, conditions that cause obvious neurologic abnormalities in multiple limbs are only discussed to the degree that they apply as a differential diagnosis for lameness. The reader is encouraged to consult other resources for further details on neurologic conditions. Similarly, the purpose of this book is not to provide a detailed anatomic description of each region but rather to limit the scope to the most clinically relevant information. Veterinary anatomic textbooks will provide a useful resource to the reader seeking more detailed anatomic descriptions. Additionally, since this book is focused on the diagnosis of lameness, treatment options are only briefly mentioned. The reader should consult other texts for detailed information on the best management of each individual condition. Recommended anatomy, surgery, and neurology resources include the following texts: Evans and De Lahunta (2013), Tobias and Johnston (2013), Dewey and Da Costa (2016), and Fossum (2018).

> The more that you read, the more things you will know. The more that you learn, the more places you'll go.
>
> *Dr. Seuss*

References

Baxter, G.M. and Stashak, T.S. (2011). Examination for lameness. In: *Adams and Stashak's Lameness in Horses* (ed. G.M. Baxter), 109–206. Hoboken: Wiley-Blackwell.

Dewey, C.W. and Da Costa, R.C. (2016). *Practical Guide to Canine and Feline Neurology*. Hoboken: Wiley-Blackwell.

Dewey, C.W., Da Costa, R.C., and Thomas, W.B. (2016). Performing the neurologic examination. In: *Practical Guide to Canine and Feline Neurology*, 3e (eds. C.W. Dewey and R.C. Da Costa), 92–137. Hoboken: Wiley-Blackwell.

Evans, H.E. and De Lahunta, A. (2013). *Miller's Anatomy of the Dog*. Philadelphia: Saunders.

Fossum, T.W. (2018). *Small Animal Surgery*. St. Louis: Elsevier Health Sciences.

Renberg, W.C. (2001). Evaluation of the lame patient. *Vet Clin North Am Small Anim Pract* 31 (1): 1–16.

Tobias, K.M. and Johnston, S.A. (2013). *Veterinary Surgery: Small Animal*. St. Louis: Elsevier Health Sciences.

Acknowledgments

Countless people have contributed to this book in such diverse ways that I am hesitant to start listing names for fear of missing someone – all were critical to creating the text in hand and I am grateful so many colleagues offered their expertise and made this book all the better through their contribution. Karyl Whitman, our tireless editor and Jeremy Delcambre, the outstanding anatomist, helped get all the fine details right. The beautiful drawings were provided by Molly Borman. Colorado State University's Orthopedic Team contributed abundant case material, insightful discussions, and exceptional photographs. My friends and family, both the two- and four-legged ones, deserve a heartfelt "Thank You" for putting up with me throughout the protracted writing process, particularly Colleen, who had avoided the topic of canine lameness throughout much of her professional career only to be subjected to an unsolicited crash course in the comfort of our own home. Many walks, rides, meals, drinks, and adventures are owed to them all. And finally, to my fantastic parents, Christa and Ulrich M. Duerr, for decades of support and encouragement to follow my passion and without whom none of this would have been possible.

Felix Duerr

Editor Biography

Felix Duerr completed his veterinary degree in Hannover, Germany, followed by internships in Saskatoon, SK, Canada, and a residency in Small Animal Surgery at Colorado State University, Fort Collins, CO, USA. He spent a number of years working as a surgeon in private practice before returning to Colorado State University in 2011. He is a Diplomate of the American College of Veterinary Surgeons (ACVS), European College of Veterinary Surgeons (ECVS), and the American College of Veterinary Sports Medicine and Rehabilitation (ACVSMR). Dr. Duerr currently oversees the Orthopedic Medicine and Mobility Program at Colorado State University and is passionate about finding new treatment options for animals with mobility concerns. He has a particular interest in injury prevention, which is what triggered the idea for this book – that establishing an accurate diagnosis early in the disease process is the key to optimizing treatment solutions.

About the Companion Website

Don't forget to visit the companion website for this book:

www.wiley.com/go/duerr/lameness

There you will find valuable video clips to enhance your learning.

Scan this QR code to visit the companion website.

Section 1

Lameness Diagnosis

Part I

Lameness Evaluation

1

Subjective Gait Evaluation

Felix Michael Duerr

Department of Clinical Sciences, College of Veterinary Medicine and Biomedical Sciences, Colorado State University, Fort Collins, CO, USA

1.1 Introduction

Lameness can be due to orthopedic, oncologic, or neurologic conditions that disrupt the tissues responsible for normal locomotion. Subjective gait analysis is one component of the orthopedic and neurologic examination and provides valuable information to assist in determining what limb(s) and structures are affected. Succeeding chapters further discuss the other components that play an important role in any canine lameness evaluation (e.g. history, orthopedic examination, etc.).

1.2 Observation at Rest

Subjective gait evaluation starts by observing the animal at rest, when it stands, or raises from a sitting or lying position. Frequently, this can be accomplished by letting the animal roam freely in the exam room during the history taking. During this time, the observer may also evaluate mental status, behavior, and posture of the patient (which is part of the neurologic exam, see Chapter 4). Many dogs will show obvious off-loading of the affected limb during standing (Video 1.1), particularly with cranial cruciate ligament disease and neurogenic (i.e. nerve root signature) lameness. Caution should be used when interpreting off-loading if the animal is not standing square. Anxious animals may be encouraged to stand still by leading them toward an exit door, pausing prior to opening the door. Most dogs will focus on the door being opened and while being distracted, the observer can judge weight-bearing in a square position.

Video 1.1:

Pelvic limb lameness – unilateral CCLD.

Difficulty in either rising, or sitting, or both suggests a problem in the hind end. For example, animals with cranial cruciate ligament disease will display a classic sitting pattern avoiding flexion of the affected stifle(s). Animals that sit "square" (Chapters 19 and 20; Video 20.2) are unlikely to suffer from cruciate disease. Animals with lumbosacral disease may have difficulty rising, while animals with bilateral cruciate disease will hesitate to sit down. Spontaneous knuckling (i.e. standing on the dorsum of their paw during stance) indicates neurologic disease.

1.3 Observation in Motion

During the subjective gait evaluation, the observer is attempting to localize and specify the type of lameness (e.g. which leg is most severely affected, neurologic versus orthopedic origin, etc.). Certain gait features, such as ataxia or dragging/scuffing of the toes, clearly indicate neurologic disease. Decreased range of motion in a joint and the associated gait changes may point toward an articular source of the lameness. Changes in stride length may indicate a musculoskeletal or neurologic problem. Increased range of motion may indicate a ligament problem (such as carpal hyperextension injury with increased carpal extension or Achilles tendon rupture with increased tarsal flexion).

The use of slow-motion video analysis for improving the observer's ability to identify a lameness has been reported in dogs and horses; however, no clinical benefit was observed in a recent canine study using dogs (He Lane et al. 2015). Although in that study the degree of lameness was not quantified. Nonetheless, in the author's experience, this technique can be extremely helpful in dogs with a subtle lameness (Video 1.2). Slow-motion videography is integrated into newer smart phone devices and numerous apps also offer this feature, thus making it easily utilized in daily practice.

Video 1.2:

Thoracic limb lameness – case examples.

1.3.1 Presentation

Ideally, the animal is presented by a dedicated handler/technician. Since most owners are not used to walking their dog without interfering with gait, this approach will allow reducing the time required to complete the lameness evaluation: the handler should allow the animal to move freely (e.g. not pulling on the leash) yet at a constant speed. Pulling on the leash makes observation of a head nod more difficult. Ideally, the animal should look straight ahead during evaluation. This can be accomplished by letting the animal walk toward the owner.

The animal should be observed at the walk and ideally at the trot if the severity of the lameness allows. In general, if animals are unable to trot, their disease should be severe enough that lameness identification can be done at a stance or walk. A flat, even surface with good traction, such as a parking lot or driveway, is ideal to avoid distractions (such as areas to sniff/mark). The gait should be viewed both from the side (to judge stride length, symmetry, and possible changes in sagittal joint range of motion) and the animal moving toward and away from the examiner (to judge head nod, pelvic tilt, and frontal plane abnormalities).

To make a lameness more detectable, the animal can be asked to trot in circles, walk stairs, go up and down hills, or perform the tasks that trigger an impaired gait or movement (e.g. such as jumping for agility dogs). For example, animals with thoracic limb disease will display a more pronounced head nod when going downstairs and will use the non-affected limb to step down first. Animals with hip dysplasia will show simultaneous advancement of the pelvic limbs (i.e. "bunny hopping") when going upstairs. Subjective gait evaluation generally is performed prior to manipulation; however, sometimes manipulation may worsen the lameness.

1.3.2 Gait Patterns

To allow the clinician appropriate evaluation of gait, an understanding of normal gait patterns is essential. Gait patterns are generally described by their beat, whether they have a suspension phase and whether they are lateral or diagonal gait patterns. The *beat* describes the number of ground impacts within each stride cycle (i.e. the walk is a four-beat gait because each limb touches the ground at different time points within the stride cycle). The *suspension phase* describes a phase where none of the feet are touching the ground, which is observed only in gaits with a high velocity like the trot and canter. The description of *diagonal versus lateral* gait describes which limb pair is supporting the animal's weight (i.e. a diagonal gait indicates that the diagonal limb pairs move simultaneously such as when trotting; whereas, in a lateral gait, the ipsilateral limb pairs move simultaneously such as when pacing). For detailed online descriptions of the footfall patterns and slow-motion animations, consult Datt and Fletcher (2012).

The dog's ambulatory motion has been described to consist of up to seven different gait patterns: walk, trot, pace, amble, canter, transverse and rotary gallop (Leach et al. 1977; Datt and Fletcher 2012). The *walk* is a four-beat gait without a suspension phase. The *amble* is an accelerated walk, maintaining the four-beat gait pattern. The *trot* is a two-beat, diagonal gait with suspension phase. The *pace* is a two-beat, lateral gait in which ipsilateral limb pairs move in synchrony (Figure 1.1 and Video 1.3). The *canter* is an asymmetric gait (i.e. a three-beat gait with different patterns on the right and left side). The *gallop* is the fastest gait. While there has been controversy whether the pace is a normal or abnormal gait, it has been described to be used by dogs without obvious orthopedic disease. Proposed reasons for dogs to pace include orthopedic pathology, tiring, confirmation such as proportionally long legs, or an acquired gait due to being forced to walk at speeds between the walk and trot (Wendland et al. 2016). Particularly if a dog switches from a regular walk to pacing, evaluation for any change in orthopedic status is indicated. However, while pacing as the only symptom (i.e. without obvious lameness) may be an early indicator of musculoskeletal disease, it should not be considered pathologic by itself. Regardless, it is important for the clinician to assess whether a dog uses the pace.

Video 1.3:

Trotting versus pacing.

Another important reason to understand gait patterns is to allow for interpretation of compensation patterns for lameness such as head nod or pelvic tilt. The trot is the most steady and rhythmic gait and therefore generally the easiest gait to identify a mild–moderate lameness. Interpretation of lameness becomes more complicated in animals that are pacing. As such, if the animal can be

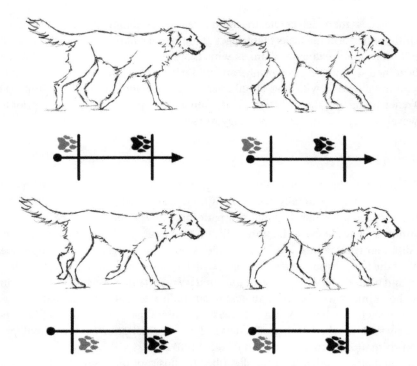

Figure 1.1 Simplification of the footfall patterns of the pace. The pace is a symmetrical lateral gait, meaning that ipsilateral limb pairs move simultaneously. Black paw prints represent thoracic limb feet and grey paw prints represent pelvic limb feet.

discouraged from pacing by choosing a different velocity (e.g. by having the handler increasing speed, see Video 1.3), this may simplify the subjective gait analysis.

1.3.3 Head Nod and Pelvic Tilt

To unload a painful limb, animals use specific adaptive strategies to reduce pain associated with weight-bearing. This is accomplished by shifting weight toward the unaffected limb(s), changes in joint angles, and alterations in foot flight. In horses, the most consistent compensatory movements are the vertical displacement and acceleration of the head in thoracic limb lameness and the vertical movement of the pelvis/tuber coxae in pelvic limb lameness (Baxter and Stashak 2011; Ross 2011). However, an overlap of these movements has been described (i.e. head movement with pelvic limb gait abnormalities particularly if lameness is severe).

Vertical head movement (i.e. the head and neck moving up and down during ambulation), also described as a head nod or head bob, is generally associated with thoracic limb lameness. It is observed because the animal attempts to off-weight the affected leg. The head is lowered when the non-affected thoracic limb touches the ground and raised when the affected thoracic limb touches the ground (Figure 1.2 and Video 1.2). To reduce the amount of weight placed on the affected limb, raising of the head happens just before the foot touches the ground. This can be observed in slow motion and in horses it has been suggested that raising of the head and neck may be easier to observe than the lowering (Ross 2011). A head nod may also be observed with severe pelvic limb lameness, because the animal is attempting to shift its body weight forward. Since the trot is a diagonal

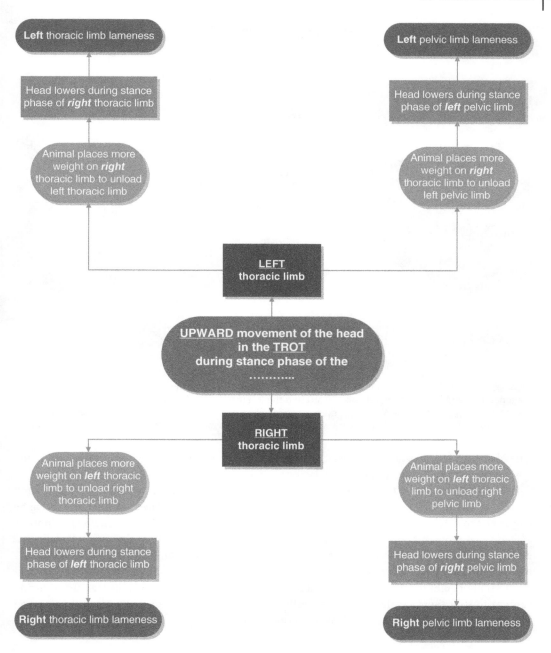

Figure 1.2 Interpretation of head movement for canine lameness during trotting (a diagonal gait), illustrating the interpretation of upward movement of the head and neck during stance phase.

gait, the head nod of a pelvic limb lameness will mimic a thoracic limb lameness of the ipsilateral side. For example, if the head is lowered during the left front stance phase, this indicates a right thoracic limb lameness or a right pelvic limb lameness (or both which would result in an exaggerated head nod). It is important to understand that these concepts only apply to a diagonal gait (i.e. the trot). When the animal paces, the opposite is true (i.e. a right thoracic limb lameness mimics a

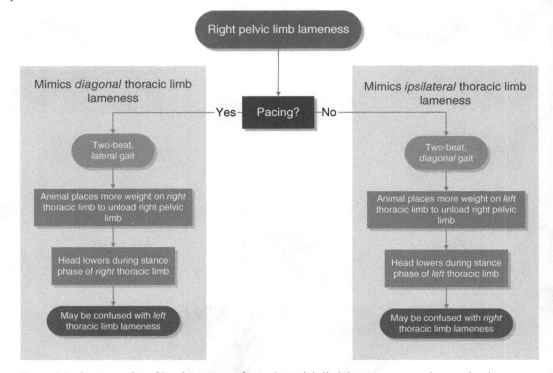

Figure 1.3 Interpretation of head movement for canine pelvic limb lameness comparing trotting (a diagonal gait) and pacing (a lateral gait), illustrating the interpretation of downward movement of the head and neck during stance phase. While this diagram is based on pelvic limb lameness, similarly the observer may confuse a left thoracic limb lameness with a right pelvic limb lameness if the dog paces (and vice versa).

left pelvic limb lameness and vice versa, see Figure 1.3). It is therefore of critical importance that the observer determines if the animal is displaying a diagonal (i.e. trot) or lateral (i.e. pacing) gait.

Pelvic movement, also termed the pelvic or hip hike, is displayed by animals with pelvic limb lameness. The animal will attempt to reduce the amount of weight placed on the affected leg by elevating the pelvis of the affected side, thereby shifting its body weight to the unaffected limb(s). This may be more difficult to observe in long-haired dogs. In dogs with a high-grade lameness, a significant drop of the pelvis is observed when the unaffected limb contacts the ground (Videos 1.1 and 1.4). In horses, it is described that the limb with the greater movement of the pelvis rather than the absolute height determines the lame leg (Baxter and Stashak 2011). Another feature allowing canines to shift their weight to the affected limb is excessive tail movement, generally observed swinging up when the affected limb contacts the ground.

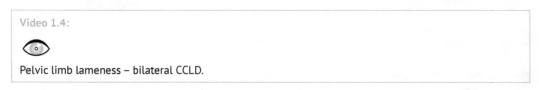

Video 1.4:

Pelvic limb lameness – bilateral CCLD.

To differentiate whether a head nod is arising from a thoracic limb or pelvic limb lameness during subjective gait analysis, the following criteria can be applied: *thoracic limb lameness* – a pelvic hike is only rarely present; *pelvic limb lameness* – generally impairment is so severe that off-weighing at the stance can also be observed, the dog's body weight is shifted forward resulting in a lower head and neck carry age than usual, and obvious clinical exam findings (e.g. stifle instability) are present.

Multiple limb lameness provides a greater diagnostic challenge. In some cases, identification of specific patterns clearly indicates that multiple limbs are involved. For example, a dog presenting with a severe right pelvic limb lameness would be expected to display a downward movement of the head on the left thoracic limb in the trot. If a downward movement is observed during weight-bearing of the right thoracic limb, this indicates that the animal is also suffering from a left thoracic limb problem. If the animal is simultaneously suffering from an ipsilateral thoracic limb and pelvic limb lameness, an exaggerated head nod will be observed. In horses, the concept of *compensatory* (also termed secondary or complementary) lameness is well established. This lameness is defined as pain secondary due to overloading of the unaffected limb. It is difficult to differentiate compensatory lameness from a primary cause. In general, the most severe lameness should be addressed primarily; however, evaluation of all affected limbs is indicated.

While the above concepts are described for a diagonal gait, similar concepts can be applied if the animal is unable to trot (i.e. during walking). The observer should look for off-loading of specific limbs, decreased stance phase, head nod, and pelvic hike. Following the simple concept, that animals will try to shift their body weight away from the lame limb, helps identify the most affected limb.

1.3.4 Lameness Characteristics

In horses, the stride is divided into the cranial and caudal phase, which is the length of the stride of the affected limb cranial or caudal to the stance position of the contralateral limb (Ross 2011). In other words, the cranial phase of the stride is the phase in front of the hoofprint of the opposite limb (Baxter and Stashak 2011). Lame horses frequently have a decreased cranial stride phase and a lengthened caudal phase; however, the overall stride length is not changed with lameness. This makes clinical sense since a unilaterally decreased stride length would not allow for movement in a straight line (Ross 2011), unless the changes are symmetric. Little is known regarding stride phases and lameness distribution in dogs and some misconceptions about it (e.g. that orthopedic disease in canines always results in a decreased stride length) have been presented in the literature. Clearly, further work in this area is needed but it is intuitive that an animal with bilateral coxofemoral arthritis will show a decreased swing phase (to avoid pain during full range of motion) resulting in the classic short-strided gait (Video 20.2). Additionally, it is important to note that decreased stride length is not pathognomonic for orthopedic disease but is also seen with neurologic conditions (e.g. lower motor neuron disease; Chapter 4). This overlap between orthopedic and neurologic causes can make differentiating the cause of lameness difficult. Therefore, careful neurologic and orthopedic examinations are critical to confirm or exclude neurologic dysfunction.

In horses, supporting limb and swinging limb lameness are further differentiated. A supporting limb lameness is observed when the foot first contacts the ground and indicates conditions of the lower limb (a parallel example in canines would be a dog with a digit fracture). In contrast, the definition of swinging limb lameness is not as clearly defined and varies between equine texts. Ross (2011), for example, describes swinging limb lameness as a non-painful lameness, rather than a lameness during swing phase. Using this definition, canine infraspinatus contracture makes for a good example of a correlate in dogs. However, some equine clinicians attribute a swinging limb lameness to conditions of the upper limb (Baxter and Stashak 2011); when using this definition, canine supraspinatus or biceps tendinopathy makes a good canine correlate.

1.3.5 Lameness Grading

While there are many grading systems to score lameness subjectively, none of them have been validated or used consistently in canine orthopedics. The most commonly used grading scale in horses is the American Association of Equine Practitioners (AAEP) system (Ross 2011): 0 = no lameness; 1 = inconsistent lameness under specific circumstances only; 2 = consistent lameness under specific circumstances only; 3 = consistent lameness at a trot; 4 = consistent lameness at a walk; and 5 = most severe lameness. While this scoring system simplifies the grading, it makes things potentially confusing because it grades lameness at both the walk and trot.

Various grading systems have been proposed to score severity of lameness in dogs, including the use of numerical rating scales (NRS) and visual analog scores (VAS). NRS describe the lameness in descriptive terms such as sound and non-weight-bearing using scales of up to 11 points (Van Vynckt et al. 2011). Although larger scales allow for differentiation of more subtle lameness, this results in less consistency between multiple observers (such as multiple veterinarians within one practice). Therefore, simple scales (Table 1.1) that allow subjective comparison within or between observers and temporal periods (i.e. if different examiners evaluate a patient at different time points) are preferable to use. VAS provide an assessment of continuous limb function. This is accomplished by asking the observer to mark the severity of lameness along a line (generally divided into 100 increments). The results are recorded as continuous variables (Quinn et al. 2007). It is well known that subjective gait analysis varies between observers and correlates poorly to objective gait analysis (Quinn et al. 2007; Waxman et al. 2008). Ideally, objective gait analysis would be used to provide a quantitative analysis; however, given the lack of its availability, an effort should be made to at least use a consistent scoring system by all healthcare professionals within one institution.

Table 1.1 Unvalidated numerical rating score used by the author to subjectively quantify canine lameness.

Score	Lameness degree	Lameness description
0	None	*No identifiable lameness* Weight-bearing at all times
1	Slight	*Inconsistent lameness* that is difficult to observe and/or it is difficult to determine the affected limb (i.e. no consistent head movement/pelvic tilt is observed) Weight-bearing at all times
2	Mild	Clearly detectable lameness associated with minor *head movement/pelvic tilt* Weight-bearing at all times
3	Moderate	Clearly detectable lameness associated with obvious *head movement/pelvic tilt* Weight-bearing at all times
4	Severe	Clearly detectable lameness associated with obvious head movement/pelvic tilt *Occasionally non-weight-bearing/toe touching*
5	Non-weight-bearing	*Always non-weight-bearing/toe touching*

This scoring system can be applied at the walk and/or the trot depending on the patient's clinical status. The patient should only be scored during motion (i.e. off-loading at a stance is not included in this assessment). To increase the sensitivity, the scoring system can be applied for both gaits. If a comparison between different time points is performed, only the scoring within one gait can be compared.

References

Baxter, G.M. and Stashak, T.S. (2011). Examination for lameness. In: *Adams and Stashak's Lameness in Horses* (ed. G.M. Baxter), 109–206. Hoboken: Wiley-Blackwell.

Datt, V.L. and Fletcher, T.F. (2012). Gait foot-fall patterns. http://vanat.cvm.umn.edu/gaits/index.html (accessed 12 February 2019).

He Lane, D.M., Hill, S.A., Huntingford, J.L. et al. (2015). Effectiveness of slow motion video compared to real time video in improving the accuracy and consistency of subjective gait analysis in dogs. *Open Vet. J.* 5 (2): 158–165.

Leach, D., Sumner-Smith, G., and Dagg, A.I. (1977). Diagnosis of lameness in dogs: a preliminary study. *Can. Vet. J.* 18 (3): 58–63.

Quinn, M.M., Keuler, N.S., Lu, Y. et al. (2007). Evaluation of agreement between numerical rating scales, visual analogue scoring scales, and force plate gait analysis in dogs. *Vet. Surg.* 36 (4): 360–367.

Ross, M.W. (2011). Movement. In: *Diagnosis and Management of Lameness in the Horse*, 2e (eds. M.W. Ross and S.J. Dyson), 64–80. Saint Louis: W.B. Saunders.

Van Vynckt, D., Samoy, Y., Polis, I. et al. (2011). Evaluation of two sedation protocols for use before diagnostic intra-articular anaesthesia in lame dogs. *J. Small Anim. Pract.* 52 (12): 638–644.

Waxman, A.S., Robinson, D.A., Evans, R.B. et al. (2008). Relationship between objective and subjective assessment of limb function in normal dogs with an experimentally induced lameness. *Vet. Surg.* 37 (3): 241–246.

Wendland, T.M., Martin, K.W., Duncan, C.G. et al. (2016). Evaluation of pacing as an indicator of musculoskeletal pathology in dogs. *J. Vet. Med. Anim. Health* 8 (12): 207–213.

2

Objective Gait Analysis

Bryan T. Torres

Department of Veterinary Medicine and Surgery, College of Veterinary Medicine, University of Missouri, Columbia, MO, USA

2.1   Introduction

The use of objective gait analysis techniques to evaluate veterinary patients has increased recently. In the past few years, gait analysis equipment has become more affordable and has begun to move from a research and specialty setting into everyday practice. Despite this, there remains little to no attention given to objective gait analysis techniques and equipment during veterinary school education. Because of this, many veterinarians begin performing gait analysis with little understanding of the fundamentals behind these techniques. Unfortunately, this can result in poor data collection and/or erroneous interpretation of results – negatively impacting patient care. Therefore, it is critical that veterinarians interested in these techniques are familiar with the basics of gait analysis.

In general, objective gait analysis can be divided into two main categories: (i) kinetics and (ii) kinematics. Kinetic gait analysis focuses on the *forces* generated during movement while kinematic gait analysis focuses on *motion* that occurs during ambulation without concern for forces.

2.2   Kinetic Analysis

Kinetic gait analysis evaluates the *forces* produced when an animal's foot is in contact with the ground. Therefore, the stance phase is the only portion of the full gait cycle where kinetic information is recorded. In many musculoskeletal or neurologic conditions, patients may have a lameness which results in reduced forces in the affected limb (e.g. reduced weight-bearing) making this a key method of detecting pathology as well as monitoring a response to therapy.

There are two major systems used in veterinary medicine to record kinetic information: (i) force plates (FPs) (or platforms) and (ii) pressure-sensitive walkways (PSWs). There are important differences between these two systems. It is important that clinicians understand the benefits as well as the limitations of each system to maximize their clinical use.

2.2.1 Force Plate Systems: The Basics

FPs measure force or more specifically *ground reaction forces (GRF)*. Put simply, GRF are the equal yet opposing force produced when an animal's foot interacts with the ground. For example, when we stand still on solid ground here on Earth, we are exerting a downward force on the ground that is equal to the product of our mass and Earth's gravity ($F = m \times g$). The reason that we do not sink into the ground is because the ground is exerting an *equal and opposite* upward force. This concept was first described by Sir Isaac Newton and is known as Newton's third law. When we move, as compared to standing still, these forces are exerted in multiple directions, not just up and down. These equal and opposite GRF produced when moving are the main focus of kinetic analysis with FP systems.

FP systems are a staple in most modern veterinary gait laboratories (Figure 2.1A) and have long been considered the gold standard in kinetic measurement of lame animals. However, there are aspects of these systems that must be considered by clinicians:

Ideal Animal Size – FPs often have a shorter working length compared to PSW systems (Figure 2.1B). Because of this, evaluating individual footfalls can be challenging in smaller animals or animals with shorter stride lengths. This makes typical FPs ideal for medium- to large-breed dogs. A method of adapting an FP for smaller animals has been described but is difficult in a clinical setting (Kapatkin et al. 2014).

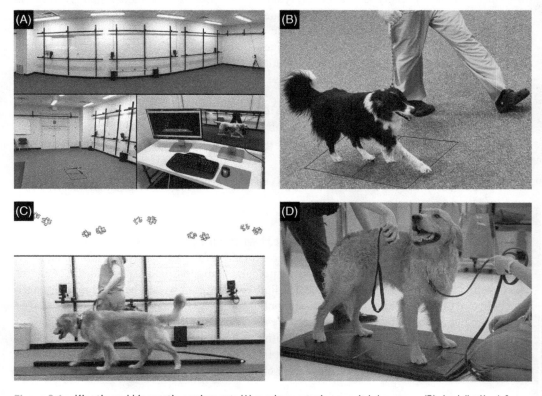

Figure 2.1 Kinetic and kinematic equipment: (A) modern veterinary gait laboratory; (B) dual (in-line) force plate system; (C) pressure-sensitive walkway (PSW) system (Tekscan Walkway™); and (D) weight distribution platform.

Portability and Storage – Most veterinary FP systems are permanently affixed to the ground in a dedicated space. The limited mobility of these systems should be considered by clinicians without dedicated space or where portability is of importance.

2.2.2 Force Plate Systems: Kinetic Measurements

FP systems measure *force* in three directions: (i) vertical force, (ii) craniocaudal force, and (iii) mediolateral force (Figure 2.2):

Vertical Force (Fz) – This is the largest and most commonly evaluated force. Graphically, it appears "bell-shaped" during a trot and "M-shaped" during a walk (Figure 2.3) due to the speed difference between trotting and walking (Decamp 1997). Changes in Fz are frequently used as measures of function and pain. Animals with lameness secondary to orthopedic disease often have a reduction in Fz values in affected limbs.

Craniocaudal Force (Fy) – This is the second largest force and is biphasic with two components that define distinct periods of forward movement – braking (deceleration) and propulsion (acceleration). Braking occurs at the beginning of stance and propulsion at the end (Figure 2.3). While these forces are less commonly reported, animals with lameness secondary to orthopedic disease can have a reduction in these components.

Mediolateral Force (Fx) – This is the smallest force in dogs moving in a straight line (Figure 2.3) and is rarely used for comparison (Torres 2018). However, with the increased interest in canine

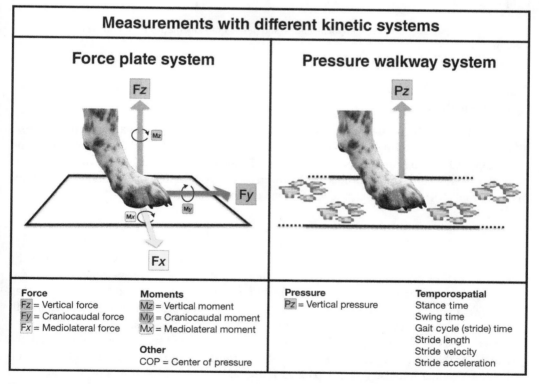

Figure 2.2 Measurements that can be obtained with different kinetic systems.

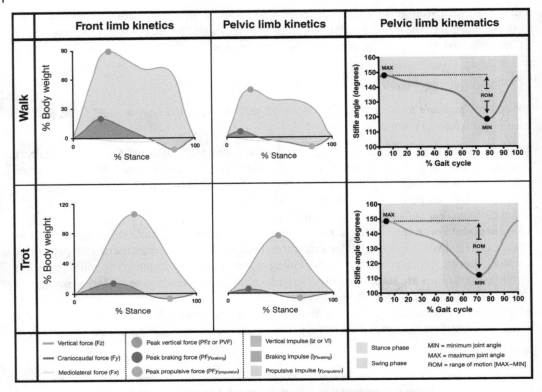

Figure 2.3 Ground reaction forces, impulse values, and pelvic limb kinematics from dogs walking and trotting.

athletics, where dogs undergo rapid directional changes, it is possible that evaluation may prove valuable in the future.

While forces are the primary measurement of clinical interest in veterinary patients, FPs also allow researchers to measure moments (Mz, My, and Mx) and to calculate the center of pressure (COP; Figure 2.2). *Moments* are the turning effect of a force (e.g. "torque"). The *COP* is where the vertical GRF is centered under the foot and has been used to evaluate balance in humans. Currently, moments and COP are infrequently evaluated in veterinary patients.

2.2.3 Force Plate Systems: Clinically Reported Values

Peak Force – This is the maximum force (Fz, Fy, and Fx) and is graphically represented as the peak or "top" of the force curve (Figure 2.3). The vertical force (Fz) has one peak referred to as the peak vertical force (PVF). The craniocaudal force (Fy) is biphasic and has a peak braking ($PFy_{braking}$) and peak propulsive force ($PFy_{propulsion}$). Reduced peak forces are associated with lameness. These are the most commonly reported and compared values.

Impulse – The impulse of any GRF is the product of that force and stance time and is simply the area under the force-time curve (Figure 2.3). The vertical impulse (VI) (Iz) is a single value and the craniocaudal impulse (Iy) is separated into braking ($Iy_{braking}$) and propulsive ($Iy_{propulsion}$) components. Reduced impulses are associated with lameness.

Body Weight Distribution (%BWD) – This is calculated from PVF and is expressed as a percentage (Table 2.1). It represents the percentage of total body weight placed on each limb. For most dogs, normal %BWD is 60% in the front limbs (30% right; 30% left) and 40% in the pelvic limbs (20% right; 20% left). Lame dogs will shift their weight to the non-lame legs and have a reduced %BWD in the affected limb. It is less common that FP software programs will automatically calculate these values. Therefore, clinicians may need to manually calculate these values.

2.2.4 Pressure-sensitive Walkway Systems: The Basics

Kinetic analysis with PSW systems is based on pressure, specifically paw pressure, instead of force (Figure 2.2). Pressure is measured by thousands of sensors embedded in the walkway. The main clinical benefit of PSWs is in reporting stride characteristics with temporospatial variables (TSVs, described below), the ability to record several consecutive foot strikes, semiautomated analysis, and improved portability. Manufacturers producing pressure-sensitive systems commonly used with companion animals include Tekscan, Inc. (Walkway™; Tekscan, South Boston, Massachusetts, USA) and CIR Systems, Inc. (GAIT4Dog®; CIR Systems, Franklin, New Jersey, USA). Systems can vary in overall physical dimension, measurement capabilities, as well as the degree of computerized automation. It is important that clinicians consider their needs before purchasing any kinetic system:

Dimensions – PSW systems often have longer working lengths than individual FPs allowing for recording of multiple footfalls in one pass over the walkway (Figure 2.1C). PSWs can be purchased in varying length, depending on clinical need (i.e. size of patient population).

Ideal Animal Size – A wide range of animal sizes can be easily evaluated due to the longer recording platform (compared to serially placed FPs). Some PSWs have sensors of varying degrees of resolution and PSWs with higher-resolution sensors are recommended for use with smaller companion animals.

Table 2.1 Commonly used calculations for gait analysis parameters.

Variable	Example formula
Body weight distribution (%BWD)	$\%BWD = \left(\dfrac{\text{PVF or Pressure from a single limb}}{\text{Total PVF or Pressure from all limbs}} \right) \times 100$
Body weight normalization (%BW)	$\text{PVF as a}\%BW = \left(\dfrac{\text{Force exerted by a limb (Newtons)}}{\text{Total weight of the dog (Newtons)}} \right) \times 100$
Percent change (%Change)	$\%Change = \dfrac{\left[\left(\bar{X}_2 \right) - \left(\bar{X}_1 \right) \right]}{\left(\bar{X}_1 \right)} \times 100$
Symmetry index (SI)	$SI = \dfrac{\bar{X}_R - \bar{X}_L}{\frac{1}{2} \left(\bar{X}_R + \bar{X}_L \right)} \times 100$
Symmetry ratio (SR)	$SR = \dfrac{\bar{X}_R}{\bar{X}_L} \times 100$

Portability and Storage – Many PSW systems can be "rolled-up" or deconstructed for storage and/or transportation. This may be an important consideration for clinicians where dedicated space is limited.

Kinetic Measurements – PSWs measure foot pressure and while sensor types can vary between systems, all measure pressure only in the vertical direction. Pressure is related to but not the same as force, measured with FPs. Clinically, vertical pressure measurements are often evaluated similarly to GRF.

Temporospatial Variables (TSV) – The rapid collection and reporting of TSVs is a major strength of PSWs. These variables (discussed later in this section) are calculated from the paw strikes recorded by the PSW.

2.2.5 Pressure-sensitive Walkway Systems: Clinically Reported Values

Kinetic Variables – Pressure (vertical direction only) is the primary kinetic variable recorded with PSWs (Figure 2.2). Some PSWs (i.e. Tekscan Walkway™) allow clinicians to use pressure measurements to indirectly calculate force (PVF and VI) through a calibration process. Because this method differs from direct force measurements obtained by FPs, these calculated force values are similar but not directly comparable to ones obtained from FPs (Lascelles et al. 2006). Clinically, this means that when evaluating patients (e.g. improved or reduced weight-bearing), all measurements for comparison should be recorded with the same system (FP system or PSW system). How pressure values are reported varies between PSW systems. Pressure values can be reported as a maximum pressure value (Tekscan Walkway™) or as a scaled pressure value called a *total pressure index* (GAIT4Dog®).

Body Weight Distribution (%BWD) – This is calculated from pressure and is automatically calculated by most PSW systems (Table 2.1). For the PSW systems that allow calculation of force values, those can be used to calculate %BWD. See the FP section for additional information.

Temporospatial Variables (TSV) – These are not kinetic variables because they do not represent force or pressure. Instead, they describe events related to time (temporo-) and distance (-spatial). For example, stance and swing time are temporal measurement and stride length is a spatial measurement. Stride velocity and acceleration involve both time and distance. Commonly reported TSVs are listed below:

Gait Cycle (Stride) Time – The combined value of the stance time + swing time represents the complete gait cycle of one leg. This occurs between each consecutive footfall (*toe-on* to *toe-off* to *toe-on*).

Stance Time – This is the total time a foot is on the ground during the gait cycle (*toe-on* to *toe-off*). This is often displayed as a percentage of the total gait cycle.

Swing Time – This is the total time a foot is off the ground during the gait cycle (*toe-off* to *toe-on*). This is often displayed as a percentage of the total gait cycle.

Stride Length – This is the distance between two consecutive footfalls of the same leg. This represents the distance a foot travels during one complete a gait cycle.

Stride Velocity – This is the velocity (i.e. speed) at which a leg completes a gait cycle.

Stride Acceleration – This is the change in velocity (i.e. speed) between two consecutive strides.

2.2.6 Static or Standing Kinetic Analysis

The previous discussion focused on the more common dynamic kinetic analysis performed when moving at a walk or trot. However, recently static kinetic analysis or "standing weight-bearing" has gained interest in veterinary medicine with the use of a weight distribution platform (WDP) or stance analyzer (Figure 2.1D). Static kinetics is not a new concept and can be performed with more complex FP and PSW systems. However, dedicated WDP equipment designed specifically to measure only standing weight-bearing has entered the veterinary market. This equipment is less expensive than complete kinetic systems and is a simple way to record basic standing weight-bearing measurements. It consists of a group of four pressure sensors that are clustered together so that dogs can stand with each of their four paws on the individual pressure sensors. Paw pressure is measured in real time and a computerized software displays the %BWD in each limb.

Advantages of WDP systems are the ease of use and that minimal skill is required (Phelps et al. 2007). However, like any gait analysis tool, pitfalls during the collection process can affect the results, such as distractions and head movement, abnormal limb position and posture, removing or replacing paws during collection or restraint, and subjective acquisition of data only during times of reduced or improved weight-bearing. Unfortunately, research regarding these areas as well as standardized and validated measurement protocols is lacking.

It is important to recognize that the role of standing weight-bearing measurements in clinical decision-making is not well defined in dogs. The clinical relevance of limb off-loading (e.g. lameness) when standing as compared to moving is not fully understood. Currently, there is limited published research regarding WDPs and there is only one recent peer-reviewed publication comparing a WDP to a more well-established kinetic system (PSW) in lame dogs (Clough et al. 2018). That study demonstrated that a WDP was able to detect an objective lameness in a small and widely varied population of dogs with various orthopedic conditions. However, the authors caution that the value of the WDP in dogs with more subtle or severe orthopedic disease is still unknown. Additionally, they note that the value of a WDP in tracking the clinical progression of orthopedic disease or therapeutic outcome has yet to be determined. For clinicians who desire to use a WDP in clinical practice, it is important to recognize these current limitations in our understanding of WDPs. Where this equipment fits in clinical practice and more importantly how to best utilize standing weight-bearing measurements in patients with clinical disease are still being explored.

2.3 Kinematic Analysis

Kinematic gait analysis is the study of motion and evaluates motion throughout the complete gait cycle. Historically, joint angles have been most commonly evaluated and, in the past, this has been limited to research facilities, universities, and large referral hospitals due to the expensive and complex equipment. However, with computer and software advancement, this method of analysis is now more widely available and affordable. This technology can vary greatly from simplistic and inexpensive to the highly advanced and costly, respectively. With proper technique, any kinematic systems can provide clinicians with valuable information to aid in the detection and treatment of musculoskeletal pathologies.

Kinematic data collection in veterinary medicine is focused on evaluating motion in one of two ways:

1) Motion occurring in a single plane (2D analysis)
2) Motion occurring in multiple planes (3D analysis)

In veterinary medicine, 2D analysis is most common. While 3D analysis provides a more complete representation of actual movement, it is complex to perform and requires advanced equipment. This consideration needs to be accounted for when deciding what is most appropriate in a particular clinical setting.

2.3.1 Description and Measurement of Joint Motion

In veterinary kinematics, joint flexion and extension are most frequently evaluated, and for appendicular joints, this is where the greatest degree of motion occurs. However, it is important that clinicians remember that true joint motion occurs in multiple planes (Figure 2.4):

Sagittal Plane – This plane of motion describes joint *flexion and extension*. It is the most common plane evaluated and is where the greatest amount of joint motion occurs.

Transverse Plane – This plane of motion describes joint *internal rotation and external rotation*.

Frontal Plane – This plane of motion describes joint *abduction and adduction*. Note: this terminology differs from the terminology used for diagnostic imaging (Chapter 10) where this plane is called dorsal plane.

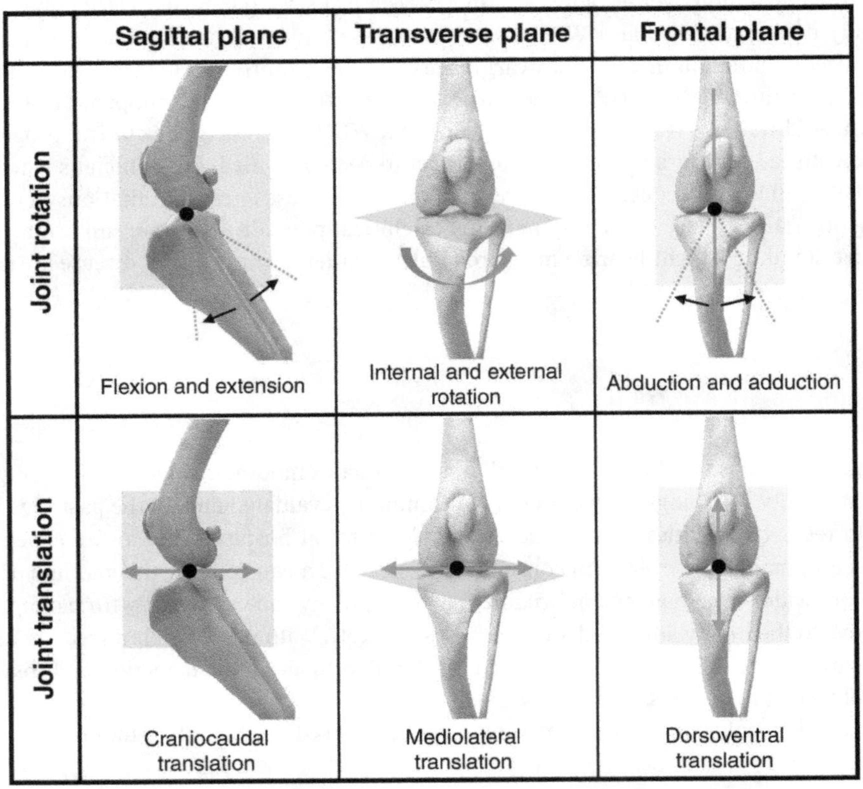

	Sagittal plane	**Transverse plane**	**Frontal plane**
Joint rotation	Flexion and extension	Internal and external rotation	Abduction and adduction
Joint translation	Craniocaudal translation	Mediolateral translation	Dorsoventral translation

Figure 2.4   Clinical joint motion in relation to the three planes of motion. Readers should note that the names of planes used to describe joint motion can differ from those in diagnostic imaging (see also Figure 10.4).

Box 2.1 Six Degrees of Freedom (6-DOF) Movement	
Joint rotations (3)	**Joint translations (3)**
Flexion and extension	Craniocaudal or "craniocaudal translation"
Internal and external rotation	Mediolateral or "mediolateral translation"
Abduction and adduction	Dorsoventral or "joint distraction"

In order to translate a complex biomechanical process like joint motion into clinically relevant terms, we must use terminology that is meaningful to researchers and clinicians. Therefore, joint motion is often discussed using the concept of six degrees of freedom (6-DOF; Grood and Suntay 1983). This describes clinical joint motion relative to three axes (x, y, and z) and associated with these axes are six distinct motions consisting of (3) rotations and (3) translations (Figure 2.4; Box 2.1).

2.3.2 Kinematic Systems

Two-Dimensional (2D) Systems – These are single camera systems that allow reliable collection of motion in a single plane. These systems are simple and inexpensive (<$1000 in most cases). Consumer grade cameras or even high-quality cellular phone cameras can be used to capture video of animals with high contrast spherical markers applied to the skin or coat (e.g. white markers on a black dog or black markers on a white dog). These markers can then be digitized by computerized software programs to determine joint or body movement. There are numerous software programs for 2D kinematics. Kinovea (www.kinovea.org), for example, is a free and open source program that is easy to use but lacks some of the more advanced and automated features of paid software. Likewise, MaxTRAQ 2D (Innovision Systems, Inc., Columbiavile, Michigan, USA) is an easy-to-use paid software program for 2D kinematics with many advanced and automated features that clinicians find useful. Regardless of software, proper camera and patient positioning is critical because 2D systems can be affected by parallax and perspective error. *Parallax error* occurs when the subject moves away from the optical axis of the camera and *perspective error* happens when the subject moves in and out of the calibrated plane of motion (Kirtley 2006). In many cases, these errors can be reduced if clinicians pay careful attention to camera and subject positioning during data collection. In general, the camera should be placed at the maximum distance allowable from the subject to provide good resolution and field of view, perpendicular to the plane interest (e.g. sagittal plane), and positioned at a height that centers the camera at the level where the markers are to be tracked (Figure 2.5). Additionally, data should be collected from patients moving along the calibrated plane without deviation (Figures 2.6 and 2.7). Clinicians wishing for further information on these types of error are directed to additional resources (Kirtley 2006; Torres 2018).

Three-Dimensional (3D) Systems – These are multi-camera systems that allow reliable collection of three-dimensional motion. In most cases, these systems consist of specialized cameras that track reflective markers placed on the skin. Unfortunately, these systems are expensive (>$100 000 in many cases) and to evaluate true 3D joint motion a more complex marker model is required. These aspects of 3D systems have restricted their use to research settings. However, one significant benefit of these systems is that they do not suffer from parallax or perspective

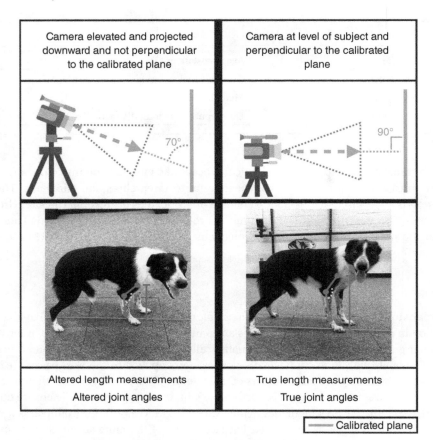

Figure 2.5   A possible source of error in 2D kinematics: camera position relative to the subject.

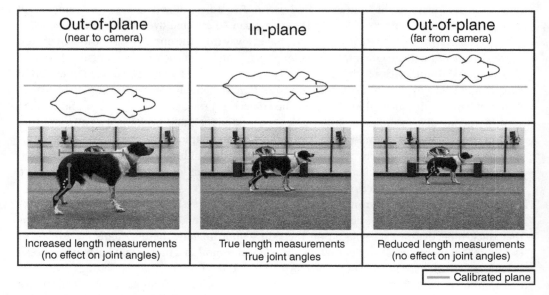

Figure 2.6   A possible source of error in 2D kinematics: subject positioning relative to the calibrated plane (*near-far*).

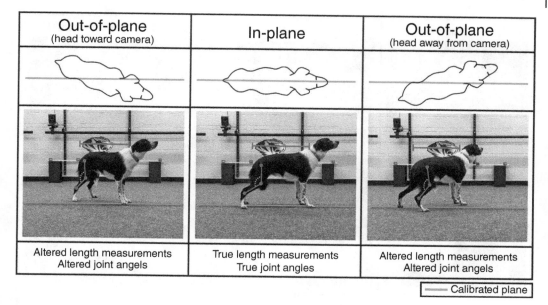

Figure 2.7 A possible source of error in 2D kinematics: subject positioning relative to the calibrated plane (*rotation*).

error, as is encountered with 2D systems. Unfortunately, even with technological advancement and the declining cost of computerized hardware, the price of these systems remains high and has limited their clinical application. Additionally, the complexity of the 3D models and operating systems makes every day clinical use challenging.

2.3.3 Kinematic Models

Clinically, kinematic analysis is most commonly performed by placing spherical markers on the skin over specific areas of the body. *The specific pattern in which these markers are placed is called a kinematic model.* The basics of these models and kinematic methods have changed very little for over 180 years (Decamp 1997; Torres 2018).

Models used with 2D kinematic systems – These are simplistic and easy-to-use models focused on one plane of motion, referred to as "planar" motion. Hence, these models are commonly called planar models. Their pattern further defines them as linear, linked, or segment models (Figure 2.8). In veterinary medicine, one of the most widely used 2D kinematic models for dogs is a full-body model (Figure 2.9).

Models used with 3D kinematic systems – In general, any model can be used with a 3D kinematic system, and historically, simple planar models described above have been used. However, evaluation of true 3D joint motion requires more complex models, often referred to as rigid body segment models (Figure 2.8). In the past few years, veterinary research has seen the use of these models and systems increases. However, they are complex and require a larger number of markers as well as advanced 3D equipment and training to obtain clinically useful results. Currently, use in a clinical setting is uncommon in veterinary medicine.

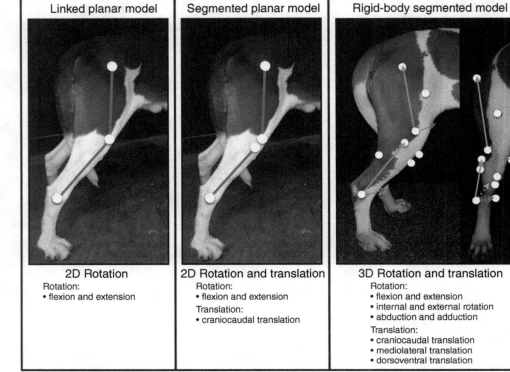

Figure 2.8   Comparison of three common kinematic models.

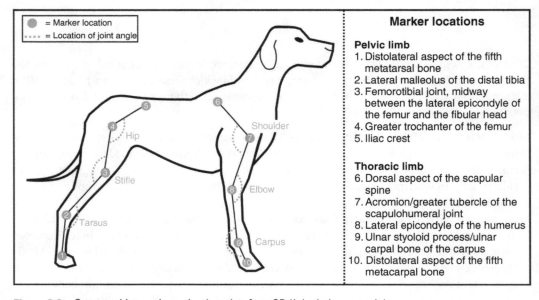

Figure 2.9   Common kinematic marker location for a 2D linked planar model.

2.3.4   Other Methods of Kinematic Analysis

The methods discussed previously are the most common methods used in clinical patients. However, there are other less common methods used mainly in a research setting that do not require markers to be placed on the skin of clinical patients:

Radiographic and advanced imaging methods (such as fluoroscopy, computerized tomography [CT], and magnetic resonance imaging [MRI]) have been used (mostly in a research setting) to evaluate kinematics. Some of these methods increase the radiation exposure to patients as well as personnel. The equipment needed for these methods is not widely available in most clinical practices and is not clinically applicable at this time.

Body-mounted inertial sensors, called inertial measurement units (IMUs), are used in human laboratories and have gained interest for use in veterinary patients (Duerr et al. 2016). This method relies on the attachment of IMUs, which contain accelerometers and gyroscopes, to provide information on 3D motion. However, attachment of these small devices to the body has proven difficult in small animal patients and therefore their clinical usefulness at this time is uncertain.

2.3.5   Kinematic Variables

Although many variables are recorded in veterinary kinematics related to joint motion, the most commonly evaluated are (Figure 2.3) as follows:

Average Joint Angle – The average or mean joint angle during movement.
Maximum Joint Angle (MAX) – The maximum (e.g. largest) joint angle during movement.
Minimum Joint Angle (MIN) – The minimum (e.g. smallest) joint angle during movement.
Joint Range of Motion (ROM) – The total range of joint motion during movement calculated by subtracting the minimum joint angle from the maximum.
Percentage of Gait Cycle – Kinematics can evaluate the entire gait cycle and therefore the stance phase and swing phase are often reported as a percentage of the total gait cycle.

Note: kinematic variables can be reported and evaluated as single point values (e.g. minimum or maximum joint angle) or as a complete gait waveform.

2.4   Making the Best of Your Gait Data Collection

Clinicians can take important steps to make the best of the gait collection process. Most of these steps help reduce error in a patient's gait data by limiting factors that contribute to data variability. Some factors are difficult to minimize, such as the small trial-to-trial or day-to-day variations, as well as the effect of skin motion artifact on kinematic analysis (Torres 2018). However, other factors discussed below are easier to address.

2.4.1   Habituation

This is the process of acclimating clinical patients to the gait collection process and environment. Clinicians should allow their patients a period of adjustment in the gait collection area prior to collecting data. However, the ideal length of time needed for this is not established and may vary between animals. In most cases, several minutes or more is recommended.

2.4.2 Animal Handlers

It has been shown that differences in handlers can affect gait data. Therefore, clinicians should try to limit the number of people who leash walk patients for gait analysis and when possible have the same person walk an individual patient at each examination time.

2.4.3 Velocity and Acceleration

Changes in movement velocity (e.g. speed) and acceleration have some of the most profound effects on both kinematic and kinetic gait data. Clinicians should select an acceptable velocity and acceleration range prior to data collection and only collect trials that conform to that range. Ideal velocity ranges for walking and trotting may vary between animals of differing sizes. In the author's experience, a walking velocity of 0.9–1.2 m/s, a trotting velocity of 1.7–2.1 m/s, and an acceleration range of −0.5 to 0.5 m/s^2 are appropriate for most medium- to large-breed dogs. Information regarding the merits of wider or narrower velocity ranges for trotting dogs can be found elsewhere (Hans et al. 2014).

2.4.4 Marker Application

Much of the easily preventable error in kinematic analysis is related to errors in initial marker placement or marker replacement (Kim et al. 2017; Torres 2018). Clinicians can minimize this by designating a point person(s) to attach the markers to animals standing in a natural position as well as establishing consistent protocols for marker placement. Standard marker locations have been established for most models and many rely on marker application over easily palpable bony landmarks to help ensure repeatability.

2.4.5 Comparing Averages

For kinetics and kinematics, single gait measurements should not be used for comparison. Instead, clinicians should compare an average value from repeated measurements. An average of five measurements or data from five trials are most commonly used for comparison. For PSW systems where multiple and repeated measurements can occur during one pass, often the results from five passes are averaged for comparison. Although the clinical benefit of using more than five passes is unclear, clinicians should avoid using less than three measurements for comparison.

2.5 Evaluating Gait Data

The appropriate analyses of data in kinetics and in kinematics often rely on similar methods. The built-in equipment software programs often can perform data comparison to varying degrees. However, it is more common that data is exported into a spreadsheet program or a stand-alone statistical program for comparison.

In veterinary medicine, single-point values such as PVF, VI, MAX, MIN, and ROM are most commonly evaluated (Figure 2.3) and provide clinicians with a single value that is easier to interpret and compare. Other methods may use the entire gait waveform for comparison (Torres 2018). However, these methods are more complex and time consuming thereby limiting their usefulness in a clinical setting.

2.5.1 Normalization to Body Weight

Comparison of kinetic data (PVF, VI, and Pressure) should be performed with data that has been normalized to an individual's current body weight at the time of testing. In doing this, values are expressed as a percentage of body weight (Table 2.1). Often, body weight normalization is performed automatically by the built-in software. However, some software programs will report data as both raw and normalized values. The use of normalized values allows clinicians to account for fluctuations in body weight when comparing different time points as well as provides a means to compare animals of differing weights and sizes.

2.5.2 Percent Change

The *Percent Change from Baseline* method is one of the most common ways that patient gait data is assessed in a clinical setting. It is most often performed by comparing the average of an initial or "baseline" measurement ($\bar{X}_1$) to a subsequent measurement ($\bar{X}_2$). For example, baseline measurements ($\bar{X}_1$) obtained prior to therapy can be compared to measurements taken at recheck examinations ($\bar{X}_2$) to evaluate the clinical changes and/or the effectiveness of therapy. Results are presented as a percentage. Using the formula in Table 2.1, a (+) percentage indicates an increase as compared to baseline and a (−) percentage indicates a reduction. Therefore, if a lame dog was evaluated with kinetic analysis before and after therapy, a (+) percentage change would indicate an improvement in weight-bearing following therapy, and a (−) percentage would indicate that the lameness worsened.

2.5.3 Gait Symmetry

The symmetry of any gait variable (kinetic or kinematic) can be evaluated. This was first introduced in small animals in the early 1990s and since then is frequently reported (Budsberg et al. 1993). The most common methods to calculate gait symmetry in veterinary medicine are called a symmetry index followed by a symmetry ratio (Table 2.1). Many PSW software programs calculate symmetry ratios. Alternatively, they can be calculated manually by comparing the average value ($\bar{X}$) from one limb (front or pelvic) to the opposite limb (front or pelvic). In this way, the animal's own limbs serve as an internal control for comparison. Because symmetry ratio and symmetry index calculations differ, the clinical interpretation of the results is different. However, clinicians should keep in mind that while it is often assumed that healthy animals are perfectly symmetrical, this is not often the case. Healthy dogs have been reported to have up to 6% asymmetry between their limbs (Torres 2018). Therefore, clinicians should interpret symmetry indices with great care in clinical patients.

References

Budsberg, S.C., Jevens, D.J., Brown, J. et al. (1993). Evaluation of limb symmetry indices, using ground reaction forces in healthy dogs. *Am. J. Vet. Res.* 54 (10): 1569–1574.

Clough, W.T., Canapp, S.O. Jr., De Taboada, L. et al. (2018). Sensitivity and specificity of a weight distribution platform for the detection of objective lameness and orthopaedic disease. *Vet. Comp. Orthop. Traumatol.* 31 (06): 391–395.

Decamp, C.E. (1997). Kinetic and kinematic gait analysis and the assessment of lameness in the dog. *Vet. Clin. North Am. Small Anim. Pract.* 27 (4): 825–840.

Duerr, F.M., Pauls, A., Kawcak, C. et al. (2016). Evaluation of inertial measurement units as a novel method for kinematic gait evaluation in dogs. *Vet. Comp. Orthop. Traumatol.* 29 (6): 475–483.

Grood, E.S. and Suntay, W.J. (1983). A joint coordinate system for the clinical description of three-dimensional motions: application to the knee. *J. Biomech. Eng.* 105 (2): 136–144.

Hans, E.C., Zwarthoed, B., Seliski, J. et al. (2014). Variance associated with subject velocity and trial repetition during force platform gait analysis in a heterogeneous population of clinically normal dogs. *Vet. J.* 202 (3): 498–502.

Kapatkin, A.S., Kim, J.Y., Garcia-Nolan, T.C. et al. (2014). Modification of the contact area of a standard force platform and runway for small breed dogs. *Vet. Comp. Orthopaed.* 27 (4): 257–262.

Kim, S.-Y., Torres, B.T., Sandberg, G.S., and Budsberg, S.C. (2017). Effect of limb position at the time of skin marker application on sagittal plane kinematics of the dog. *Vet. Comp. Orthop. Traumatol.* 30 (06): 438–443.

Kirtley, C. (2006). *Clinical Gait Analysis: Theory and Practice*. Edinburgh: Elsevier Health Sciences.

Lascelles, B.D., Roe, S.C., Smith, E. et al. (2006). Evaluation of a pressure walkway system for measurement of vertical limb forces in clinically normal dogs. *Am. J. Vet. Res.* 67 (2): 277–282.

Phelps, H.A., Ramos, V., Shires, P.K., and Werre, S.R. (2007). The effect of measurement method on static weight distribution to all legs in dogs using the quadruped biofeedback system. *Vet. Comp. Orthop. Traumatol.* 20 (2): 108–112.

Torres, B.T. (2018). Gait analysis. In: *Veterinary Surgery: Small Animal* (eds. S.A. Johnston and K. Tobias), 1385–1396. St. Louis: Elsevier.

3

The Orthopedic Examination

Dirsko J.F. von Pfeil[1,2] and Felix Michael Duerr[3]

[1] Small Animal Surgery Locum, PLLC, Dallas, TX, USA
[2] Sirius Veterinary Orthopedic Center, Omaha, NE, USA
[3] Department of Clinical Sciences, College of Veterinary Medicine and Biomedical Sciences, Colorado State University, Fort Collins, CO, USA

3.1 Introduction

The orthopedic examination plays a crucial role in determining the source of lameness and appropriate diagnostic and therapeutic steps. Orthopedic examination findings should always be interpreted in conjunction with the findings from the general physical examination and if available the myofascial (Chapter 6), rehabilitation (Chapter 5), and neurological examinations (Chapter 4), as well as subjective (Chapter 1) and objective gait evaluation (Chapter 2). This chapter outlines essential steps useful in assessing the overall orthopedic health of a dog. Additional information and more detailed instructions on regional orthopedic examinations are further discussed in the specific regional chapters contained within this book.

Early diagnosis of musculoskeletal conditions in animals is critical to improve a patient's final outcome by instituting appropriate treatment or preventative strategies early in the disease progression. Hence, at the minimum, a *brief* orthopedic exam should be performed on every animal presenting to a veterinary health professional. A *thorough* orthopedic exam should be performed on any patient with signs of musculoskeletal abnormalities or if orthopedic treatment interventions are intended. A systematic approach to the orthopedic exam is important to ensure evaluation of all structures and therefore, the exam should always be performed in the same order.

3.2 The Orthopedic Examination

The orthopedic examination includes the following steps (Table 3.1):

1) History and signalment
2) Visual exam
3) Subjective gait analysis (Chapter 1)
4) Palpation

Table 3.1 Summary of the components of the orthopedic examination.

Component	Variable	Comments
Signalment	Breed, age, and sex	Inherited dog database can be consulted to determine likely differential diagnoses (Sargan 2004)
History	Onset of lameness Inciting cause Progressiveness Response to treatment	To narrow down most likely diagnosis (e.g. geriatric patient with progressive lameness = higher suspicion of neoplasia and arthritis)
Visual examination	Conformational or anatomical abnormalities	Off-loading of limb during standing/at rest indicates affected limb
Limb palpation	Bones	Possible observations include pain, swelling, and crepitus (fracture)
	Muscles	Possible observations include atrophy, pain, and swelling
	Joints	Possible observations include periarticular swelling, pain, crepitus, joint effusion, increased or decreased range of motion, and abnormal end-feel
	Ligaments	Possible observations include varus and valgus instability

3.2.1 History and Signalment

Prior to performing a specific orthopedic examination, the *history* of lameness, previous diagnostics (radiographs, other imaging, and laboratory tests), previous treatment attempts (medications, rehabilitation, etc.) and their effect, goals of the owner for their pet, any other systemic disease present, travel history, vaccination and preventative medications given, diet, and any supplements administered should be recorded. Whether a pet or a working or sporting dog is examined is also important since certain conditions have been associated with specific sporting activities, for example, supraspinatus tendinopathy in agility dogs (Canapp et al. 2016) or specific orthopedic injuries in marathon sled dogs (von Pfeil et al. 2015). Additionally, onset, possible causes such as trauma, timing, and progression of lameness, will help narrowing down the diagnosis. For example, soft tissue injuries frequently improve or resolve within days. However, an animal presenting with chronic, progressive lameness is more likely to suffer from diseases such as chronic ligamentous instability, arthritis, or neoplasia. If the lameness is worse in the morning or after longer periods of rest, this may indicate degenerative disease. A lameness that improves with exercise is more likely to be a chronic soft tissue problem or osteoarthritis, whereas a lameness that worsens is more likely to be related to neoplasia or neurologic disease.

In general, caution is advised when trusting owners' identification of a lameness. Owners frequently misinterpret a head nod (i.e. identifying the incorrect limb as lame). But owner-recorded videos (when available) of the lameness can help the practitioner to identify the affected limb, particularly if the lameness is inconsistent. Yet, a non-weight-bearing lameness can be correctly identified by owners and hence this information is valuable and needs to be clearly teased out during history taking. It is advisable to have owners point out the limb that they believe to be impaired and specifically ask whether the animal has shown a non-weight-bearing lameness. Note that the term "favoring," although commonly used to describe a lameness, is somewhat confusing and as such should be avoided – it is better to use the terms "using less" or "lame."

Pertinent questions that should be included in the history are as follows:

1) Was the inciting cause of the lameness observed?
2) How long has the lameness been observed?
3) What was/is your dog's activity level before/since the onset of lameness?
4) Has the lameness worsened, stayed the same, or improved?
5) Does the lameness improve or worsen with exercise?
6) Have any diagnostics been performed?
7) What treatment(s) has been initiated (including rest and pharmacologic management) and what was the response?

Knowing the patient's *signalment* and taking a thorough history in combination with knowledge of predisposed breeds is very useful in establishing a diagnosis. Many patients presenting to the veterinary health professional for lameness are suffering from inherited diseases. It is therefore advisable to consider these diseases as highly likely differential diagnoses. Online resources are available to provide this information for purebred dogs (Sargan 2004). For example, a frequent diagnosis for an eight-month-old Labrador Retriever with a two-month history of bilateral thoracic limb lameness is elbow dysplasia (ED) or shoulder osteochondrosis dissecans.

3.2.2 Visual Exam

The distant, visual examination is an important part of the orthopedic exam and many conditions can be suspected without physical palpation. As mentioned in Chapter 1, dogs will frequently show off-loading at a stance clearly indicating the affected limb, which is best observed from a distance (Video 1.1). During the visual exam, conformational abnormalities such as angular limb deformities, joint instabilities (e.g. valgus deviation with medial collateral ligament injury of the carpus), and other osseous deformities can be identified. Periarticular swelling (which may indicate joint effusion or chronic degenerative changes), soft tissue masses or swelling (such as Achilles tendon swelling; Figure 18.8), or other obvious pathology (such as traumatic digit injuries; Figure 12.8) can be noted. In shorthaired dogs, muscle atrophy can be visible. Standing joint angles should be assessed and compared between contralateral limb pairs or to reported normal values (Milgram et al. 2004) if bilateral abnormalities are present. For example, carpal hyperextension (Video 13.1) and Achilles tendon rupture (Video 18.1) can be suspected based on the visually increased joint angles.

3.2.3 Palpation

The examination can be performed with the patient in a standing or recumbent position, using restraint as needed. However, because restraint affects the ability to interpret subtle responses of the patient, its usage should be minimized. In general, a combination of standing and recumbent positions is ideal. It is important to compare contralateral limbs to determine whether detected abnormalities are normal or pathologic, keeping in mind that many diseases are bilateral. This is best accomplished during a standing examination – if dogs are unable or unwilling to stand, an assistant may support the dog's weight by gently lifting from below the abdomen. The recumbent position is necessary to perform certain specific tests (e.g. Ortolani) and helpful to allow more detailed palpation of the affected limb. Recumbent versus standing position may also elicit a different response from the animal and as such may be helpful if pain responses are difficult to interpret in an individual patient.

Following a consistent approach to the orthopedic examination is recommended because doing so can avoid omitting important steps during the evaluation and subsequently missing a diagnosis. A full neurologic examination (Chapter 4) should be performed in any dog suspected to have neurologic disease. However, a few components of the neurologic examination should be included in every orthopedic examination (i.e. paw replacement, paraspinal palpation, tail lift, and neck range of motion). The text below, Table 3.2, and Video 3.1 outline the approach to the orthopedic examination regularly performed by the authors.

Video 3.1:

Complete orthopedic examination.

Starting the orthopedic examination with palpation of the pelvic limbs maintains distance from the front of the animal, thus permitting an assessment of the patient's demeanor in a safe manner. The first step is to evaluate proprioception of both pelvic limbs by performing the paw replacement test (Video 4.2). If there is uncertainty about which pelvic limb is affected, the examiner can gently pull back on both legs simultaneously to compare weight-bearing to identify the impaired leg (Video 3.1). Subsequently, palpating the pelvic limbs simultaneously (comparing left to right) will detect any muscle asymmetry, masses, or soft tissue swelling. The tarsus and stifle are also evaluated for presence of joint effusion. Next, the examiner should lift the tail (a pain response may indicate lumbosacral disease) and then perform paraspinal palpation (in between dorsal spinous processes and the paraspinal musculature). This is followed by examining neck range of motion (ventroflexion, dorsoflexion, and lateral movements). The thoracic limbs are palpated in a similar fashion and compared for any asymmetry (e.g. muscle mass, soft tissue masses, etc.) and evaluated for joint effusion of the elbow and carpus, ending at the distal limb whereupon proprioceptive testing is performed (e.g. paw replacement test). To identify the lame thoracic limb, legs are lifted alternatingly while standing over the animal.

Following this general palpation, a more detailed evaluation of the musculoskeletal structures of the limbs is performed. While the above outlined steps 1–13 (Table 3.2) should be performed in a standing position (to allow a comparative assessment), the following steps 14–44 may also be performed in lateral recumbency. In general, the detailed palpation consists of *long bone palpation* (e.g. evaluation for swelling, heat, pain, and crepitus), *muscle palpation* (e.g. evaluation for swelling, hypertrophy, atrophy, and pain), *collateral ligament assessment* (e.g. applying varus/valgus stress), *joint assessment* (e.g. performing flexion, extension for all joints, and abduction for shoulder and hip joint in addition to evaluation for periarticular swelling, crepitus, joint effusion, and pain), and *specific tests* (e.g. drawer motion for cruciate disease). Of important note is that while the detection of pain is an important feature of determining the source of lameness, it is not necessary to elicit frequently referenced symptoms of pain (e.g. biting and vocalizing) to make this determination. The authors prefer to use more subtle signs, such as resistance to range of motion, head turning, licking, widening of the pupillae, swallowing, muscle twitching, or moving away from the evaluator (during standing exam). This approach maintains a positive relationship with the patient, facilitating further diagnostics and treatment. Furthermore, it allows to follow a systematic, consistent approach to the orthopedic exam (rather than evaluating the affected limb last as frequently recommended).

Table 3.2 Individual steps of the orthopedic examination.

Region	Step	Examination procedure/ structure	Comment
Pelvic limbs	1	Evaluate weight distribution	Pulling caudally on the limbs can detect the affected limb
	2	Paw replacement	Delayed response indicates neurologic disease
	3	Palpation for asymmetry (muscle mass/soft tissue swelling/masses, etc.)	Muscle atrophy can be disuse or neurogenic (i.e. secondary) Pain, swelling, and masses indicate local pathology (e.g. trauma, infection, neoplasia, etc.)
	4	Tarsal joint effusion	Indicates articular disease
	5	Stifle joint effusion	Indicates articular disease, most frequently cranial cruciate ligament disease (CCLD)
Spine	6	Tail lift	Pain indicates lumbosacral disease
	7	Paraspinal palpation	Pain indicates neurologic disease
	8	Neck range of motion	Pain indicates neurologic disease
Thoracic limbs	9	Evaluate weight distribution	Lifting up on the limbs can detect the affected limb
	10	Palpation for asymmetry (muscle mass/soft tissue swelling/masses, etc.)	Muscle atrophy can be disuse or neurogenic (i.e. secondary) Pain, swelling, and masses indicate local pathology (e.g. trauma, infection, neoplasia, etc.)
	11	Elbow joint effusion	Indicates articular disease, most frequently ED
	12	Carpal joint effusion	Indicates articular disease
	13	Paw replacement	Delayed response indicates neurologic disease
Distal pelvic limb	14	Evaluate nails, webbing, and paw pad	Frequent source of trauma, foreign bodies, etc.
	15	PROM of all digits	Pain indicates digit pathology – if painful, perform PROM of individual digit/joints
	16	Sesamoid palpation (#2, 7)	Pain indicates sesamoid disease
Metatarsals	17	Long bone palpation	Pain may indicate neoplasia, fracture
Tarsus	18	PROM	Pain, reduced or increased range of motion, indicates disease of the joint or surrounding soft tissue structures
	19	Varus and valgus stress	Instability indicates collateral ligament disruption
	20	Achilles tendon insertion	Swelling at insertion indicates tendinopathy
Tibia	21	Long bone palpation	Pain may indicate neoplasia (proximal and distal tibia), fracture, and panosteitis
Stifle	22	PROM	Pain, reduced or increased range of motion, indicates disease of the joint or surrounding soft tissue structures
	23	Varus and valgus stress	Instability indicates collateral ligament disruption
	24	Evaluate for signs of CCLD	Palpate for presence of medial buttress, pain on hyperextension, and perform drawer and tibial compression test. Note: effusion (evaluated in step 5) is also an indicator of CCLD

(Continued)

Table 3.2 (Continued)

Region	Step	Examination procedure/ structure	Comment
	25	Assess location of patella	Medial luxation generally in extension, lateral in flexion
Femur	26	Long bone palpation	Pain may indicate neoplasia (proximal and distal femur), fracture, and panosteitis
Hip	27	Hip flexion	Indicates pathology of the hip joint or muscle pathology (e.g. semimembranosus pathology)
	28	Hip extension	Indicates pathology of the hip or stifle joint, neurologic disease (e.g. lumbosacral disease), or muscle pathology (e.g. iliopsoas myopathy)
	29	Hip abduction	Indicates pathology of the hip joint
Distal thoracic limb	30	Evaluate nails, webbing, and paw pad	Frequent source of trauma, foreign bodies, etc.
	31	PROM of all digits	Pain indicates digit pathology – if painful, perform PROM of individual digit/joints
	32	Sesamoid palpation (#2, 7)	Pain indicates sesamoid disease
Metacarpals	33	Long bone palpation	Pain may indicate neoplasia, fracture
Carpus	34	PROM	Pain, reduced or increased range of motion indicates disease of the joint or surrounding soft tissue structures
	35	Varus and valgus stress	Instability indicates collateral ligament disruption
	36	Flexor carpi ulnaris tendon insertion	Swelling at insertion indicates tendinopathy
Radius	37	Long bone palpation	Pain may indicate neoplasia (distal radius), fracture, and panosteitis
Elbow	38	PROM	Pain, reduced or increased range of motion, indicates disease of the joint or surrounding soft tissue structures
	39	Varus and valgus stress	Instability indicates collateral ligament disruption
	40	Campbell's test	Pain indicates medial compartment disease
Humerus	41	Long bone palpation	Pain may indicate neoplasia (proximal humerus), fracture, and panosteitis
Shoulder	42	PROM	Pain, reduced or increased range of motion, indicates disease of the joint or surrounding soft tissue structures
	43	Shoulder abduction	Pain or increased abduction angle indicates pathology of the medial stabilizers of the shoulder
	44	Biceps and supraspinatus palpation	Pain during stretching and/or palpation of the insertion indicates myotendinopathy

Steps 1–13 should be performed in a standing position joint (to allow comparison to the contralateral limb), and steps 14–44 maybe be performed in either standing or recumbent position.
PROM, passive range of motion, i.e. flexion/extension.

Long bone palpation is important not only in geriatric dogs (to detect potential primary bone tumors), but also in any dog because other diseases, such as panosteitis (in younger patients) or fractures, can be present.

Muscle atrophy is an important indicator of pathology in the affected limb. Neurogenic atrophy is generally severe and can develop in as little as a week, while disuse atrophy from orthopedic disease is generally less severe and develops over multiple weeks. Notably, a severely atrophied leg may not necessarily be the most impaired limb. For example, a dog with chronic left cruciate disease may acutely rupture the right cruciate ligament which would result in a severe right pelvic limb lameness but left-sided muscle atrophy. Measurement of limb circumference to assess atrophy is subjective and generally performed by palpation or use of a Gulick tape measure (please refer to Chapter 5 for further details).

Joint crepitus is defined as a grinding or grating sensation or sound that is caused by severe degeneration of the joint or intra-articular fractures. As such, joint disease has to be severe and therefore should be radiographically detectable. It is not uncommon to palpate a popping sensation during elbow flexion-extension, which can be observed in dogs without radiographic changes. This should be differentiated from joint crepitus since it is likely due to flexor tendons passing over the medial epicondyle. Similarly, shoulder abduction may cause a popping noise which is likely due to cavitation (i.e. the formation of gas bubbles within the joint cavity). Clicking or popping of tendons over bony prominences and cavitation has been described in people (Unsworth et al. 1971) but these concepts have not yet been confirmed in dogs. Regardless, the term (joint) crepitus should be reserved for animals with substantial joint disease.

Specific tests (e.g. testing for cranial drawer, goniometry, Ortolani maneuver, etc.) are crucial to determine the diagnosis for various conditions. These are described in the individual region chapters.

3.2.3.1 Pelvic Limb Palpation

The palpation starts with observation and palpation of the distal limb: flexion and extension of all digits together should be performed to assess if a problem is present, as indicated by signs of discomfort or abnormal anatomy. If an impairment is detected, further evaluation of each individual digit is performed to assess potential collateral ligament injuries or other pathology. The nails, webbing, and pads should also be examined for any injuries, foreign bodies, or masses. The sesamoid bones are located just distal to the tarsal pad (Figure 12.7) and should be palpated carefully for swelling and pain. Swelling of the tarsal joint is best felt by palpating the area just proximal to and on each side of the calcaneus. Because long and short collateral ligaments stabilize the tarsus, assessment of this joint must include applying varus and valgus stress in flexion and extension. The insertion of the common calcanean tendon should be evaluated carefully for any swelling or pain and followed proximally to the musculotendinous junction. The muscles surrounding the tibia should also be palpated. The stifle should be evaluated for signs of cruciate ligament disease or patellar luxation. Frequent signs of cruciate disease include joint effusion, medial buttress, pain on hyperextension, positive drawer (Figure 19.7) and tibial compression (Figure 19.8) test, and a meniscal click. Medial patellar luxation is diagnosed by extending the stifle while rotating the limb internally. The thumb of one hand is placed on the lateral aspect of the patella, and the patella is pushed medially out of the femoropatellar joint. The opposite (i.e. stifle flexion and external rotation while pushing the patella laterally) is performed for lateral patellar luxations. The collateral ligaments of the stifle should also be evaluated by applying medial and lateral stress in extension. The tibial and femoral diaphysis should be carefully palpated for any signs of pain to assess for bone pathology. The muscle groups around the femur should be palpated as for other areas.

Of important note is that pain on hyperextension of the hip joint is *not* pathognomonic for hip dysplasia/arthritis: other diseases, frequently mistaken for hip pathology (because of pain on "hip extension"), include iliopsoas injury, lumbosacral disease (Chapter 16), and most frequently, cruciate disease. Cruciate disease can be ruled out by palpation of the stifle and evaluation of abduction of the hip joint. If abduction is not painful, hip pathology is less likely (Figure 20.8). In juvenile animals, the hip should be evaluated for a positive Ortolani sign (Figure 20.9).

3.2.3.2 Thoracic Limb Palpation
Digital palpation of the thoracic limb is performed as for the pelvic limb. The carpus should be carefully evaluated for joint effusion. Namely, just below the distal end of the radius, the carpal joint is easily palpated (Figure 13.3) and any swelling is considered abnormal. Palpation of the distal radius and proximal humerus is extremely important due to the high incidence of primary bone tumors in this region. The muscles surrounding the radius and ulna (with particular emphasis on the flexor carpi ulnaris muscle; Figure 13.10) should be carefully palpated along with the distal aspect of the flexor tendons. The elbow should be evaluated for hyperextension, pain during flexion, joint effusion, and medial compartment palpation (i.e. Campbell's test; Figure 14.6). Hyperextension of the joint is performed by pushing cranially at the level of the elbow joint while keeping the shoulder in a consistent position (i.e. the range of motion of the shoulder should not change when the elbow is extended, Video 14.2). Pain on flexion can be tested while the animal is standing by simply flexing the elbow joint and evaluating for symptoms of pain and whether the dog "moves" away and hops toward the contralateral side (Video 14.2).

The muscles surrounding the humerus should be carefully palpated and the axillary region should be examined to assess for possible discomfort arising from the brachial plexus. Shoulder range of motion should be evaluated ideally without performing any range of motion in the elbow, which is difficult particularly for extension testing. Abduction of the shoulder can be estimated during stance (Figure 15.7) but accurate abduction angle measurement requires sedation. All regional shoulder muscles should be carefully palpated and evaluated for a pain response or spasm. The biceps tendon can be palpated just medial to the greater tubercle (Figure 15.11). The supraspinatus insertion tendon is palpated at its attachment to the greater tubercle. Pain can usually be elicited when palpating and stretching the muscle at the same time (shoulder flexion and elbow extension). Palpation of the axillary area in older animals is advised to assess for possible brachial plexus tumors.

3.2.3.3 Other Techniques for Lameness Detection
If the above-listed examinations do not reveal a source of discomfort, the cause of lameness may be secondary to muscle injury, neurologic disease, or non-painful conditions (such as muscle contractures), or because the examiner was unable to locate the painful area, or a result of the dog not displaying a detectable pain response despite best attempts localizing the source of pain. In such cases, several examination steps can be taken to identify the source of lameness. Specifically, evaluation of the muscles including *myofascial exam and stretching* (Chapters 5 and 6) facilitates identification of myopathies. If no other abnormalities of a specific joint (such as decreased passive range of motion, see Chapter 5) are identified, all muscles of the affected thoracic limb should be thoroughly palpated and this should include passive flexibility testing. Neurologic disease that causes subtle lameness can be difficult to diagnose on palpation; however, a full *neurologic exam* may identify neurologic deficits and should therefore be performed (Chapter 4).

In some cases, although a substantial lameness associated with structural musculoskeletal disease is observed during movement, no obvious pain response is identified during palpation.

For example, dogs with significant elbow pathology (such as coronoid disease or incomplete ossification of the humeral condyle) may show no pain response during joint range of motion. This may be explained by the fact that weight-bearing causes a much different force than range of motion (perhaps displacing a coronoid fragment or causing micromotion in the condyle). Therefore, *joint compressions* (i.e. manual compression of the joint performed by pushing the distal bone forming the joint against the stabilized proximal bone) may be an examination method that can mimic these forces and be utilized in cases when lameness is difficult to localize with routine palpation techniques.

In horses, *flexion tests* are used frequently to further isolate the source of a lameness by holding a joint in flexion for 30–60 seconds and evaluating any worsening of lameness during motion immediately after its release (Baxter and Stashak 2011). Many normal horses demonstrate a positive response to flexion tests, which makes interpretation challenging. However, flexion tests have not been validated as a reliable indicator of musculoskeletal pathology in dogs. Nevertheless, when performing this test on dogs, a difference between the affected and unaffected side can be helpful in further narrowing the differential list (i.e. if a difference in response between contralateral limbs is identified, this suggests that the source of lameness is localizing to the joint and associated soft tissue structures stretched). In general, dogs will display two possible positive responses to flexion testing: Some dogs show varying degrees of discomfort when the sustained joint flexion is performed (i.e. in some dogs, it may not be feasible to hold the joint in flexion for 30 seconds), whereas others show a substantial difference in lameness degree after flexion is released. Again, since this test has not been validated in dogs, it must be performed in exactly the same manner for both limbs and even if a difference between sides is identified, the results need to be interpreted with caution.

References

Baxter, G.M. and Stashak, T.S. (2011). Examination for lameness. In: *Adams and Stashak's Lameness in Horses* (ed. G.M. Baxter), 109–206. Hoboken: Wiley-Blackwell.

Canapp, S.O., Canapp, D.A., Carr, B.J. et al. (2016). Supraspinatus tendinopathy in 327 dogs: a retrospective study. *Veterinary Evidence* 1 (3) https://doi.org/10.18849/ve.v1i3.32.

Milgram, J., Slonim, E., Kass, P.H., and Shahar, R. (2004). A radiographic study of joint angles in standing dogs. *Veterinary and Comparative Orthopaedics and Traumatology* 17 (2): 82–90.

Sargan, D.R. (2004). Idid: inherited diseases in dogs: web-based information for canine inherited disease genetics. *Mammalian Genome* 15 (6): 503–506.

Unsworth, A., Dowson, D., and Wright, V. (1971). "Cracking joints". A bioengineering study of cavitation in the metacarpophalangeal joint. *Annals of the Rheumatic Diseases* 30 (4): 348–358.

von Pfeil, D.J.F., Lee, J., Thompson, S., and Hinchcliff, K., 2015. *Musher and Veterinary Handbook*, 3. Raleigh, NC: International Sled Dog Veterinary Medical Association/Lulu Press.

4

The Neurologic Examination

Lisa Bartner

Department of Clinical Sciences, College of Veterinary Medicine and Biomedical Sciences, Colorado State University, Fort Collins, CO, USA

4.1 Introduction

The most common cause of a gait abnormality is orthopedic disease, yet gait irregularities can also be associated with neurologic causes. Gait abnormalities resulting from neurologic dysfunction can be broadly categorized into three components that may be observed in combination or as an isolated component depending on the nervous structures involved: neurogenic lameness, paresis, and ataxia (Box 4.1).

Neurogenic lameness is attributable to discomfort caused by pathology affecting the nerve roots and surrounding meninges (e.g. from a lateralized disc herniation). Thus, this is frequently referred to as "nerve root signature lameness" (Dewey et al. 2016). These patients commonly have a weight-bearing lameness, although in more severe cases, the limb may be held up. This lameness can easily be confused with orthopedic causes of lameness (Video 4.1).

Video 4.1:

Brachial plexus tumor causing neurogenic lameness and partial Horner syndrome.

Paresis describes a partial loss of voluntary movement that is due to disruption of the signal transmission from either the level of the upper motor neuron (UMN) or lower motor neuron (LMN). A UMN paresis results from loss of normal signal transmission from higher motor centers to the LMN and causes the inability to initiate gait voluntarily (i.e. decrease in voluntary movement). An LMN paresis results from loss of normal signal transmission from the LMN to the muscle and causes the inability to support weight (i.e. decrease in muscle "power"). Lesions causing UMN paresis generally affect multiple limbs, whereas those causing LMN paresis can involve only a single limb (monoparesis), which is commonly confused with lameness (Figure 4.1). Some texts use the term weakness synonymously with paresis; however, since systemic conditions can also

---

Box 4.1   Neurologic Components of Gait Abnormalities

- Neurogenic lameness (= Nerve root signature lameness)
  ○ UMN lesion
    ▪ Not commonly associated with neurogenic lameness
  ○ LMN lesion
    ▪ = Pathology affecting the afferent (*dorsal*) nerve root or meninges (=pain)

- Paresis (= Partial loss of voluntary movement)
  ○ UMN lesion (brain, spinal cord: C1–C5, T3–L3)
    ▪ = Disruption of signal transmission from brain to LMN resulting in inability to initiate gait voluntarily (= spastic paresis)
    ▪ = Pathology affecting brain or spinal cord
  ○ LMN lesion (spinal cord: C6–T2, L4–S3; nerves, neuromuscular junction, and muscle)
    ▪ = Disruption of signal transmission from LMN to muscle resulting in inability to support weight (= flaccid paresis)
    ▪ = Pathology affecting spinal cord, efferent (*ventral*) nerve roots, muscles, or neuromuscular junction

- Ataxia (= Incoordination)
  ○ UMN lesion
    ▪ = General proprioceptive (brainstem, spinal cord: C1–5, T3–L3)
    ▪ = Vestibular
    ▪ = Cerebellar
  ○ LMN lesion
    ▪ Not associated with ataxia

---

cause weakness (e.g. profound anemia, electrolyte disturbances, and nutritional deficits); in this text, paresis will be used when referring to primary neurologic causes.

Ataxia is characterized by uncoordinated movement and originates from within the central nervous system (CNS). Since it generally affects multiple limbs, it is not commonly confused with orthopedic causes of lameness.

Animals with neurologic disease may display a combination of neurogenic lameness, paresis, and/or ataxia. For example, a disc compressing the nerve roots can result in both monoparesis and neurogenic lameness, which can be explained by involvement of ventral and dorsal nerve roots (due to their close anatomic proximity), respectively. If the disc herniation is also compressing the spinal cord white matter, ataxia will be evident caudal to the lesion.

4.2   Neuroanatomy Related to Limb Function

4.2.1   Anatomical Components of the Nervous System

There are three main components of the nervous system: the CNS, peripheral nervous system (PNS), and autonomic nervous system (ANS). The CNS consists of the brain and spinal cord. The cell bodies of the neurons are located throughout and synapse on LMNs of the PNS or ANS. The ANS unconsciously regulates important body functions including the respiratory and circulatory system and as such is not relevant to lameness. Most causes of lameness or paresis related to the

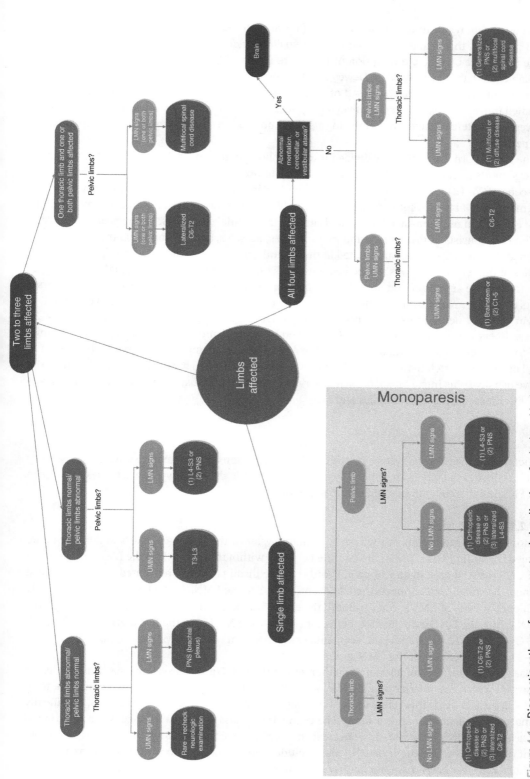

Figure 4.1 Diagnostic pathway for neuroanatomic localization of spinal cord lesions based on motor function in the affected limb(s). Lesions causing upper motor neuron (UMN) paresis generally affect multiple limbs, whereas those causing lower motor neuron (LMN) paresis can involve only a single limb and, hence, are commonly confused with lameness. PNS, peripheral nervous system; C, cervical; T, thoracic; L, lumbar; S, sacral; and Cd, caudal.

nervous system result from conditions of the PNS although some can involve the CNS (i.e. spinal cord). As such, this chapter focuses on these two components and the aspects relevant to canine lameness. More complete description of the entire neuroanatomy and neurologic conditions are available (De Lahunta et al. 2015; Dewey and Da Costa 2016).

Nerve cells (neurons) are composed of a cell body and the nerve fibers (axons). The axons are bundled into either *sensory* tracts conveying *afferent* information from peripheral regions to higher processing centers or *motor* tracts relaying *efferent* information from the motor planning centers to the periphery.

The spinal cord is functionally divided into the following regions, defined by the normal spinal enlargements (intumescences) in the cervical and lumbar areas: cervical (C1–C5), cervical intumescence (C6–T2), thoracolumbar (T3–L3), lumbar intumescence (L4–S3), and caudal regions (segments caudal to S3; Figure 4.2). In dogs, the spinal cord ends around the sixth or seventh lumbar vertebrae in medium–sized individuals and further caudal (e.g. L7, S1) in dogs of small size.

The *PNS* consists of the sensory and motor nerves, muscles, and neuromuscular junctions. The cell bodies of motor neurons are located in the ventral gray matter of the spinal cord, while the cell bodies of the sensory neurons are located outside the spinal cord in the spinal ganglia. The respective fibers arise as *ventral* and *dorsal nerve roots* on each side of the spinal cord. Thus, the dorsal roots convey primarily sensory information, while the ventral roots carry motor nerve fibers. The origin of these nerve roots from the spinal cord defines each *spinal cord segment* (Figure 4.2). Motor fibers can be somatic, innervating skeletal (striated) muscle in the PNS, or autonomic, innervating smooth and cardiac muscle in the ANS. The dorsal and ventral nerve roots fuse at the level of the intervertebral foramen and form a *spinal nerve*. Distal to the intervertebral foramen, the nerve usually splits into a *dorsal branch* innervating the epaxial muscles and skin, as well as a *ventral branch* supplying limb muscles and skin.

4.2.2 Functional Components of the Nervous System

Functionally, the nervous system can be divided into the sensory and motor systems. The sensory system conveys sensory information toward the CNS, while the motor system activates muscles in the PNS and thereby initiates and controls motion.

4.2.2.1 Motor Systems

Motor neurons are distributed within two motor systems, the UMN and LMN systems, and are named accordingly. The UMNs are confined entirely within the CNS, while the LMNs originate in the CNS (ventral grey matter of spinal cord) but the distal portions are located in the periphery. Hence, the spinal cord connects the UMNs in the CNS to the LMNs in the PNS. The UMNs greatly influence activity of LMNs so accordingly, the entire function of the CNS is manifested through the LMN. Thus, the LMNs are the motor effector cells of the PNS. Using the five divisions of the CNS, the C1–C5 and T3–L3 spinal cord segments are components of the UMN system, and C6–T2 and L4–S3 are components of the LMN system (Figure 4.2).

Based on the location of a lesion (whether within the LMN or UMN system), specific deficits are observed which are referred to as UMN or LMN signs (Table 4.1). For example, when the term *UMN disease* is used, this refers to the UMN signs produced by diseases of the CNS, specifically spinal cord white matter and/or brain. The term *LMN disease* is sometimes used when referring to diseases of the PNS. However, this can create confusion since the LMNs are the true motor component of the PNS while the term PNS also includes the sensory portions (sensory nerves). Thus, this text will use *LMN disease* when referring to conditions affecting the motor arm of the PNS specifically and *PNS disease* when referring to dysfunction of the entire PNS. The nomenclature

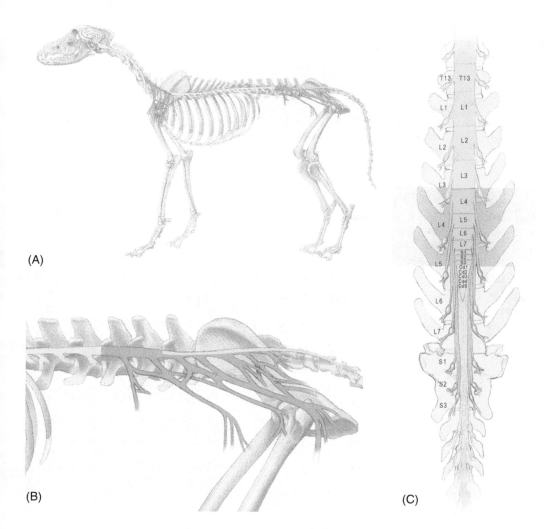

Figure 4.2 Schematic representation of neural organization of (A) spinal cord anatomy and (B, C) magnification of the lateral and dorsal aspect of the lumbar, and sacral vertebrae and coinciding nervous tissue. Components of the UMN system (yellow), residing completely within the central nervous system, include the intracranial structures, C1–C5 and T3–L3 spinal cord segments. The LMN system (purple), with only cell bodies residing within intumescences of the central nervous system, includes the C6–T2 and L4–S3 spinal cord segments and the spinal nerves forming the brachial and lumbosacral plexuses. Most noteworthy, the L4–S3 spinal cord segments (purple) lie within the third to fifth lumbar vertebral bodies.

"neuromuscular disease" is also often used in other texts as yet another synonym for PNS disease since the muscle and neuromuscular junction are considered part of the PNS.

As a rule, LMN deficits will dominate at the level of a lesion and UMN signs will predominate caudal to the lesion. Unless the lesion is at an intumescence, the LMN deficits may not be clinically recognizable. For example, a disc herniation compressing the C3 spinal nerve may cause an LMN paresis to the group of epaxial muscles innervated by that nerve, which may not be clinically evident; whereas a disc herniation of the same severity compressing the spinal nerve of C6 would be more likely to cause LMN paresis to the group of muscles innervated by the radial nerve and result in a lameness and/or monoparesis of the ipsilateral thoracic limb.

Table 4.1 Comparison between neuroanatomy and clinical signs from lower motor neuron (LMN) and upper motor neuron (UMN) lesions.

	LMN	UMN
Neuroanatomy		
Neuroanatomic origins	Peripheral nervous system: spinal cord gray matter (cell bodies) and brainstem (cranial nerves)	Central nervous system (cerebral cortex, basal nuclei, brainstem, and spinal cord white matter)
Spinal cord segments	C6–T2 L4–S3 S4–Cd segments	C1–C5 T3–L3
Neuroanatomic components	Neuron (cell bodies and nerve fibers form nerve root, spinal nerve, and named nerve) Neuromuscular junction Muscle	Neuron (cell bodies and nerve fibers form UMN tracts)
Clinical signs		
Quality of paresis or paralysis	Flaccid (i.e. loss of muscle "power")	Spastic (i.e. loss of voluntary movement)
Ataxia type	None	General proprioceptive (GP)
Posture	Crouched stance Limbs more centered under the trunk to help support weight-bearing Collapse of limbs when weight-bearing Ventral neck flexion (generalized conditions) Inability to support weight (paresis) Off-weighting a limb(s) (nerve pain)	Normal to slightly crouched May vary between base-wide and base-narrow stances Limbs may be in an awkward state (e.g. crossed over, more toward, or away from midline) Standing on dorsum of the paw (spontaneous knuckling)
Gait	Gait characterization: • "Regularly irregular" gait LMN paresis: • Shortened stride • Nails or foot pads may drag • Shuffling gait • ± "Bunny hopping" in pelvic limbs • May prefer to walk rather than stand • Normal initiation phase with shortened protraction phase • ± Muscle fasciculations • Inability to support weight (paresis) Neurogenic lameness: • Shortened stride • Nails or foot pads may drag • Unwillingness to support weight (nerve pain)	Gait characterization: • "Irregularly irregular" gait UMN paresis and GP ataxia[a]: • Lengthened stride • Nails may drag • Stiff • Delayed initiation and protraction phase • May vary between base-wide and base-narrow gait
Segmental spinal reflexes	Usually decreased or absent at respective anatomic segment (unchanged for others)	Normal or may be increased caudal to respective segment
Muscle mass	Denervation atrophy within 7–10 days (i.e. neurogenic atrophy) Usually severe	Disuse atrophy after 30 days Usually mild to moderate; severe with chronicity

Table 4.1 (Continued)

	LMN	UMN
Muscle tone	Decreased to absent	Normal to increased
Sensory	Perceives noxious stimulus but may not be able to withdraw	Normal or abnormal if there is complete anatomic or functional spinal cord transection
Postural reaction deficits	Normal, delayed, or absent (especially those relying on strength, e.g. hopping)	Delayed or absent

[a] UMN paresis and GP ataxia are considered collectively since it is difficult to clinically separate the gait deficits. C, cervical; Cd, caudal; L, lumbar; LMN, lower motor neuron; PNS, peripheral nervous system; S, sacral; T, thoracic; UMN, upper motor neuron.

Since the vertebral column grows more rapidly during development than the spinal cord, the relationship of the spinal cord segments to the vertebrae is altered (Figure 4.2). Paramount to the LMN system, the C6–T2 spinal cord segments reside within the fifth cervical to the first thoracic vertebrae, while the L4–S3 segments lie within the third to fifth lumbar vertebral bodies; some individual variability exists between different breeds and dog sizes. This becomes clinically relevant when determining the expected neurologic dysfunction associated with a specific lesion location. For example, a lateralized disc herniation at the L4–L5 disc space is likely to affect the spinal nerve of L4 supplying the femoral nerve. However, if that disc material herniated on midline, causing more severe compression to the spinal cord instead of the nerve, the caudal lumbar spinal cord segments (e.g. L6, L7, and S1) supplying the sciatic nerve would be impaired.

4.2.2.2 Sensory System

The sensory portions of the nervous system most relevant when diagnosing gait abnormalities are nociception (also called somatic afferent) and proprioception (specifically general proprioception [GP]).

4.2.2.2.1 Nociception

The nociceptive system has receptors near the body surface that receive their stimuli from the external environment. The information is conveyed through specialized receptors which include mechanoreceptor for touch, thermoreceptors for temperature, and nociceptors for noxious stimuli. In dogs, nociception is most readily evaluated since they are unable to communicate on more subtleties, such as heat.

Nociceptors found in the skin can be activated by pinching the skin, which is useful to localize neurologic lesions. A *dermatome* is the region of skin innervated by an individual dorsal spinal nerve branch (e.g. nerve fibers of C7). These have been mapped in the dog. The *cutaneous area* is the total area of skin innervated by a cutaneous nerve (e.g. a specific nerve that originates from two or more spinal nerves, for example C7–T2 for the radial nerve). Neighboring dermatomes and cutaneous areas can overlap but areas do exist where there is no overlap; these are called *autonomous zones*. Thus, the *autonomous zone* is the most specific when localizing lesions.

4.2.2.2.2 Proprioception

The ability to recognize and sense the location of limbs in relation to the rest of the body is called *general proprioception (GP)*. The neurons of the GP system detect position and movement of the muscles and joint via specialized mechanoreceptors called proprioceptors. After receptor stimulation, information entering the spinal cord is either processed directly on LMNs to complete a reflex arc (e.g. patellar reflex) or is projected to the brain (i.e. conscious and unconscious proprioception). Clinically, it is difficult to accurately separate unconscious from conscious proprioception and as such, the term *general proprioception* is preferred and will be used in this text.

4.3 The Neurologic Examination

The neurologic examination is always performed in combination with a full history and physical exam. This allows the clinician to first identify clues that are indicative of a neurologic problem (e.g. worn toe nails indicating proprioceptive deficits; Figure 4.3 and Box 4.2) and then determine the level and extent of the nervous system dysfunction. Doing so establishes the anatomical diagnosis, a critical step in the approach to a neurologic patient.

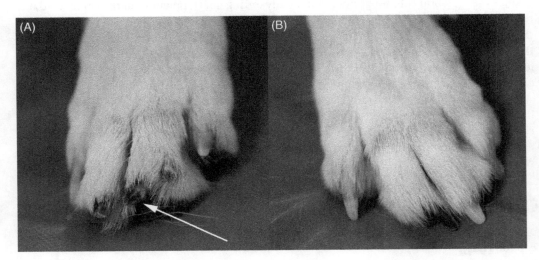

Figure 4.3 Toe nail wear commonly seen on the weight-bearing toes in patients with (A) neurologic disease (white arrow) and (B) normal digits for comparison.

Box 4.2   Clinical Findings Indicating Neurologic Causes of Lameness or Monoparesis

- Unprovoked, intermittent, or sudden vocalization
- Focal pain (e.g. nerve root signature)
- Neurologic deficits:
  - Paresis or paralysis and ataxia (including knuckling)
  - Postural reaction deficits
  - Rapid muscle atrophy
- Paresis that worsens with activity
- Other neurologic signs (Horner syndrome with thoracic limb lameness)
- Uneven nail wear
- Hyper- or hypoesthesia
- Lack of orthopedic examination abnormalities

The neurologic examination can be divided into eight parts: (i) mentation status and behavior, (ii) posture, (iii) gait, (iv) cranial nerves, (v) postural reactions, (vi) muscle mass and tone, (vii) spinal reflexes, and (viii) perception of sensory stimuli and pain (Table 4.2). This sequence is the order which the author feels most logically evaluates the nervous system while considering patient comfort. However, the specific order is far less important than having a systematic way of

Table 4.2 Components of the neurologic examination and interpretation of the patient with lameness and/or paresis.

	Findings/observations	Interpretation
Mentation status and behavior	Normal	UMN or LMN; some intracranial
	Abnormal	Intracranial
Posture	Neck guarding	Cervical pain (muscle, joints, meninges, nerve root, and bone/disc) or referred (e.g. intracranial)
	Kyphosis	Congenital or acquired malformation, spinal pain, and abnormal muscle tone
	Scoliosis	
	Lordosis	
	Head turn	Prosencephalon or cervical pain
	Head tilt	Vestibular or cervical pain
	Spontaneous knuckling	UMN (GP ataxia)
Gait	Lameness	Orthopedic or LMN
	Paresis/paralysis (general)	UMN (spastic or normal) or LMN (flaccid)
	Monoparesis/-paralysis	*LMN (focal disease)*
	Hemiparesis/-paralysis	*UMN more likely*
	Paraparesis/-paralysis	*UMN or LMN (multifocal)*
	Tetraparesis/-paralysis	*UMN or LMN (generalized)*
	Ataxia	All UMN; cerebellar, vestibular, and/or GP ataxia
Cranial nerves	Normal	UMN or LMN; some intracranial
	Abnormal	Brainstem; LMN (CNs VII, IX, X, XII most common), focal or multifocal (e.g. polyneuropathy)
Postural reactions	Normal	Orthopedic disease
		Some LMN (e.g. NMJ, muscle, and cauda equina)
	Delayed or absent	UMN (intracranial or spinal cord), LMN, other (e.g. sedation and systemic illness)
Muscle mass and tone	Normal tone	Orthopedic or UMN
	Hypertonic	UMN
	Hypotonic or atonic	LMN
	Muscle atrophy	
	Acute; severe	*LMN (neurogenic)*
	Chronic; mild, moderate, or severe	*Orthopedic or UMN*

(Continued)

Table 4.2 (Continued)

	Findings/observations	Interpretation
Spinal reflexes	Normal	Orthopedic or UMN; less commonly some LMN (e.g. muscle or NMJ)
	Increased/exaggerated	UMN, excitement, pseudohyperreflexia
	Clonus	UMN
	Decreased	LMN, limited joint mobility, age-related (patellar), and excitement (tense; activation of extensor muscles)
	Absent	LMN, limited joint mobility, age-related (patellar), and less commonly UMN (i.e. spinal shock or myelomalacia)
	Cutaneous trunci reflex	Cutoff: UMN, transverse thoracolumbar spinal cord
		Unilaterally absent: LMN (C8–T1 spinal cord segments or lateral thoracic nerve), ipsilateral
		Bilaterally absent: usually equivocal
	Perineal	LMN (S1–S3 spinal cord segments or nerves)
Perception of sensory stimuli and pain	Normal	
	Increased sensitivity (hyperesthesia)	Orthopedic or neurologic
	Reduced or absent sensitivity (anesthesia)	Neurologic
	Reduced nociception (hypalgesia)	Neurologic
	Absent nociception (analgesia)	Neurologic

CN, cranial nerves; GP, general proprioceptive; LMN, lower motor neuron; NMJ, neuromuscular junction; UMN, upper motor neuron.

approaching every neurologic examination. Observation of a patient's mentation, behavior, and posture should begin while taking a history and the dog is able to freely move about the room. Observations should continue throughout the examination to catch subtleties as the patient is moved from one position to another.

Certain components, for example postural reactions (Box 4.3), should be assessed for any patient as "screening" tests. For patients presenting with a lameness, Box 4.3 displays the minimal components of the neurologic examination that should be performed. However, if the patient or history is suggestive of neurologic dysfunction, a full neurologic examination should be completed.

4.3.1 Mentation Status (Awareness) and Behavior

Mentation is recorded in terms of *level of consciousness* as alert, dull, obtunded, stuporous, or comatose, and in terms of the *content or quality of consciousness* (e.g. inappropriate behavior). Since most neurologic conditions causing a monoparesis or lameness will involve the PNS, mentation

---

Box 4.3 Key Components of the Neurologic Examination that Should Be Performed in a Given Patient

- All patients:
  - Gait and posture evaluation
  - Postural reactions: Proprioceptive placement and hopping
  - Sensory palpation
  - Muscle mass and tone

- Patients with thoracic limb lameness:
  - Assess for Horner syndrome
  - Assess for neck pain
  - Withdrawal reflexes (thoracic and pelvic limb)
  - Cutaneous trunci reflex

- Patients with pelvic limb lameness:
  - Tail lift
  - Paraspinal palpation
  - Withdrawal reflexes (thoracic and pelvic limb), patellar reflexes, and anal tone
  - Perineal reflex
  - Cutaneous trunci reflex

---

and behavior should be unaffected unless multiple lesions (e.g. vehicular trauma causing brachial plexus avulsion and traumatic brain injury) are present.

4.3.2 Posture

The neural organization of gait and posture is complex and involves all levels of the nervous system. Posture evaluation is a subjective assessment of the position of the head, neck, trunk, and limbs. An example of an abnormal posture that may be associated with a lameness includes *neck guarding*. This term refers to a patient where the head and neck are held in a fixed position, even when walking around a turn. When thoracic limb paresis accompanies cervical pain, the back may be arched (kyphosis), and the nose kept close to the ground in an effort to off-weight the thoracic limbs.

Spontaneous knuckling of a foot (i.e. without an observer flipping the paw), causing the dog to stand on the dorsum of the paw, is generally caused by proprioceptive deficits, indicating neurologic origin, not orthopedic. Off-weighting a single limb can be seen with nerve pain (i.e. nerve root signature), but it can also be seen in orthopedic conditions.

4.3.3 Gait

Initial gait assessment allows the clinician to determine which limb(s) is/are affected and to get an impression of the nature (i.e. orthopedic versus neurologic), location, extent, and severity of the lesion. Please refer to Chapter 1 for further details regarding subjective gait analysis.

Specific to the patient with neurologic disease, abnormal gait patterns can be grouped into six components: (1, 2) two qualities of *paresis* (UMN and LMN), (3) *neurogenic lameness*, and (4–6) three qualities of *ataxia* (cerebellar, vestibular, and GP). Understanding the difference between paresis and ataxia is very important to establish a neuroanatomic diagnosis. While ataxia is not

---

Box 4.4   Loss of Voluntary Motor Terminology

- Paresis = partial loss of voluntary motor function (i.e. disruption of UMN signal transmission or LMN implementation of movement)

- Plegia/paralysis = complete loss of voluntary motor function (i.e. severe paresis)
  - Mono- = Single limb
  - Hemi- = Thoracic limb and pelvic limb of one side
  - Tetra- = All limbs
  - Para- = Only pelvic limbs

---

present with LMN dysfunction, it is a key feature localizing to a UMN lesion (Box 4.1). Severe paresis with complete loss of voluntary movements is termed *plegia or paralysis* (Box 4.4). The only difference between paresis and paralysis is the severity of the lesion, and it cannot be used to differentiate between UMN and LMN lesions. Further, in a paralyzed patient, ataxia cannot be assessed.

Paresis, or paralysis, can result from UMN or LMN lesions. UMN lesions disrupt the signal transmission and therefore result in a *loss of voluntary movement* thus producing a spastic paresis (i.e. increased muscle tone). LMN lesions disrupt execution of the movement by the muscle due to *loss of muscle power* producing a flaccid paresis (i.e. decreased muscle tone). The degree of LMN paresis can range from shortened stride length to partial or complete inability to support weight. If the animal is ambulatory, the shortened stride length or partial inability to supporting weight can appear as lameness making the gait in LMN disease similar to that of a patient with orthopedic disease. Stride length in UMN paresis is typically lengthened due to both delayed initiation and completion of the protraction (swing) phase. Determining the quality of paresis or paralysis is critical in differentiating LMN from UMN lesions and is made through evaluating muscle mass, muscle tone, and reflexes.

Gait abnormalities usually result from injury or disease to musculoskeletal components, nerve roots, or the LMN. As mentioned above, gait abnormalities are more commonly associated with orthopedic disease and are typically the result of pain or abnormal anatomy. Orthopedic disease is not usually associated with paresis or paralysis nor should the patient be ataxic. However, gait abnormalities can occur from neurologic lesions, from pain associated with compression or inflammation of a nerve root, for example from a disc extrusion or a nerve sheath tumor (Video 4.1). This "neurogenic lameness" is called *nerve root signature lameness* (i.e. pain from irritation of the nerve root that is referred down the limb). Signs of nerve root signature vary in severity where some animals will hold up the limb completely while standing, presumably to minimize stretching of the irritated nerve, and others show only off-weighting or a minor weight-bearing lameness.

Ataxia is a hallmark of UMN disease and does not accompany pure LMN lesions nor orthopedic diseases. As such, if ataxia is present, the animal has UMN dysfunction. Given the location of the UMN, ataxia generally affects at least two limbs (unless a severely lateralized lesion is present which is rare). There are three types of ataxia in veterinary neurology, the name of each indicating the level of the lesion: cerebellar, vestibular, and GP ataxia. Animals with cerebellar and vestibular ataxia generally display obvious gait abnormalities in all four limbs (such as hypermetria, base-wide gait, or loss of balance), which can be symmetric or asymmetric, respectively. Animals with GP ataxia can demonstrate various degrees of scuffing and knuckling of the nails or footpads, limbs crossing midline, stumbling, and a base-wide or base-narrow gait (Table 4.1). The swing phase is prolonged (from loss of inhibition) producing a longer stride than normal and many times, an overreaching quality is noticed at the end of the swing phase, sometimes described as "soldier marching." If these symptoms are subtle, they may be confused with an orthopedic problem.

In many cases, by observing gait alone, the examiner can determine, not only if a patient has a gait abnormality due to orthopedic disease or a neurologic lesion but for the latter, whether a UMN or LMN lesion is present. However, patients with bilateral limb pain (e.g. hip disease or ruptured cruciate ligaments) may "appear" ataxic, making the distinction challenging. Similarly, some dogs with marked bilateral paresis due to an LMN lesion can appear uncoordinated, but as a function of the severity of the paresis limiting the rate and range of foot placement. Gait abnormalities due to orthopedic disease can also be difficult to differentiate from paresis, especially a monoparesis. LMN lesions causing paresis are manifested as a gait with a shortened stride length (from inability to support body weight) or a limb(s) that buckles under the weight of the dog and may be accompanied by increased fatigability and decreased muscle tone. In contrast, if the alteration of stride phases is caused by orthopedic disease, muscle tone is maintained, and fatigability is often not evident. Orthopedic lameness may also improve after activity, depending on the disease. To decide if a dog is truly ataxic, using descriptions of cardiac arrhythmias as an analogy for gait can be a helpful guide. Dogs that are ataxic will have foot placement that is *irregularly* irregular, implying neurologic origin. A rhythmic, *regularly* irregular gait is more consistent with lameness, monoparesis (e.g. a nerve sheath tumor affecting the radial nerve), or symmetric paresis (e.g. an intervertebral disc herniation in the lumbar intumescence lesion causing paraparesis). The presence of uneven nail wear (Figure 4.3) supports a nervous system lesion causing paresis and/or ataxia; orthopedic conditions do not typically have uneven nail wear.

4.3.4 Cranial Nerves

Cranial nerve dysfunction, if present, is a clear indicator of neurologic disease. Of particular importance to the patient with lameness is evaluation of the patient for evidence of Horner syndrome, a disruption of the sympathetic innervation of the eye. This innervation is complex and involves several neurons. The neurons initially travel from the brainstem to the spinal cord and synapse on LMNs in the cranial thoracic spinal cord, typically at the level of T1–T3 spinal cord segments, before redirecting and coursing cranially to provide sympathetic innervation to the eye (Penderis 2015). Sympathetic stimulation keeps the eyeball positioned normally within the orbit, widens the palpebral fissure, and dilates the pupils. Disruption of this pathway may result in Horner syndrome, characterized by retraction of the eye ball (enophthalmos), pupillary constriction (miosis), narrowing of the palpebral fissure (ptosis), and third eyelid protrusion; protrusion of the third eyelid occurs passively with enophthalmos. The finding of Horner syndrome indicates an ipsilateral lesion in the nervous system along the sympathetic pathway at any number of locations of the sympathetic pathway. In a dog presenting with thoracic limb lameness, the finding of Horner syndrome not only confirms a neurologic lesion but more specifically points to a lesion involving the first to third thoracic spinal cord segments or LMNs as they exit (e.g. lateralized disc protrusion or a brachial plexus tumor, Videos 4.1 and 16.1). Commonly, only ipsilateral miosis (i.e. partial Horner syndrome) is seen with lesions at this level.

4.3.5 Postural Reactions

Postural reactions test the same neurologic pathways already evaluated in gait assessment, namely the proprioceptive and motor systems. They help identify which limb or limbs is/are affected and confirm that a nervous system disorder is present. However, since all components of both the CNS and PNS must be functioning normal to have a normal response, these tests do not provide precise localizing information. In this respect, they can detect nervous system dysfunction but are not specific to localize within a region of the nervous system.

Postural reactions (Figure 4.4 and 4.2) are response tests; they are not spinal reflexes. When performing an initial screening examination, at minimum proprioceptive placement (paw replacement) and hopping should be performed on each patient. If they are normal, the other reactions

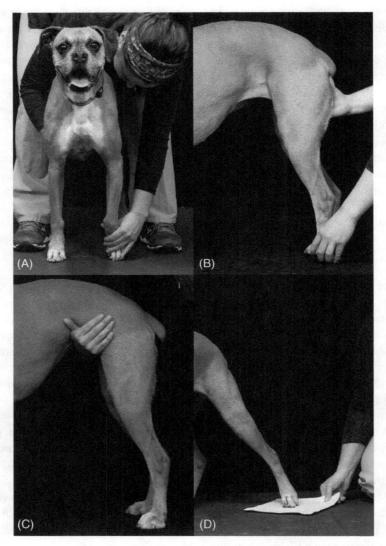

Figure 4.4 Testing postural reactions using proprioceptive placement (paw replacement) in the (A) thoracic and (B) pelvic limbs. The examiner places one hand under the sternum or pelvic symphysis to support the patient's body weight and maintain a midline center of gravity, while the hand on the same side as the limb being tested, flips the paw onto its dorsum. Placing a hand under the (C) caudal abdomen should be avoided since replacement of the paw tends to be less consistent. (D) For placing reactions or the "paper test," a sheet of paper or cardboard is placed beneath each of the patient's limbs beginning in a neutral weight-bearing position. The paper is then steadily and slowly pulled laterally until the patient repositions the limb.

are also likely to be normal. In animals where the paw replacement and/or hopping reactions are equivocal or difficult to interpret, other postural reactions should be performed. Likewise, if the nature or the size of the dog precludes accurate assessment of these tests, hemiwalking, for example, can be helpful.

Video 4.2:

Neurologic examination – postural reactions.

4.3.5.1 Proprioceptive Positioning and Placing Reaction

During testing of proprioceptive placement, the animal's weight is supported by the examiner while the foot is slowly flipped, and the dorsum is gently placed on the ground. The animal should return the foot to a normal position immediately. Supporting most of the animal's weight is important since this makes it easier to eliminate weakness and orthopedic disease as a reason for a delayed test. When testing the thoracic limb, the supporting hand is placed under the sternum (Figure 4.4). More reliable assessment of pelvic limb paw replacement is generally achieved when a hand is placed ventral and parallel to the pubic symphysis, rather than under the caudal abdomen.

A similar test, called placing reaction, can be performed by placing the foot on a sheet of cardboard or paper that is slowly pulled laterally ("paper test"). Once an abnormal limb position is reached, the animal should reposition the foot for normal weight-bearing. The paw replacement test is more sensitive for proprioception in the distal extremity, whereas this paper test detects abnormalities in the proximal limb.

In compressive diseases, abnormalities in proprioceptive placing may be apparent before paresis, because of the superficial position of these pathways. Dogs with PNS disease, on the other hand, can have normal postural reactions if they still have voluntary motor. They may be too weak to correct, but if some of the body weight is supported, they can correct normally unlike in instances of spinal cord lesions, where the animal will be unable to correct even with adequate support.

Distractions, excitement, or a highly compliant patient can delay paw replacement. In these situations, hopping reactions should be performed. Dogs with orthopedic disease may appear to have delayed proprioceptive placing (thought to be due to limb or joint pain that would be associated with shifting weight or flexing joints) when their body weight is not supported by the examiner. If orthopedic disease is severe (e.g. femur fracture or severe joint instability) and animals are not weight-bearing voluntarily, a lack of correction can be observed even when their body weight is supported appropriately (Video 4.3). Other factors that can falsely influence results of paw replacement, such as systemic illness or sedation, must be considered during interpretation. Hopping may be more reliable in these cases.

Video 4.3:

Orthopedic disease mimicking neurologic disease.

4.3.5.2 Hopping Reaction

The hopping reaction of the thoracic limb is tested with the animal facing in the same direction as the examiner and one thoracic limb lifted off the ground (Video 4.2). As the weight is increased on the tested limb, the animal's ability to maintain full limb extension is observed (evaluating muscle tone/strength). The patient's weight is then shifted laterally and the appropriateness of repositioning the foot (i.e. hopping) is interpreted. Important components of the response that are evaluated include initiation, movement, and support throughout the test. Testing in the pelvic limbs is completed in a similar fashion but with the examiner facing away from the patient (Video 4.2).

Hopping response testing is more sensitive than other postural reactions, especially when minor deficits are present. Not only is proprioception tested – indicated by how quickly the patient moves the limb as the examiner moves the shoulder or hip laterally – but strength and muscle tone are assessed as the patient bears weight on the limb. Poor initiation of correction suggests sensory deficits (i.e. proprioceptive) while weak follow-through suggests motor deficits (i.e. paresis).

If pain is a component of the clinical picture, it may affect postural reactions that rely on muscle strength such as hemiwalking, wheelbarrowing (Video 4.2), and hopping. In these situations, the results should not be overinterpreted.

4.3.6 Muscle Mass and Tone

Muscle mass will be affected differently depending on the underlying disease. If innervation to the muscle is compromised, there is disruption in trophic factors and *neurogenic* (i.e. *denervation*) *atrophy* occurs. These changes take place very rapidly, starting within several hours of injury, and become most noticeable in 7–10 days. Conversely, mechanical unloading of the muscles, seen with either musculoskeletal or UMN disease, can cause *disuse atrophy*. This atrophy occurs very slowly and becomes apparent only after several weeks to months following onset. Knowing how rapid muscle atrophy occurred can greatly influence the list of differential diagnoses. For example, rapid focal muscle atrophy occurring in the thoracic limb with an associated lameness should alert the clinician to a higher likelihood of a neurogenic origin, such as a nerve sheath tumor.

Muscle tone, along with gait assessment, will help differentiate UMN from LMN lesions. Through passive manipulation of the limb, the degree of muscle tone is assessed, especially of extensor muscles. Dysfunction in the UMN system can cause muscle hypertonicity appearing as a *spastic* paresis/paralysis; however, normal muscle tone is present frequently. LMN dysfunction causes muscle hypotonicity and a *flaccid* paresis/paralysis. Decreased muscle tone is a key feature specifically localizing to the LMN system.

4.3.7 Spinal Reflexes

Normally during gait and posture, spinal reflexes (also called segmental spinal reflexes) maintain the limbs in extension to support the animal's weight. Evaluation of these reflexes should be considered a continuum of gait evaluation and postural reaction testing; not as a sole entity. Disruption of sensory input, the associated spinal cord segments, or LMN output will result in decrease or loss of reflex activity. Spinal reflexes are a dominant factor in differentiating UMN from LMN disease. A normal sensorium (consciousness) is not required to elicit these reflexes; they will remain intact as long as the local reflex arc (i.e. the cell bodies and sensory and motor nerves) is intact, even if the spinal cord cranial to the lesion is completely transected.

Two types of reflexes are evaluated in the limbs (Table 4.3): myotatic and flexor reflexes. *Myotatic reflexes* are monosynaptic (two neuron pathways; i.e. one synapse) stretch reflexes and include the

Table 4.3 Myotatic and flexor reflexes of the thoracic and pelvic limbs.

Reflex site	Reflex name	Spinal cord segments	Named nerve(s) tested	Efferent fibers	Normal response
Thoracic limb	Flexor withdrawal	C6–T2	Axillary, median, musculocutaneous, radial, thoracodorsal, suprascapular, and ulnar	Flexor muscles of the shoulder, elbow, carpus, and digits	Shoulder, elbow, and carpal flexion
	Biceps[a]	C6–C8	Musculocutaneous	Biceps muscle group	Elbow flexion
	Triceps[a]	C7–T2	Radial	Triceps muscle group	Elbow extension
	Extensor carpi radialis[a]	C7–T2	Radial	Extensors of the carpus and digits	Carpal extension
Pelvic limb	Flexor withdrawal	L4–S1	Sciatic and femoral	Femoral nerve – rectus femoris muscle ± psoas muscles Sciatic nerve – flexor muscles of the stifle, hock, and digits	Hip, stifle, and hock flexion
	Patellar	L4–L6	Femoral	Quadriceps muscle	Stifle extension
	Gastrocnemius[a]	L7–S1	Tibial branch of sciatic	Caudal thigh muscles: tarsal extensors and digital flexors	Hock extension
	Cranial tibial[a]	L6–S1	Fibular (peroneal) branch of sciatic	Tarsal flexors, digital extensors	Hock flexion
Anus	Perineal	S1–S3 and caudal	Caudal and Perineal and caudal rectal branches of pudendal	Caudal nerves – tail depressor muscles Pudendal nerve – anal sphincter	Anal sphincter contraction and tail flexion
Skin overlying thoracolumbar vertebrae	Cutaneous trunci[a]	C8–T1	Lateral thoracic	Cutaneous trunci muscles	Skin twitch

[a] Sometimes may not be able to elicit in normal.

extensor carpi radialis, biceps, triceps, patellar, cranial tibial, and gastrocnemius reflexes. The *flexor* (i.e. withdrawal or pedal) reflex of the thoracic and pelvic limb has a multisynaptic (i.e. multiple neuronal pathways) reflex arc and is the more consistent reflex.

Spinal reflexes are graded on a scale of from 0 to +4: Absence (0) or diminished (1+) reflexes indicate a complete or incomplete lesion, respectively, in the sensory or motor component of the reflex arc. This would indicate an LMN lesion, although differentiation between lesions of the nerve (neuropathy), neuromuscular junction (junctionopathy), and muscle (myopathy) are not always feasible based on the reflex assessment. In general, loss of reflexes in one muscle group indicates a neuropathy (e.g. the femoral nerve). Bilateral reflex deficits are more common with a segmental spinal cord lesion that affects the motor neuron in the gray matter, such as a midline compressive L4–L5 lesion causing reduced bilateral patellar reflexes. If multiple myotatic reflexes are diminished or absent, then a spinal cord lesion, polyneuropathy, myopathy, or abnormalities in the neuromuscular junction may be suspected. Normal (2+), exaggerated (3+), and clonic (4+) reflexes occur when there is loss of the inhibitory UMN pathways resulting in myotatic reflexes being increased. Increased muscle tone usually accompanies these exaggerated reflexes. Clonus is more often seen in chronic lesions. Exaggerated reflexes should not be overinterpreted. If gait and postural reactions are normal, then reflexes are usually normal. If the reflexes appear exaggerated in this case, this is most likely examiner error or increased muscle tension (e.g. due to patient anxiety).

4.3.7.1 Myotatic (Stretch) Reflexes

A plexor (pleximeter) is used to perform the myotatic reflexes. Generally, the flat surface is used when striking tendons while the pointed edge is used on muscle bellies. In small or chondrodystrophic dogs, the handle can provide a focal contact on tendons. Reflexes will be easiest to interpret in the relaxed dog lying in lateral recumbency.

4.3.7.1.1 *Pelvic Limb Myotatic Reflexes*

The *patellar (quadriceps) reflex* tests are the most reliable myotatic reflex of the pelvic limb. However, neurologically normal dogs, 10 years of age or older may have reduced or absent patellar reflexes in one or both limbs (Levine et al. 2002). In these dogs, gait and postural reactions should be normal. The reflex is performed with the patient lying in lateral recumbency. A supportive hand is placed under the femur, allowing the stifle to flex slightly. Excessive flexion or extension of the stifle joint can falsely influence the appearance of the reflex. The patellar ligament is struck crisply using the flat surface of the plexor and the stifle briskly extends. The normal response is for the stifle to extend.

The cranial tibial and gastrocnemius reflexes are less reliable and therefore less frequently performed. Interpretation of the results should be performed with caution (Lorenz et al. 2011; Dewey and Da Costa 2016). The *cranial tibial reflex* is performed with the patient in lateral recumbency, and the limb is held parallel to the ground while the belly of the cranial tibial muscle is struck with the plexor, midway along its length. To elicit the *gastrocnemius reflex*, the metatarsal area is grasped so that the tibiotarsal joint is held in flexion while the common calcanean tendon is struck with the pleximeter above the calcaneus.

4.3.7.1.2 *Thoracic Limb Myotatic Reflexes*

There are no reliable myotatic reflexes for the thoracic limb. The biceps and triceps reflexes are difficult to elicit and while the extensor carpi radialis reflex can be easily elicited, there is debate of its value since it can be elicited in limbs with a transected radial nerve. If these reflexes are performed, they should be interpreted with caution and in context with other findings and compared to the unaffected (if available) limb.

Similar to the pelvic limb, all reflexes of the thoracic limb are performed in lateral recumbency. The *biceps reflex* is elicited by placing an index finger firmly on the tendinous insertion of the biceps muscle on the radius. While extending the elbow and pulling the thoracic limb caudally, the index finger is gently struck with the plexor. To elicit the *triceps reflex*, the antebrachium is held with the elbow maintained in flexion and rotated slightly outward (elbow abducted). The triceps tendon is struck with the plexor, just above the olecranon. To elicit the *extensor carpi radialis reflex*, the antebrachium is supported with the elbow and carpus resting passively in flexion. The muscle belly of the extensor carpi radialis is struck with the pleximeter, just distal to the elbow on the medial aspect.

4.3.7.2 Flexor (Pedal and Withdrawal) Reflexes

In the normal animal, the flexor reflex is meant to serve as protection against noxious stimuli that would be potentially damaging to the skin. For example, if the animal steps on a sharp object, the foot is immediately withdrawn even before pain is consciously perceived. The flexor withdrawal reflex is more complex than myotatic reflexes; because the response involves flexion of all the muscles in the limb, several spinal cord segments are activated. The receptors of the withdrawal reflex are specialized nociceptors that respond only to noxious stimuli (pressure, heat, and cold). As such, the stimulus used during reflex testing must be strong enough to discharge these nerves. A sufficient noxious stimulus applied to a digit should cause the joints to flex (i.e. the limb withdraws). Which afferent nerve is assessed depends on the specific area of skin being stimulated (for applicable cutaneous areas, please refer to Table 4.4). The flexor reflex is a spinal reflex and there-

Table 4.4   Cutaneous sensory testing and autonomous zones used in the pelvic and thoracic limbs.

Nerve tested	Cutaneous sensation	Site used for testing autonomous zone
Thoracic limb		
Radial	Dorsal surface of the paw Dorsal surface of digits 1, 2, 3, and 4	Dorsal surface of digits 1, 2, 3, and 4
Musculocutaneous	Medial aspect of the antebrachium	Medial aspect of the antebrachium
Ulnar	Caudal and palmar surfaces of the antebrachium and paw; including digit 5	Caudal aspect of the antebrachium and lateral aspect of digit 5
Median	Palmar surface of the paw	None exist
Pelvic limb		
Lateral cutaneous femoral	Craniolateral surface of the thigh	Craniolateral surface of the thigh
Caudal cutaneous femoral	Caudal aspect of the proximal thigh	Caudal aspect of the proximal thigh
Genitofemoral	Proximal medial surface of the thigh and prepuce/vulva	Proximal medial surface of the thigh and prepuce/vulva
Saphenous	Medial aspect stifle to hock Digits 1 and 2	Medial aspect; stifle to hock
Sciatic	Caudal aspect of the distal thigh and caudal surface of the tarsus	Caudal aspect of the distal thigh and caudal surface of the tarsus
Tibial	Plantar surface of the paw Plantar surface of digits 3, 4, and 5	Plantar surface of digits 3, 4, and 5
Fibular (peroneal)	Dorsal surface of the paw Dorsal surface of digits 3, 4, and 5	Dorsal surface of digits 3, 4, and 5

fore requires no activation from the brain. It is critical not to confuse reflex withdrawal with conscious perception (such as vocalizing, head turning, etc.). Withdrawal of the limb is not a behavioral response; it is merely a reflex and not a sign that nociception is intact. As long as the LMN system is intact, the flexor reflex will always be present. Testing for the flexor reflex however provides the clinician the ability to assess two components of the neurologic examination: the reflex arc and conscious perception of pain (nociception). If the reflex is present and a conscious response is observed, both are intact.

4.3.7.2.1 Pelvic Limb Flexor Reflex

To test the flexor reflex of the pelvic limb, the limb is extended, and using the fingers, the examiner pinches the interdigital skin. Both medial and lateral digits, e.g. between digits 2 and 3 and digits 4 and 5, should be tested since they have different cutaneous areas (Table 4.4). The least noxious stimulus should be used at first but can be slowly increased in intensity if there is no reaction. Finding the area where the skin becomes thicker at the distal edge and applying the stimulus there generally yields a more consistent response. If no response is noted, then hemostats can be used by applying gradually increased pressure of stimulus accordingly, taking care not to damage the skin. If still no reflex is elicited, hemostats can be repositioned to squeeze across the nail bed, the digit, and finally the metatarsal or metacarpal bones.

The normal response for this reflex is flexion of the hip, stifle, and hock. Reduced flexion of the tarsus indicates a lesion in the sciatic nerve, nerve roots of sciatic nerve, or spinal cord segments (L6–S1); the hips and stifle are flexed normally since the femoral nerve remains intact. Reduced flexion of all joints indicates a lesion in the L3–S1 spinal cord, the respective nerve roots, or the femoral and sciatic nerves. An exaggerated reflex indicates a UMN lesion.

4.3.7.2.2 Thoracic Limb Flexor Reflex

The thoracic limb is tested in the same manner as the pelvic, taking the same care to test medial and lateral digits. The normal response is flexion of the shoulder, elbow, and carpus. Diminished or absent reflexes indicate a lesion in the C6–T2 spinal cord segments, the respective nerve roots, or the named nerves. Decreased flexion of the elbow and/or carpus during testing of the withdrawal reflex indicates deficits in the musculocutaneous and median nerves, respectively. An exaggerated reflex would indicate a UMN lesion, occurring either in the C1–C5 spinal cord or caudal brainstem. However, although this is the most reliable thoracic limb reflex, some dogs with reduced thoracic limb flexor reflexes can still have a C1–C5 spinal cord lesion and vice versa, where normal flexor reflexes can be evident when a C6–T2 spinal cord lesion has been confirmed (Forterre et al. 2008).

4.3.7.3 Perineal Reflex

The perineal reflex tests the integrity of the S1–S3 spinal cord segments as well as the caudal nerves. The skin of the perineum is stimulated using forceps or a cotton-tip applicator. Both right and left sides should be tested. This reflex may be diminished in patients that have lesions affecting the sacral spinal cord or cauda equina, especially if urinary bladder dysfunction is present, for example degenerative lumbosacral stenosis. The normal response is ipsilateral contraction of the perineum.

4.3.7.4 Cutaneous Trunci ("Panniculus") Reflex

The cutaneous trunci (previously called *panniculus)* reflex tests the sensory integrity of all dermatomes over the thoracolumbar vertebral column, which are supplied by the dorsal branches of each spinal nerve in the region. Like cutaneous areas of peripheral nerves, dermatomes are areas of skin innervated by one spinal nerve. These sensory nerves synapse on both sides of the cord but predominantly on the *contralateral* side, before coursing cranially. Thus, this is a *bilateral* reflex. The efferent portion is mediated by the C8–T1 spinal cord segment, the lateral thoracic nerve, and the cutaneous trunci muscle. As such, this reflex is useful in detecting C8 and T1 spinal cord lesions, the lateral thoracic nerve, and locating the level of a transverse thoracolumbar spinal cord lesion.

To test this reflex, the dog should be either standing squarely or lying straight in sternal recumbency. This reflex is present in the thoracolumbar region but is absent in the cervical and sacral regions. Testing should begin at the level of the fourth or fifth lumbar vertebra. The skin just lateral to midline of one side is gently grasped and pinched. Hemostats positioned perpendicular to the vertebral column work best, especially those with curved tips directed downward. As with the withdrawal reflex, only enough pressure should be applied to elicit the reflex. The normal response is *bilateral* contraction of the skin overlying the cutaneous trunci muscle along the dorsal and lateral trunk. If a normal reflex is elicited caudally, then there is no need to continue cranially; since the nerves course in a cranial direction, the entire pathway must be intact. If an abnormal reflex response is encountered, testing up to the level of the first thoracic vertebra is performed and the location where the reflex becomes normal (*cutoff point*) is noted. The opposite side is then tested in the same manner.

Similar to the flexor reflexes, two responses can be observed in the normal patient, a twitch of the skin and/or a behavioral response. Contraction of the cutaneous trunci muscle indicates the reflex arc is intact; a behavioral response indicates perception of discomfort. A lateral thoracic nerve lesion will result in a diminished or absent reflex on the affected side (i.e. LMN dysfunction) and a transverse spinal cord lesion in the thoracolumbar region will result in a bilateral *cutoff* whereby the muscle contraction caudal to the level of a spinal cord lesion (approximately 1–4 spinal segments) will be diminished or absent. Similarly, a lesion affecting the brachial plexus causes an LMN lesion to the ipsilateral lateral thoracic nerve and results in loss of the ipsilateral cutaneous trunci reflex. For example, in a patient with a right brachial plexus injury, the muscle contraction will be elicited only on the left side of the trunk, regardless of where the skin is tested (Video 16.1).

In some normal animals, a cutaneous trunci reflex will not be elicited. In these circumstances, it should be interpreted as equivocal since no localizing information can be inferred if there is no cutoff.

4.3.8 Sensory Testing and Palpation

At this point in the neurologic examination, some information has already been gathered about the patient's sensory system, for example during testing of cranial nerves, proprioceptive positioning, and spinal reflexes. The last portion of the neurologic examination is further evaluation of the sensory component. This includes nociception (perception of pain), spinal and limb palpation, and cutaneous sensory testing. To maintain accuracy in localizing the source of pain or abnormal sensation, sensory testing should be completed prior to administering sedation. The age, breed, and temperament can also influence a patient's level of response.

4.3.8.1 Nociception

Many publications describe testing for superficial and deep pain by varying the degree of compression applied to the skin, implying there are different pathways carrying information about each.

In animals, however, one nociceptive pathway predominates (spinothalamic tract) making the distinction between deep and superficial pain very difficult. In this text, the term *nociception* will be used to infer the patient's perception of a noxious stimulus.

In patients with severe transverse spinal cord lesions (i.e. paraplegic or tetraplegic), nociception should only be assessed in limbs that have absent voluntary motor and where the presence of sensation has not already been established. Any noxious stimulus that elicits a behavioral response may be used to confirm the presence of pain sensation. Pinching the digit or interdigital webbing may be adequate in some animals. When a response is more difficult to elicit, hemostats should be used. If there is no response to a noxious stimulus applied to the toes, then the same stimulus can be applied to the metacarpal/-tarsal bones. If there is no motor present in the tail, nociception can be assessed in a similar caudal to cranial direction.

4.3.8.2 Spinal and Limb Palpation

Palpation of the limbs and vertebral column is performed from distal to proximal and caudal to cranial, respectively. Palpation should always begin using a light touch to prevent more forceful than necessary maneuvers near a painful or unstable region, which could be dangerous to the patient (e.g. unstable vertebral fracture) or the examiner (e.g. aggression provoked from pain or fear). Details of lumbosacral and cervical palpation are described in the respective Chapters 16 and 21.

It is important to consider that pain assessment is subjective, as well as examiner and patient dependent. Also, pain can be referred from other sources (e.g. abdominal pathology or intracranial disease causing spinal hyperesthesia) or transfer to appendicular skeletal structures. For example, a patient may react or sit when pressure is applied, downward onto the caudal lumbar spine, if some of this pressure is conveyed onto painful stifle or coxofemoral joints.

4.3.8.3 Cutaneous Sensory Testing

Nervous system lesions typically cause loss of sensation caudal or distal to the lesion, and in many cases, sensation will be *increased at* the site of injury. Therefore, the distribution of cutaneous sensory loss provides great localizing information as lesions can be pinpointed to a specific nerve or two to three spinal cord segments. For this purpose, areas of increased sensitivity (hyperesthesia), decreased sensation (hypoesthesia, also called hypesthesia), or absent sensation (anesthesia) are evaluated and mapped out. This concept is also used during the flexor withdrawal and cutaneous trunci reflex testing as described above. Similarly, testing can be performed along the other zones described, such as autonomous zones of the limbs (Figures 4.5). Testing is generally performed using a hemostat (as described above) and is started caudally or distally and advanced cranially or proximally, respectively. The direction can be reversed to better map the specific point where decreased sensation transitions to normal sensation. If the patient displays a behavioral response at any point during the exam, then sensation is present, and giving a more severe stimulus is not necessary.

The autonomous zones most commonly tested in the thoracic limb include the skin of the dorsal paw for the radial nerve, the medial surface of the antebrachium for the musculocutaneous nerve, and the caudal surface of the antebrachium for the ulnar nerve (Table 4.4, Figure 4.5). Due to overlap from the ulnar nerve, the median nerve does not have an autonomous zone. In the pelvic limb, sites for testing autonomous zones include the craniolateral surface of the thigh for the lateral cutaneous femoral nerve, the caudal aspect of the proximal thigh for the caudal cutaneous femoral nerve, the proximal medial surface of the thigh and prepuce or vulva for the genitofemoral nerve,

(A)

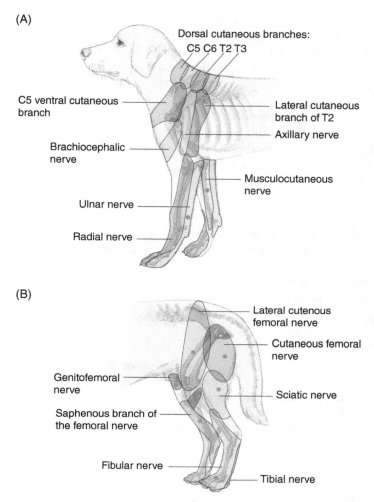

Dorsal cutaneous branches:
C5 C6 T2 T3

C5 ventral cutaneous branch

Lateral cutaneous branch of T2

Axillary nerve

Brachiocephalic nerve

Musculocutaneous nerve

Ulnar nerve

Radial nerve

(B)

Lateral cutenous femoral nerve

Cutaneous femoral nerve

Genitofemoral nerve

Sciatic nerve

Saphenous branch of the femoral nerve

Fibular nerve

Tibial nerve

Figure 4.5 Cutaneous innervation of the (A) thoracic and (B) pelvic limbs: autonomous zones (i.e. areas innervated by a single nerve; shaded regions) and the recommended sites for testing (red dots) are shown.

the medial surface of the tarsus and stifle for the saphenous nerve (branch of the femoral nerve), the caudal aspect of the distal thigh and caudal surface of the tarsus for the sciatic nerve, the plantar surface of the paw for the tibial nerve, and the dorsal surface of the paw for the fibular (peroneal) nerve. Cutaneous testing in the cervical region is unreliable in localizing lesions (Table 4.4, Figure 4.5).

4.4   Diagnostic Tests

The division between musculoskeletal and neurologic disorders is not always straightforward. Nonetheless, this distinction is important since the diagnostic approaches and therapeutic plans can vary considerably depending on the cause. To add further confusion, the same patient may have both orthopedic and neurologic disease. Some patients presenting early in a neurologic disease process, such as a nerve sheath tumor, may only display lameness as a sole deficit, making differentiation from orthopedic disease very difficult. Typically, orthopedic causes are easiest to exclude first with an orthopedic examination, and if any identified abnormalities are nonexplanatory or no abnormalities are found, neurodiagnostics (e.g. neuroimaging) are then pursued.

General considerations regarding diagnostic imaging technologies are discussed in Chapter 10. Multiple abnormalities may be found on neuroimaging, and the clinician will need to determine their clinical significance. Any abnormality needs to be interpreted in light of the clinical history and corroborated with the neurologic examination.

4.4.1 Survey Radiographs

Orthogonal spinal radiographs can be used to assess vertebral structures, intervertebral disc spaces, and intervertebral foramina. To accomplish ideal positioning, sedation is generally advised. Mineralized intervertebral discs may be evident in the foramen or canal and occasionally neoplastic lesions can cause enlargement of the intervertebral foramen from pressure atrophy. Bone lysis due to discospondylitis or neoplasia may also be seen, depending on chronicity.

4.4.2 Myelography

Myelography is an imaging examination where contrast material is injected into the subarachnoid space followed by either radiographs or computed tomography (CT). The images, called myelogram, can provide information on the spinal canal, spinal cord, meninges, subarachnoid space, and nerve roots. It is helpful in detecting extramedullary compressive lesions, but it is frequently not useful in identifying intramedullary, foraminal, nerve root, or nerve lesions.

4.4.3 Computed Tomography

CT has the advantage of being a fast imaging modality but does have limitations regarding its ability to diagnose neurologic lesions. Similar to myelography, CT is useful in detecting compressive extramedullary lesions, such as mineralized intervertebral discs. However, compared to magnetic resonance imaging (MRI), CT images provide limited information on the nerves and intramedullary diseases, such as neoplasia and fibrocartilaginous emboli (FCE). If a herniated intervertebral disc is not mineralized, it will not be easily detectable on CT. CT can be combined with myelography and/or an intravenous contrast agent to increase the diagnostic accuracy.

4.4.4 Magnetic Resonance Imaging

MRI is the imaging modality of choice for the CNS and PNS. MRI is valuable in identifying inflammation or regions of edema, which signify pathology. Structural lesions (such as intervertebral disc herniation), soft tissue proliferation secondary to discospondylitis or spondylomyelopathy, neoplasia, and intramedullary pathology (e.g. FCE) are also detectable by MRI. Intravenous contrast can be administered and may accentuate some lesions, especially those outside of, or disruptive to, the blood–brain barrier, e.g. certain neoplasms, meningitis, and discospondylitis.

4.4.5 Electrodiagnostic Examination

Electrodiagnostic studies assess the integrity of muscles and nerves through recording action potentials. The two most commonly performed electrodiagnostic studies include electromyography (EMG), which measures spontaneous electrical activity of muscles, and nerve conduction velocity (NCV), which evaluates the function of a motor or sensory nerve by measuring the velocity of an evoked action potential along its length. General anesthesia is required for most electrodiagnostic tests to minimize both movement artifacts and patient discomfort. A detailed discussion of electrodiagnostic testing can be found in the literature (Cuddon 2002; Dickinson and Lecouteur 2002).

Collectively, electrodiagnostic studies are useful screening tests to confirm dysfunction in the muscle or nerve. Although these tests do not diagnose specific PNS disorders, because orthopedic disease will not cause abnormalities on electrodiagnostic studies, they can aid in distinguishing if equivocal signs of lameness (e.g. pain or atrophy) are caused by neurologic or orthopedic disease. For example, if muscle atrophy is present, EMG will be normal if the cause is disuse atrophy rather than neurogenic. Thus, the distribution of abnormalities can be mapped out through testing of specific muscles and nerves, the results of which guide additional testing needed, like muscle and nerve biopsies, so that only tissue from abnormal regions is collected.

4.4.6 Cerebrospinal Fluid Analysis

Cerebrospinal fluid (CSF) is contained in the ventricular system and subarachnoid space, where it bathes the brain and spinal cord, including nerve roots. It is produced in the ventricles by the choroid plexus and ependymal cells as well as the brain tissue.

Analysis of CSF often contributes to a diagnosis but rarely gives a specific diagnosis, much like abnormal complete blood count (CBC) or serum chemistry results. Thus, it is very sensitive for detecting CNS disease but in most cases, it is not very specific. Indications for CSF collection include any disease affecting the brain, a spinal cord lesion not definitively diagnosed on advanced imaging, and lesions suspected to affect the spinal nerve roots (radiculopathies), which are the only portion of the PNS still enclosed in meninges.

Collection of CSF is performed either from the cerebellomedullary or lumbar cistern; typically, the location that is nearest or caudal to the suspected location is selected. A normal CSF does not exclude neurologic disease. For example, if a disease process does not involve the meninges, it may not be evident on CSF analysis. Descriptions of how to perform and interpret CSF fluid analysis can be found elsewhere (Di Terlizzi and Platt 2009; Dewey and Da Costa 2016).

References

Cuddon, P.A. (2002). Electrophysiology in neuromuscular disease. *Vet Clin North Am Small Anim Pract* 32 (1): 31–62.

De Lahunta, A., Glass, E., and Kent, M. (2015). *Veterinary Neuroanatomy and Clinical Neurology.* St. Louis: Elsevier.

Dewey, C.W. and Da Costa, R.C. (2016). *Practical Guide to Canine and Feline Neurology.* Hoboken: Wiley-Blackwell.

Dewey, C.W., Da Costa, R.C., and Thomas, W.B. (2016). Performing the neurologic examination. In: *Practical Guide to Canine and Feline Neurology*, 3e (eds. C.W. Dewey and R.C. Da Costa), 92–137. Hoboken: Wiley-Blackwell.

Di Terlizzi, R. and Platt, S.R. (2009). The function, composition and analysis of cerebrospinal fluid in companion animals: Part II—Analysis. *Vet J* 180 (1): 15–32.

Dickinson, P.J. and Lecouteur, R.A. (2002). Muscle and nerve biopsy. *Vet Clin North Am Small Anim Pract* 32 (1): 63–102.

Forterre, F., Konar, M., Tomek, A. et al. (2008). Accuracy of the withdrawal reflex for localization of the site of cervical disk herniation in dogs: 35 cases (2004-2007). *J Am Vet Med Assoc* 232 (4): 559–563.

Levine, J.M., Hillman, R.B., Erb, H.N., and De Lahunta, A. (2002). The influence of age on patellar reflex response in the dog. *J Vet Intern Med* 16 (3): 244–246.

Lorenz, M.D., Coates, J.R., and Kent, M. (2011). *Handbook of Veterinary Neurology*. St. Louis: Elsevier/ Saunders.

Penderis, J. (2015). Diagnosis of Horner's syndrome in dogs and cats. *In Practice* 37 (3): 107–119.

5

The Rehabilitation Examination

Sasha Foster

James L. Voss Veterinary Teaching Hospital, Colorado State University, Fort Collins, CO, USA

5.1 Introduction

Canine rehabilitation modifies human physical therapy evaluation and treatment techniques into the canine model with the goal of improving functional outcomes for patients. Mobility depends on the health and quality of many tissues, from the deepest part of the joint, the articular cartilage, to the superficial muscles, fascia, and skin. When tissues are injured, these attributes deteriorate which may produce painful and abnormal function. For example, if cartilage is no longer smooth and pliable, joint surface movement becomes restricted; this in turn may shorten the joint capsule, leading to secondary tightening of muscles, which may then cause weakness and atrophy. What rehabilitation brings to the lameness exam is the ability to clinically differentiate which tissues (e.g. joint, muscle, ligament, and fascia), based on their normal and abnormal attributes, may be contributing to lameness. The evaluation techniques used to clinically differentiate these tissues are subjective, manual evaluation techniques consisting of (i) passive range of motion (PROM), (ii) joint play, (iii) flexibility testing, (iv) strength testing, and (v) special tests (Box 5.1). The latter entail specific maneuvers that evaluate a specific condition (such as cranial drawer for cruciate ligament instability). This chapter will focus on the first four components of the rehabilitation exam (please refer Chapters 12–22 for special tests regarding individual regions).

When completing manual therapy evaluations, the available scientific evidence needs to be considered before determining a diagnosis and establishing a treatment plan. Only few canine studies exist to support the use of manual evaluation techniques, such as PROM and limb circumference evaluation (Millis and Ciuperca 2015). Even studies in people (who have the capacity to communicate pain to an evaluator) show that the reliability of manual evaluation techniques is variable (May et al. 2010). Yet, results of manual therapy evaluation can be useful to the evaluator to develop and further define a differential diagnosis list, particularly regarding muscle injuries. Nonetheless, the systematic application of established diagnostics such as radiographs, ultrasound, CT, and MRI

Box 5.1   Components of the Rehabilitation Exam

---

1) Passive Range of Motion (PROM)
   a) End-feel
   b) Osteokinematics (goniometry)

2) Joint Play
   a) Arthrokinematics

3) Flexibility
   a) Passive flexibility (muscle stretching)
   b) Myofascial exam (Chapter 6)

4) Strength
   a) Canine Muscle Test (C-MT)

5) Special tests (see Chapters 12–22 for specific regions)

---

continues to be the gold standard for determining the underlying cause of lameness. Therefore, if diagnostics are not available, care should be taken when using clinical exam findings for the purpose of treatment planning.

5.2   Passive Range of Motion

PROM testing comprises the foundation of the rehabilitation manual evaluation for the purpose of determining if osteokinematic abnormalities contribute to a canine patient's lameness. *Osteokinematics* describe the movement between two bone segments (i.e. flexion and extension, abduction and adduction, and external and internal rotation of a joint). PROM testing includes two components that provide important pieces of clinical information: (i) the subjective description of the end-feel and (ii) the objective goniometric measurement. *End-feel* is the subjective description of the sensation that the observer experiences at the end of joint range of motion (i.e. the "end-feel limiting structure" of the joint). The end-feel provides the tester with information about which tissues should be evaluated further (Figure 5.1), while the goniometric measurements determines if PROM is normal, restricted, or excessive.

Various classifications, terminology, and descriptions have been used to describe different end-feel observations (Petersen and Hayes 2000; Marcellin-Little and Levine 2015). The purpose of assessing end-feel is to determine which tissue type may be allowing excessive PROM or restricting it. Some end-feels can be normal or pathologic, depending on the joint and the point at which during motion they are observed (Table 5.1 and Figure 5.2). As such, the observer needs to be aware of the normal end-feels for each joint (Table 5.2). If PROM testing detects an abnormal amount of motion (decreased or increased) between the two bone segments, the type of end-feel may indicate which tissues are causing this finding and isolate those that require further evaluation as seen in Figure 5.1. With the end-feel in mind, the objective goniometric measurement is taken to determine if range of motion is normal. Reference ranges are available (Figure 5.3, Tables 5.3 and 5.4) but because they may vary between breeds (Thomas et al. 2006; Hady et al. 2015), the contralateral limb should be used for comparison (if unaffected).

Passive range of motion (PROM) end-feels

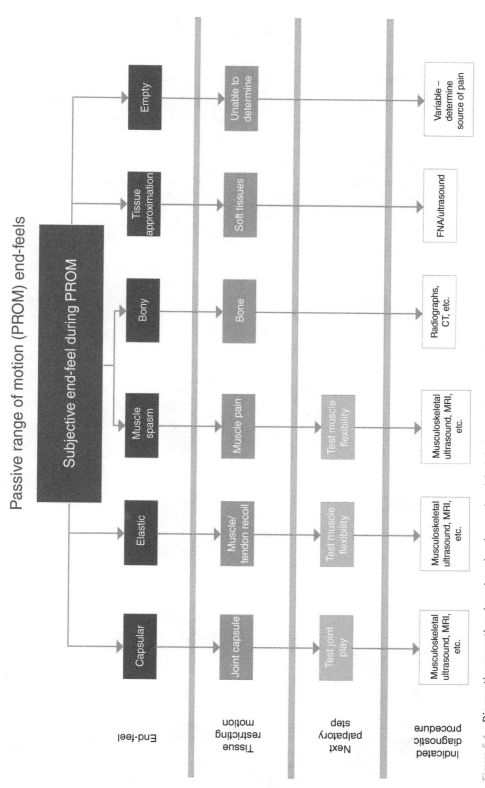

Figure 5.1   Diagnostic suggestions based on the observed end-feel during passive range of motion.

Table 5.1 Description of end-feels with normal and abnormal examples.

End-feel	Description	Example normal	Example abnormal
Capsular	Firm and yielding: joint capsule restricts motion and resistance is not abrupt	Shoulder and hip extension	Loss of hip extension PROM with hip osteoarthritis
Elastic	Yielding with recoil: muscle and tendons restrict motion	Tarsal flexion	Patellar tendonitis, carpal hyperextension
Bony	Hard and unyielding: bone restricts motion and resistance is abrupt	Elbow extension (or capsular)	Advanced elbow osteoarthritis, loss of elbow flexion, and extension PROM
Muscle spasm	Resistance with pain and visual and palpable muscle spasm: muscle pain restricts motion	None	Myotendinopathies
Tissue approximation	Soft tissue limits motion	Shoulder or stifle flexion	Large lipoma interfering with motion
Empty	No end-feel noted: unable to determine end-feel due to pain	None	Intra-articular fracture, unable to evaluate

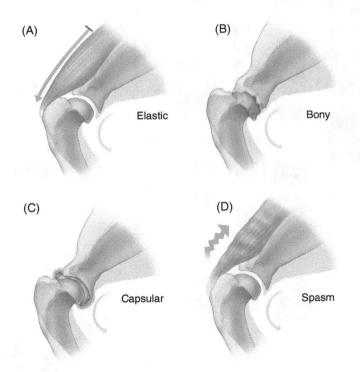

Figure 5.2 Illustration of selected end-feels: (A) an *elastic* end-feel describes the sensation that is observed when muscle or tendon are limiting range of motion, for example, with a supraspinatus tendinopathy; (B) a *bony* end-feel can be observed if severe osteophyte production in an arthritic joint is reducing range of motion; (C) similarly, a *capsular* end-feel may be observed with osteoarthritis; however, the limiting tissue in this case is the thickened capsule rather than osteophytes; (D) *muscle spasm* end-feel limits range of motion because of muscle pain.

Table 5.2 Normal passive range of motion (PROM) limiting structures and end-feel description (used by author) for the major canine joints.

Joint PROM	Normal end-feel	Normal limiting structure
Shoulder extension	Capsular	Joint capsule
Shoulder flexion	Tissue approximation	Triceps muscle group on body wall
Elbow extension	Capsular/bony	Joint capsule/oblique ligament
Elbow flexion	Tissue approximation	Carpal extensor muscle group on biceps brachii muscle
Carpus extension	Elastic	Carpal flexor muscle group
Carpus flexion	Capsular	Joint capsule
Hip extension	Capsular	Joint capsule
Hip flexion	Tissue approximation	Quadriceps muscle group on body wall
Stifle extension	Capsular	Cranial cruciate ligament
Stifle flexion	Tissue approximation	Gastrocnemius on hamstring muscle group
Tarsal extension	Capsular	Joint capsule
Tarsal flexion	Elastic	Gastrocnemius stretch

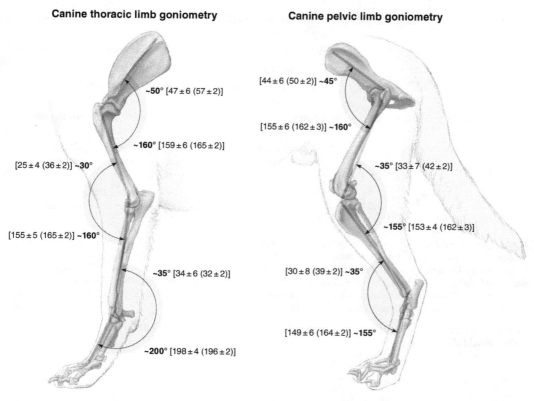

Canine thoracic limb goniometry

~50° [47 ± 6 (57 ± 2)]

~160° [159 ± 6 (165 ± 2)]

[25 ± 4 (36 ± 2)] ~30°

[155 ± 5 (165 ± 2)] ~160°

~35° [34 ± 6 (32 ± 2)]

~200° [198 ± 4 (196 ± 2)]

Canine pelvic limb goniometry

[44 ± 6 (50 ± 2)] ~45°

[155 ± 6 (162 ± 3)] ~160°

~35° [33 ± 7 (42 ± 2)]

~155° [153 ± 4 (162 ± 3)]

[30 ± 8 (39 ± 2)] ~35°

[149 ± 6 (164 ± 2)] ~155°

Figure 5.3 Rounded approximation (in bold) of published angles (goniometry) and normal measurements of the canine thoracic and pelvic limb. Bracketed reference values of the mean (±SD) measurements are provided for German Shepherd Dogs followed by those for Labrador Retrievers, in parentheses. *Source:* Adapted from Thomas et al. (2006).

Table 5.3 PROM and flexibility testing for the thoracic limb.

Joint	Normal PROM	Muscle(s) inhibiting	Flexibility testing
Shoulder	Flexion (47–57°)	Supraspinatus	Shoulder flexion
		Biceps brachii	Shoulder flexion and elbow extension
	Extension (159–165°)	Deltoids	Shoulder extension, adduction, and internal rotation
		Infraspinatus	Shoulder flexion or extension[a], adduction, and internal rotation
		Latissimus dorsi/teres major/deep pectoralis	Shoulder extension, abduction, and external rotation
		Triceps long head	Shoulder extension and elbow flexion
	Abduction (30–32°)	Subscapularis	Shoulder abduction or shoulder flexion with external rotation
		Superficial pectoralis	Shoulder abduction
Elbow	Flexion (25–36°)	Triceps long head	Shoulder extension and elbow flexion
	Extension (155–165°)	Biceps brachii	Shoulder flexion and elbow extension
Carpus	Flexion (32–34°)	Common and lateral digital extensor	Elbow extension, carpus flexion, digit flexion
		Extensor carpi radialis	Elbow extension and carpus flexion
	Extension (196–198°)	Flexor carpi radialis	Carpus extension
		Flexor carpi ulnaris (humeral head)	Elbow flexion and carpus extension
Digits (thoracic)	Flexion (N/A)	Common and lateral digital extensor	Elbow extension, carpus flexion, and digit flexion
	Extension (N/A)	Superficial digital flexor	Elbow flexion, carpus extension, and proximal interphalangeal joint extension
		Deep digital flexor	Elbow flexion, carpus extension, and distal interphalangeal joint extension

Normal goniometric measurements for each joint are outlined in the second column, the "inhibiting" muscle (i.e. muscle that could decrease the PROM measurements) in the third column, and the joint positions to stretch the muscle are outlined in the fourth column. If the observer detects decreased PROM, an elastic end-feel and/or pain while performing goniometric measurements, flexibility testing of the "inhibiting" muscles should be performed. The normal PROM measurements are the mean measurements described for German Shepherd Dogs and Labrador Retrievers. *Source:* Adapted from Thomas et al. (2006).

[a] Depending on the position of the shoulder joint, this muscle can be an extensor or flexor and as such flexibility testing should also include both.

Table 5.4 PROM and flexibility testing for the pelvic limb (see Table 5.3 for column descriptions and how to use this table).

Joint	Normal PROM	Muscle(s) inhibiting	Flexibility testing
Hip	Flexion (44–50°)	Deep and middle gluteal	Hip flexion and adduction
		Superficial gluteal and piriformis	Hip adduction
	Extension (155–162°)	Sartorius, cranial head, and rectus femoris	Hip extension and stifle flexion
		Iliopsoas	Lumbar spine extension, ventral pelvic tilt, hip extension, and hip internal rotation
	Abduction (N/A)	Pectineus and adductor	Hip abduction
Stifle	Flexion (33–42°)	Quadriceps complex	Stifle flexion
		Sartorius, cranial head, and rectus femoris	Hip extension and stifle flexion
	Extension (153–162°)	Biceps femoris	Hip flexion, adduction, internal rotation, and stifle extension and tarsal flexion
		Semitendinosus	Hip flexion, external rotation, and stifle extension and tarsal flexion
		Semimembranosus	Hip flexion, slight abduction, and stifle extension
		Gracilis	Hip flexion, abduction (greater degree than semimembranosus), external rotation, and stifle extension and tarsal flexion
Tarsus	Flexion (30–39°)	Gastrocnemius	Stifle extension and tarsal flexion
	Extension (149–164°)	Long digital extensor	Stifle flexion, tarsal extension, and digit flexion
		Cranial tibialis	Tarsal extension
Digits (pelvic)	Flexion (N/A)	Long digital extensor	Stifle flexion, tarsal extension, and distal interphalangeal joint flexion
	Extension (N/A)	Superficial digital flexor	Tarsal flexion and proximal interphalangeal joint extension
		Deep digital flexor	Tarsal flexion and distal interphalangeal joint extension

5.2.1 How to Perform Passive Range of Motion Testing

PROM testing is a skill set that requires basic knowledge of joint osteokinematics, awareness of muscle origins and insertions, manual handling skills, and correct choice and use of a goniometer. A frequently neglected factor causing incorrect PROM angles is improper positioning of the limb. PROM testing should be an evaluation of the motion between two bone segments, avoiding the influence of muscle tension across the joint. This can be accomplished by placing all muscles that surround the joint, especially muscles that cross more than one joint, in a slacked (non-taut) position. Knowledge of muscle anatomy and function is crucial to accomplish this task. However, as a rule when testing flexion PROM, the proximal and distal joints should be positioned in flexion; when

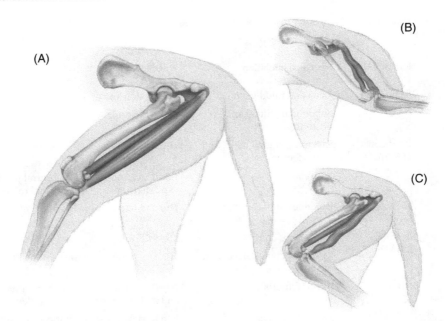

(A)

(B)

(C)

Figure 5.4   Flexibility versus PROM of the hamstrings/stifle joint: when testing stifle extension PROM and end-feel, the muscles resisting stifle extension (i.e. the hamstring group) must be on slack to eliminate their influence on osteokinematic end-feel and goniometric measurements. This is accomplished by positioning the hip in extension. If the hip is placed in flexion, flexibility of the hamstrings is tested. This concept is illustrated using the semimembranosus muscle as an example (*this muscle has two bellies: the cranial belly, a hip extender and the caudal belly, a hip extender and stifle flexor*). Given that flexibility testing means performing the opposite joint motion of the concentric contraction of a muscle, if (A) the hip is placed in flexion and the stifle in extension, the flexibility of both semimembranosus bellies is evaluated. If (B) all joints are placed in extension PROM of the stifle and hip joint can be accurately measured, since both bellies are on slack. If (C) the hip and stifle are placed in flexion, the flexibility of the cranial semimembranosus belly only is tested.

testing extension, the joints should be positioned in extension. For example, when testing stifle extension and osteokinematic end-feel, the tester must place the hamstring muscle group on slack (i.e. by extending the hip joint). If this is not performed, hamstring flexibility, rather than PROM of the stifle joint, is tested (Figure 5.4). PROM testing positions for all major joints, current published measurements and flexibility testing positions for the common muscles that may influence PROM at each joint can be found in Tables 5.3 and 5.4.

It is important to note that there are ranges of motion where single-joint muscles cannot be placed on slack – this will always influence subjective end-feel and objective goniometric measurements. For example, both the supraspinatus and biceps brachii muscles cross the cranial aspect of the shoulder joint (i.e. act as shoulder extenders). However, the supraspinatus is unable to be placed on slack when testing flexion PROM of the shoulder joint because it crosses only a single joint. The biceps brachii, on the other hand, can be placed on slack by flexing the elbow during shoulder flexion PROM testing. Similarly, other muscles that cross multiple joints such as the humeral head of the flexor carpi ulnaris and the gastrocnemius cannot be placed on slack when testing for PROM of carpus extension or tarsal flexion, respectively.

The second confounding factor in PROM testing is improper use and placement of the universal goniometer. Steps necessary to perform accurate goniometry are outlined in Figure 5.5 and

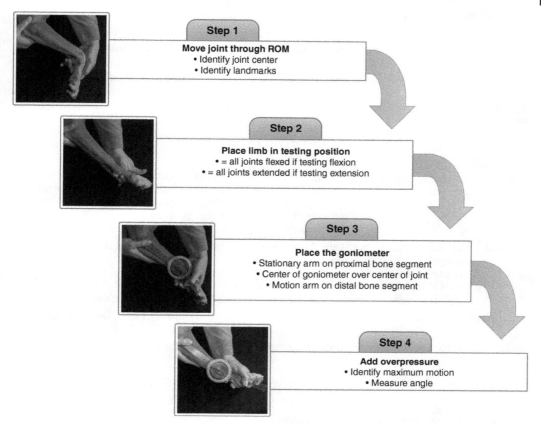

Figure 5.5 Passive range of motion (PROM) for carpus *extension* is completed in a series of four steps. *First*, the patient is relaxed in lateral recumbency and the joint is moved through range of motion to identify the joint center and landmarks. *Second*, the limb is positioned for testing by placing the multi-joint muscles on slack; in this, this case by ensuring the elbow is extended and the subjective end-feel is determined. *Third*, the goniometer is placed over the joint with the stationary arm on the proximal bone, the axis on the point of rotation of the joint, and the mobile arm on the distal bone. *Fourth*, with the goniometer in place, the joint is moved into the testing range of motion applying overpressure at end range to achieve full range of motion of the joint.

previously published landmarks for goniometer positioning (Jaegger et al. 2002; Freund et al. 2016) should be considered to standardize goniometric measurements (Table 5.5). In veterinary medicine, all PROM measurements should be measured on the flexion side of the joint (i.e. on the cranial aspect for the elbow, hip, and tarsus, and on the caudal aspect for the shoulder, carpus, and stifle; Figure 5.3). Current evidence suggests that canine goniometric measurements are more accurate when using a universal goniometer compared to digital, electronic, and smart phone devices/apps (Thomas et al. 2006; Freund et al. 2016).

PROM testing of the peripheral limbs can be completed with the patient in a standing or recumbent position, but only if they are performed consistently when measurements between time points are compared. If the patient reacts to any of the testing positions while standing, or if the tester subjectively feels hypo- or hypermobility in any joint, PROM testing with the patient in lateral recumbency is indicated. This position will allow the antigravity muscles to relax. The muscles

Table 5.5 Previously published landmarks for placement of goniometer arms.

	Stationary (=proximal) arm		Motion (=distal) arm	
	Distal landmark	Proximal landmark	Distal landmark	Proximal landmark
Shoulder	Spine of scapula		Lateral epicondyle of the humerus	Insertion of the infraspinatus muscle on the greater tubercle of the humerus
Elbow	Lateral epicondyle of the humerus	Insertion of the infraspinatus muscle on the greater tubercle of the humerus	Cranial to caudal midpoint of the antebrachium at the level of the ulnar styloid process	Lateral epicondyle of the humerus
Carpus	Cranial to caudal midpoint of the antebrachium at the level of the ulnar styloid process	Lateral epicondyle of the humerus	Long axis of metacarpal bones III and IV	
Hip	Tuber sacrale	Tuber ischiadicum	Lateral epicondyle of the femur	Greater trochanter
Stifle	Lateral epicondyle of the femur	Greater trochanter	Lateral malleolus of the fibula	Craniocaudal midpoint of the proximal aspect of the tibia at the level of the tibial crest
Tarsus	Lateral malleolus	Craniocaudal midpoint of the proximal aspect of the tibia at the level of the tibial crest	Long axis of metatarsal bones III and IV	

Source: Adapted from Jaegger et al. (2002) and Freund et al. (2016).

will therefore have less of an influence on the PROM evaluation. Also, it is important to note that PROM testing in a standing position must be differentiated from measuring standing angles; the latter has recently been described and evaluates the posture of a dog rather than range of motion of a joint (Sabanci and Ocal 2018).

5.2.2 How to Interpret Passive Range of Motion Testing

PROM testing determines whether joint range of motion is abnormal and which tissue type restricts range of motion. This information can be helpful in determining appropriate subsequent diagnostic steps. For example, when testing a patient's shoulder extension PROM, if the end-feel is elastic and the PROM goniometric measurement is 140°, the observer should conclude that PROM may be decreased because of muscle pathology (as indicated by the elastic end-feel; Table 5.1). Several muscles limit shoulder extension (Table 5.3), including the latissimus dorsi, teres major, deep pectoralis, deltoids, infraspinatus, and the long head of the triceps. Flexibility testing of these muscles and thorough evaluation for pain should then be performed. These findings may then lead the tester to determine that further diagnostics (e.g. ultrasound) of the area may be indicated (Figure 5.1).

5.3 Joint Play

While testing range of motion is commonly taught in veterinary school, testing of motion within the joint is only taught for very specific examples (such as "cranial drawer" motion with rupture of the cranial cruciate ligament). These small amplitude movements at the level of the joint are defined as *arthrokinematics, joint play, or accessory motions*. The concept of arthrokinematic testing has been described for assessment of the canine spine, where it is known as the chiropractic evaluation (Taylor and Romano 1999). Although there is a lack of research supporting the use of chiropractic evaluations and treatments in veterinary medicine (Rome and Mckibbin 2011), there are several examples of arthrokinematic assessments being applied in veterinary orthopedics. Such examples include the testing for hip laxity (Ortolani maneuver; Chapter 20) and evaluation of cranial or caudal drawer motion of the stifle. While these examples are well-known applications of arthrokinematics in small animal orthopedics, the rehabilitation exam aims to use the same concept to identify more subtle abnormalities for all joints. In other words, the chiropractic examination includes arthrokinematic evaluation of the spine, whereas joint play is the arthrokinematic evaluation of appendicular joints.

When goniometric measurements are increased or decreased, further evaluation of joint arthrokinematics is warranted. PROM tests osteokinematic motion, whereas joint play (i.e. arthrokinematics) tests the subjective quality and quantity of movement between two articular surfaces (Figure 5.6). Joint play occurs between two joint surfaces and may include a combination of three primary types of motion: rolling, spinning and gliding (sliding) which can be associated with specific osteokinematic motions. For example, carpus extension and carpus flexion PROM are associated with the carpal bones gliding caudally and cranially respectively on the radius and ulna. If carpus PROM measurement is abnormal, further evaluation of joint play of the carpal bones on the radius and ulna is indicated.

Because the primary PROM limitations diagnosed during canine lameness exam are the osteokinematic motions of flexion and extension, the remainder of this section is devoted to further rehabilitation manual evaluation of the joint play gliding which is associated with these specific motions. However, the same concepts also apply for evaluating the motion of abduction and adduction.

5.3.1   How to Perform Joint Play Testing

Joint play testing is the subjective evaluation of two components of arthrokinematics – the quality and quantity of motion. This test is passive and should be completed with the dog resting in lateral recumbency. The testing joint should be placed in a neutral position (approximately midrange between end range flexion and extension) slacking the joint capsule and ligaments to allow the distal joint surface to glide on the proximal surface with the least interference from these joint stabilizing structures. To prepare to test joint play, the tester manually stabilizes the proximal bone as close to the joint surface as possible without painfully compressing soft tissues. To initiate the

(A)   (B)

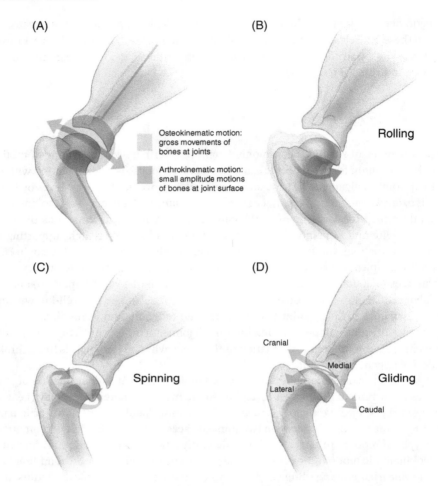

Osteokinematic motion:
gross movements of
bones at joints

Arthrokinematic motion:
small amplitude motions
of bones at joint surface

Rolling

(C)   (D)

Spinning

Cranial

Medial

Lateral

Gliding

Caudal

Figure 5.6 Osteokinematics and arthrokinematics are related to each other and are used to accurately assess and describe joint range of motion. (A) Osteokinematics describe the gross movements of bones as manifested at the joint by a change in joint angle (e.g. flexion and extension through range of motion). Arthrokinematics describe small changes at the level of the joint surface itself (e.g. accessory motions). Arthrokinematic motions include (B) *rolling*, which is a rotary movement (i.e. one bone is "rolling" off the other which would for example cause flexion of the shoulder); (C) *spinning*, which is also a rotary movement, however rather than rolling one bone is "spinning" on the other like a top, causing internal or external rotation; and (D) *gliding or sliding*, which is a translatory movement that can happen in four directions (i.e. one bone gliding on the other which may be part of normal range of motion or pathologic, such as a drawer motion).

test, the tester manually mobilizes the distal bone (again, as close to the joint as possible) parallel to the proximal bone joint surface in one direction at a time – cranially, caudally, medially, and laterally. As the distal surface of the joint is gliding on the proximal surface, the tester feels for joint surface quality and notes descriptions such as crepitus or pain (Cookson and Kent 1979). Since this testing is subjective, it is ideal for the tester to compare findings to the contralateral, unaffected joint. If no unaffected joint is available, breed-to-breed comparison may be considered. This information can then be used to determine if the joint surface quality is normal and if the joint surface gliding motion is restricted or excessive.

5.3.2   How to Interpret Joint Play Testing

Joint play testing determines the quality and quantity of joint surface gliding motion. In addition to PROM testing, this information can be helpful in determining appropriate subsequent diagnostic steps. For example, if shoulder flexion PROM is restricted with a capsular end feel, joint play evaluation is indicated. If joint play in the medial direction is increased, disruption of the medial shoulder stabilizers (i.e. the medial glenohumeral ligament and subscapularis muscle) is suspected. If joint play in the cranial direction is abnormal, then pathology of the cranial structures is suspected (e.g. the supraspinatus and biceps brachii muscles). A decrease in cranial glide may indicate adaptive shortening of the biceps brachii muscle. On the other hand, an increase in cranial glide may be noted with complete disruption of the biceps brachii muscle. These observations may aid in selecting appropriate further diagnostics (e.g. sedated examination, MRI and/or ultrasound). This concept can be applied to any joint; knowledge of the common diseases affecting the region helps dictate the most appropriate next diagnostic step. For example, if carpus extension PROM end-feel is elastic (i.e. normal) but the goniometric measurement is 215° (i.e. increased), further evaluation with joint play testing is indicated. If the amount of glide is excessive, indicating the carpal bones move beyond normal arthrokinematic motion, the observer may consider diagnostics for joint hypermobility (e.g. stress radiographs of the carpus).

5.4   Flexibility Testing

Flexibility testing is evaluation of muscle extensibility, in other words, the ability of the muscle to *stretch* or passively elongate when an external manual force is applied. This flexibility testing is generally combined with the myofascial exam (Chapter 6). Flexibility testing is an evaluation of the passive extensibility of the contractile and connective tissue components of the muscle. The purpose of flexibility testing is to determine whether flexibility is increased (e.g. indicating a rupture), decreased (e.g. indicating a contracture), or normal and whether it is painful (e.g. indicating inflammation). The answer to these questions may lead the tester to determine that further diagnostics of a specific muscle or muscle groups may be needed (e.g. ultrasound).

Flexibility testing is frequently confused with PROM testing. The difference between the two tests lies in the positioning of the entire limb. For PROM, the goal is to put muscles on slack (to isolate the joint), whereas for flexibility testing the goal is to stretch the muscles to isolate them. Unfortunately, this is not possible for single-joint muscles; however, the concept becomes clear with the example of two-joint muscles (Figure 5.4).

During the rehabilitation evaluation, flexibility testing is indicated in three instances: (i) PROM is normal; (ii) PROM is limited with an elastic or muscle spasm end-feel; or (iii) PROM is excessive with an elastic or muscle spasm end-feel.

If PROM is normal, flexibility testing is completed to determine if a muscle is contributing to the lameness and if so, to what extent the muscle may be injured. An example is lameness due to acute tenosynovitis of the biceps brachii muscle for which PROM of shoulder flexion may be normal (i.e. shoulder flexion with the elbow flexed to place the biceps brachii on slack), but flexibility testing of the biceps brachii (i.e. shoulder flexion with elbow extension placing the bicep brachii on taut) is decreased and painful.

In the second instance, if PROM is limited with an elastic or muscle spasm end-feel, flexibility testing is completed to determine which muscle is contributing to the abnormal PROM. An example is supraspinatus tendinopathy for which PROM shoulder flexion has an elastic end-feel (the normal end-feel should be "tissue approximation"; Table 5.1 and Figure 5.2) and the tester can palpate and see muscle spasms during testing. In this instance, because the supraspinatus is a single-joint muscle, the PROM position and the stretched position are the same; the tester would further evaluate the muscle for pathology by direct palpation (Chapter 6).

In the third instance, if PROM is excessive with an elastic or muscle spasm end-feel, flexibility testing is completed to determine which muscles are injured. For example, when tarsal hyperflexion is observed, flexibility testing of the tarsal extensor muscles (e.g. gastrocnemius) should be completed to determine which muscles may be contributing to the excessive PROM and to what extent they are injured as described in the first instance above.

5.4.1 How to Perform Flexibility Testing

To test flexibility of a specific muscle, the patient should be placed in lateral recumbency and relaxed. The observer needs to be familiar with the origin (the most proximal aspect) of the muscle as well as the insertion (the most distal aspect) of the muscle. The observer then manually stabilizes the bone on which the origin of the muscle is located and slowly guides the insertion of the muscle away from the origin placing the muscle on a passive stretch (i.e. performing the opposite joint motion as a concentric contraction would elicit; Figure 5.4). While holding the stretch, the observer notes the amount of flexibility (in comparison to the contralateral side), the patient's response to flexibility (e.g. pain and pulling away), and the body's response to flexibility (e.g. muscle spasms).

While goniometric normal values have been described for PROM testing, such values have not been described for flexibility testing in dogs. To use goniometric measurements for flexibility testing, the joint angle of the muscle origin must remain static while the tester is measuring the insertion joint angle. For example, when measuring flexibility of the gastrocnemius muscle with a goniometer, the joint angle of the stifle must remain consistent during the test, as well as from one test to another (e.g. maintaining that the stifle is positioned and held at 140° while tarsal flexion is measured each time). Because goniometric measurements of muscle flexibility have not been evaluated in the canine model, in clinical practice, the degree of flexibility is most commonly compared to the other limb.

5.4.2 How to Interpret Flexibility Testing

Flexibility testing is completed to determine if a muscle is contributing to lameness and if so, to what extent the muscle may be injured. A minor muscle injury may have associated normal to mildly decreased flexibility with pain and muscle spasm. For instance, in the earlier example of acute tenosynovitis of the biceps brachii muscle, PROM of shoulder flexion may be normal, but flexibility of the biceps brachii is decreased and painful. In comparison, a moderate muscle injury may produce increased flexibility due to fiber disruption with associated pain and muscle spasm. An example is lameness due to a partial biceps brachii rupture for which PROM of shoulder flexion may be normal, but flexibility of the biceps brachii is excessive with pain and muscle spasms. Flexibility testing after a severe muscle injury may result in extreme flexibility without pain due to absent of intact muscle fibers. For example, PROM of shoulder flexion due to a complete biceps brachii rupture may be normal, but flexibility of the biceps brachii is grossly excessive and pain free. Findings such as these from flexibility testing can be used to determine specifically which muscle and to what extent it may be injured, which may assist with developing a diagnostics plan (e.g. ultrasound).

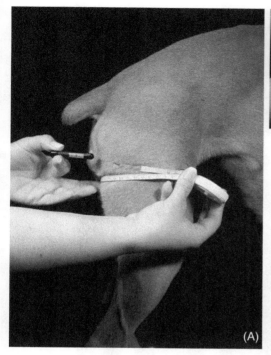

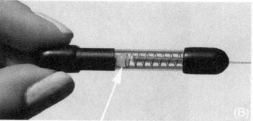

Figure 5.7 (A) The Gulick tape measure is used to measure limb circumference. (B) The device contains a 4-oz spring-loaded tension indicator that allows the tester to standardize the amount of tension applied. The appropriate tension is applied when one red bead is visible (white arrow).

5.5 Strength Testing

Whereas flexibility testing evaluates the passive extensibility, or stretch of a muscle, strength testing evaluates the force-producing capacity of the muscle to determine if weakness is contributing to lameness. Strength testing can only tell the tester if the muscle is strong or weak, not the underlying reason why. If the evaluator finds muscle weakness during the strength test, further diagnostics to determine the cause should be pursued.

Prior to strength testing, the quantity of muscle bulk should be estimated to determine if muscle atrophy has occurred, even though muscle circumference is not necessarily directly correlated with muscle strength. Muscle mass can be estimated by direct palpation or by measuring the limb circumference with a Gulick tape measure. Direct palpation certainly is subjective, and several authors have also called into question the validity and reliability of Gulick measurements. Namely, the ability to replicate positioning of the tape measure on the limb (particularly from one session to another), hair regrowth (if used during convalescence from surgery), and systemic weight gain or loss is a factor that influences these measurements (Smith et al. 2013; Bascuñán et al. 2016). Therefore, the clinician should understand the correct use of a Gulick device and take note of the area measured to improve the accuracy of subsequent measurements (Figure 5.7).

5.5.1 How to Perform Strength Testing

Strength testing in people is performed using validated tests, such as the manual muscle test (MMT) to determine hip extensor muscle strength (Perry et al. 2004). These tests rely on communication with the patient (e.g. asking the patient to maintain a certain joint or limb position while

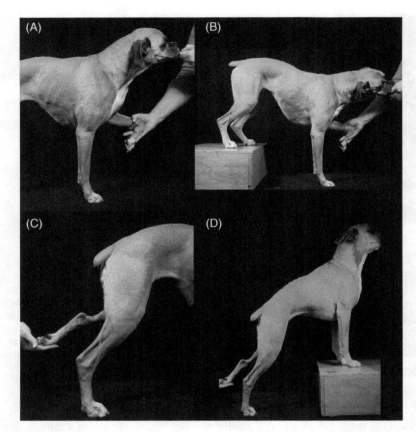

Figure 5.8 Canine Muscle Test (C-MT): to test strength, the contralateral limb is lifted off the ground and the patient is observed for signs of breaking the isometric hold for approximately 30 seconds. This is first performed on a flat surface, and if the patient can maintain the isometric standing position, the front or pelvic limbs are placed on a box and the test is then repeated. For example, for thoracic limb strength testing, the tester lifts (A) the contralateral thoracic limb while the patient is standing on a flat surface; or (B) the pelvic limbs are placed on a box. Similarly, for testing of pelvic limb strength, the patient is first observed while (C) lifting the contralateral hind limb on a flat surface before (D) placing the thoracic limbs on a box.

manual forces are applied), which are difficult to duplicate in dogs. The Canine Muscle Test (C-MT; Figure 5.8) developed by the author evaluates strength by observing the ability of a limb to maintain a static standing position, when the contralateral limb is lifted off the ground (similar to the first phase of testing postural reactions with the hopping test; Chapter 4). To differentiate different degrees of strength, the test is completed in two different standing positions, first on the floor and then on an incline (i.e. the limbs that are not evaluated on an approximately elbow height box) whereby both are scored on a 0–5 scale (Box 5.2).

5.5.2 How to Interpret Strength Testing

The results of strength testing provide the tester with general information about the degree of muscle weakness and with specific information about which areas are most affected. Generalized weakness (from systemic causes) is expected to affect all limbs equally, while osteoarthritis would only affect the diseased limb. Weakness in the absence of decreased PROM or flexibility is more

---

Box 5.2   Canine Muscle Test (C-MT) Scores

Scoring of the patient's ability to maintain a standing position of the tested limb (i.e. the limb on the ground) for approximately 30 seconds when the contralateral limb is lifted (i.e. the ability to isometrically brace against gravity):

- 5 (Normal) = Able to maintain on an incline
- 4 (Good) = Able to maintain on an incline, but shows compensation[*]
- 3 (Fair) = Able to maintain on neutral ground
- 2 (Poor) = Able to maintain on neutral ground, but shows compensation[*]
- 1 (Trace) = Failure to maintain on neutral ground
- 0 (Zero) = Non-weight-bearing on tested limb on neutral ground

[*] Compensation is defined as breaking the isometric hold by shifting weight to another limb, failing to maintain the standing position or muscle trembling.

---

likely to be associated with a neurological cause. Weakness in the presence of decreased PROM or flexibility may be related to each other. For example, hip osteoarthritis is associated with muscle weakness in people (Loureiro et al. 2013). A similar finding has been observed in dogs by the author and seen as a strength score of 2 and a hip drop during the C-MT. This may be due to hip joint pain and gluteal muscle weakness secondary to decreased joint range of motion (since a muscle weakens when it cannot contract through the full range of motion). In this instance, specific diagnostics of the gluteal muscle group may not be indicated, but the strength score will be beneficial for the purpose of rehabilitation treatment planning and monitoring. Specific areas of weakness can be used to develop more specialized diagnostic plans. For example, the evaluator can look for particular signs that indicate pelvic limb weakness such as a pelvic drop (gluteal weakness), increased tarsal flexion angle (Achilles complex weakness), and digital pads directed forward (deep digital flexor weakness). If increased tarsal flexion is noted during the C-MT, the tester would go on to further evaluate the tarsal extenders with flexibility testing and palpation. Findings from these specific muscle evaluations can be used to determine which diagnostics may be beneficial for determining the underlying cause of lameness (e.g. ultrasound).

References

Bascuñán, A.L., Kieves, N., Goh, C. et al. (2016). Evaluation of factors influencing thigh circumference measurement in dogs. *Veterinary Evidence* 1 (2) https://www.veterinaryevidence.org/index.php/ve/article/view/33.

Cookson, J.C. and Kent, B.E. (1979). Orthopedic manual therapy – an overview. Part I: the extremities. *Physical Therapy* 59 (2): 136–146.

Freund, K.A., Kieves, N.R., Hart, J.L. et al. (2016). Assessment of novel digital and smartphone goniometers for measurement of canine stifle joint angles. *American Journal of Veterinary Research* 77 (7): 749–755.

Hady, L.L., Fosgate, G.T., and Weh, J.M. (2015). Comparison of range of motion in Labrador Retrievers and Border Collies. *Journal of Veterinary Medicine and Animal Health* 7 (4): 122–127.

Jaegger, G., Marcellin-Little, D.J., and Levine, D. (2002). Reliability of goniometry in Labrador Retrievers. *American Journal of Veterinary Research* 63 (7): 979–986.

Loureiro, A., Mills, P.M., and Barrett, R.S. (2013). Muscle weakness in hip osteoarthritis: a systematic review. *Arthritis Care & Research* 65 (3): 340–352.

Marcellin-Little, D.J. and Levine, D. (2015). Principles and application of range of motion and stretching in companion animals. *The Veterinary Clinics of North America. Small Animal Practice* 45 (1): 57–72.

May, S., Chance-Larsen, K., Littlewood, C. et al. (2010). Reliability of physical examination tests used in the assessment of patients with shoulder problems: a systematic review. *Physiotherapy* 96 (3): 179–190.

Millis, D.L. and Ciuperca, I.A. (2015). Evidence for canine rehabilitation and physical therapy. *The Veterinary Clinics of North America. Small Animal Practice* 45 (1): 1–27.

Perry, J., Weiss, W.B., Burnfield, J.M., and Gronley, J.K. (2004). The supine hip extensor manual muscle test: a reliability and validity study. *Archives of Physical Medicine and Rehabilitation* 85 (8): 1345–1350.

Petersen, C.M. and Hayes, K.W. (2000). Construct validity of Cyriax's selective tension examination: association of end-feels with pain at the knee and shoulder. *The Journal of Orthopaedic and Sports Physical Therapy* 30 (9): 512–527.

Rome, P.L. and Mckibbin, M. (2011). Review of chiropractic veterinary science: an emerging profession with somatic and somatovisceral anecdotal histories. *Chiropractic Journal of Australia* 41 (4): 127–139.

Sabanci, S.S. and Ocal, M.K. (2018). Categorization of the pelvic limb standing posture in nine breeds of dogs. *Anatomia, Histologia, Embryologia* 47 (1): 58–63.

Smith, T.J., Baltzer, W.I., Jelinski, S.E., and Salinardi, B.J. (2013). Inter- and intratester reliability of anthropometric assessment of limb circumference in Labrador Retrievers. *Veterinary Surgery* 42 (3): 316–321.

Taylor, L.L. and Romano, L. (1999). Veterinary chiropractic. *The Canadian Veterinary Journal* 40 (10): 732–735.

Thomas, T.M., Marcellin-Little, D.J., Roe, S.C. et al. (2006). Comparison of measurements obtained by use of an electrogoniometer and a universal plastic goniometer for the assessment of joint motion in dogs. *American Journal of Veterinary Research* 67 (12): 1974–1979.

6

The Myofascial Examination

Rick Wall[1,2]

[1] Animal Clinics of The Woodlands, The Woodlands, TX, USA
[2] Center for Veterinary Pain Management and Rehabilitation, The Woodlands, TX, USA

6.1 Introduction

Myofascial pain syndrome (MPS) is defined as muscle, sensory, motor, and autonomic nervous system symptoms caused by stimulation of myofascial trigger points (MTPs; Stecco et al. 2013). Because many definitions exist for MPS, so as to avoid confusion, within this chapter, the definition of MPS will be used to describe a form of myalgia that is characterized by the presence of MTPs. MPS is a common cause of pain and disability in people (Weller et al. 2018) and lameness associated with canine MPS has been reported by several authors (Janssens 1991, 1992; Frank 1999; Wall 2014). Yet, identification and treatment of MPS is not commonly performed in veterinary practice.

A simple definition of myofascial examination would be examination of muscles for pain and dysfunction. More specifically it could be defined as the examination of skeletal muscle to identify MTPs. The goal of this chapter is to provide the current status of knowledge and an introduction to the myofascial examination.

6.2 Characteristics of Myofascial Trigger Points

In human healthcare, MTPs are defined as discrete, focal, hyperirritable spots located in a taut band of skeletal muscle (Alvarez and Rockwell 2002). These spots are painful when pressed and have been associated with referred pain, motor dysfunction, and autonomic phenomena. As such, MTPs have been described to have three major characteristics: *sensory, motor, and autonomic.*

The *sensory* component includes local pain, referred pain, as well as both peripheral and central sensitization. The muscle pain or myalgia associated with MTPs is described in people as diffuse and is difficult to localize with defined referred pain patterns. A common referred pain pattern found in people is pain down the back of the thigh and calf from MTPs in the caudal portion of the deep gluteal muscle.

The *motor* component includes the development of the taut band within the muscle, a local twitch response, and muscle weakness:

The *taut band* is a localized, linear, discrete band of hardened muscle within the softer, homogeneous muscle that runs parallel to muscle fibers. The MTP is located within the taut band and is what distinguishes it from other painful areas within muscle. The contractile properties of this group of taut fibers is not the result of alpha motor neuron initiating activity at the motor endplate (like in muscle spasm), but rather due to intrinsic causes. Taut bands result in muscle shortening and reduced joint range of motion.

The *local twitch* response is an additional motor component of the MTP. It is a unique spinal cord reflex resulting in a rapid contraction of the taut band following manual stimulation via direct palpation or insertion of a needle (Gerwin 2010). The presence of a local twitch response can serve as validation of the presence of a MTP.

Weakness is recognized in muscles with MTPs. This weakness is without muscle atrophy and is not related to neuropathy or myopathy. Weakness is often rapidly reversed following inactivation of the MTP suggesting that weakness from MTPs is due to inhibition of muscle activation. A MTP in one muscle can also inhibit effort or contractile forces in another muscle, suggesting a central inhibition process (Gerwin 2010). Additional motor or muscle dysfunction from MTPs is the result of disordered muscle recruitment or activation patterns in muscles during movement or specific action.

In people, several conditions such as coryza, lacrimation, salivation, changes in skin temperature, piloerection, and erythema have been identified as *autonomic* manifestations of myofascial pain (Lavelle et al. 2007). However, such conditions remain difficult to observe in the canine patient.

6.3 Etiology and Pathophysiology of Myofascial Trigger Points

The etiology as to the formation of the taut bands and MTPs is unknown. However, the *Integrated Trigger Point Hypothesis* postulates that muscle injury leads to motor end plate dysfunction and excessive release of acetylcholine. This excessive release of acetylcholine results in extended release of calcium from the sarcolemma resulting in sarcomere shortening and sustained muscle fiber contraction (Gerwin 2010; Wall 2014). This sarcomere shortening has been observed histopathologically (Simons and Stolov 1976).

More recently the role of fascia and hyaluronic acid in the pathophysiology of MTPs has been theorized. The muscle fascia receives innervation with both mechanoreceptors that detect changes in length and tension as well as nociception. Hyaluronic acid is present in abundance in the body's connective tissues and serves as a lubricant and reservoir for electrolytes and nutrients. However, alterations in the conformation of hyaluronic acid can result in adhesion rather than lubrication. It has been proposed that increased temperature and massage may allow reversal of the pathologic configurations of hyaluronic acid (Stecco et al. 2013).

Other possible mechanisms that have been suggested to cause muscle injury and the development of MTPs and MPS are thought to be related to muscle overload or stress due to direct trauma, unaccustomed eccentric contractions, eccentric contractions in unconditioned muscle, or maximal or submaximal concentric contractions (Wall 2014; Gerwin 2016). MTPs can be observed in limbs that are not primarily affected as well as in muscles of the affected limb that are overused. An example would be the formation of MTPs in the coxofemoral flexors of the affected limb in dogs that are non-weight-bearing due to cranial cruciate ligament rupture. These dogs maintain the non-weight-bearing posture by continuous flexion of the coxofemoral joint. The muscles that induce flexion of the coxofemoral joint are therefore required to continuously contract, which may result in the metabolic overload and the formation of MTPs (please refer to the MPS patterns below for more detail).

6.4 The Myofascial Examination

Myopathies are a frequent cause of lameness, yet, examination of the muscles for pain and/or dysfunction is not generally part of the standard physical, orthopedic, or neurologic examination in the canine. In the author's opinion, it is imperative that the myofascial examination be included in any lameness workup to avoid missing a source of lameness and allowing for appropriate treatment.

Anatomical understanding as to the functional muscle units (i.e. muscles that activate a joint) of a joint is crucial and can assist in examination for additional areas of pain and dysfunction. Identification of taut bands and hypersensitive MTPs within muscle is an acquired skill that requires practice and an understanding of muscular anatomy, especially muscle fiber direction.

The myofascial examination begins in the examination room, usually with the patient standing. This portion of the examination is to identify areas of myalgia and patterns (Table 6.1). The myofascial examination is not completely separate from the orthopedic examination but rather complimentary to it. Once the areas of myalgia have been identified, examination of the muscles in a relaxed state is preferred. This portion of the examination is usually performed with the patient in a lateral recumbent position.

There are two basic palpation techniques (Figure 6.1) employed in a myofascial examination (Wall 2014):

- *Flat palpation*: Examination by finger pressure across muscle fibers in a perpendicular direction to the muscle fibers while compressing them against a firm underlying structure such as bone. This technique is employed for muscles such as the supraspinatus, infraspinatus, and psoas major.
- *Pincer palpation*: Examination of a part of a muscle by holding it in a pincer grasp between the thumb and fingers. Groups of muscle fibers are rolled between the tips of the digits to detect taut bands. This technique is used for muscles such as the triceps, sartorius, and tensor fasciae latae.

Table 6.1 Common myofascial pain syndrome patterns.

Clinical problem	Clinical exam findings	MTP locations
Chronic CCLD or slow recovery post-Tibial Plateau Leveling Osteotomy (TPLO) or Femoral Head and Neck Ostectomy (FHO)	Non-weight-bearing or limited weight bearing in surgical limb	Stifle flexors, extenders, and adductors as well as in thoracic limb due to weight shifting
C6–T2 lesion	Neurologic signs typical for radiculopathy	Triceps and any muscles innervated by the innervated nerve
Hip dysplasia	Weight-bearing lameness	Pectineus, gluteal musculature, and hip flexors as well as in thoracic limb due to weight shifting

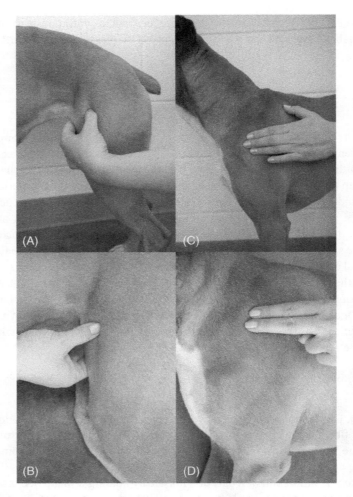

Figure 6.1 Palpation techniques for myofascial examination. Palpation is performed initially while the patient is (A, C) standing but examination of the muscle in the relaxed state requires palpation in (B, D) lateral recumbency. (A, B) *Pincer palpation* is used for muscles that are distant from an underlying firm structure. (C, D) *Flat palpation* is used for muscles that can be compressed against a firm underlying structure (e.g. bone).

Palpation of an MTP in the canine can result in a pain response (such as vocalization and/or withdrawal) as pressure is applied. Therefore, when performing the myofascial examination, the use of an assistant to provide gentle patient restraint is recommended. With experience, palpation techniques to locate MTPs require less pressure and produce minimal to no patient response.

6.5 Myofascial Pain Syndrome Patterns Associated with Lameness

MTPs are categorized as "active" MTP and "latent (passive)" MTP (Shah and Gilliams 2008). Active MTPs spontaneously produce pain whereas latent MTPs only produce pain when examined by palpation. However, with the exception of pain, all other MTP characteristics are shared by active and latent MTPs. This is of clinical importance since latent trigger points also cause muscle shortening and the other above-described changes and thereby affect function (Janssens 1991).

MPS has been categorized as primary (unrelated to other medical conditions) or secondary (associated with a comorbid medical condition; Weller et al. 2018). An acute muscle strain injury that results in the formation of MTPs is an example of the former, whereas an example of the latter includes the formation of MTPs in the functional unit muscles secondary to any articular dysfunction (Table 6.1).

Chronic cranial cruciate ligament disease (CCLD) is a good example of secondary MPS in the functional muscle units. In this scenario, the functional muscle units are those that flex and extend the stifle joint. Pelvic limb muscles that assist in stifle extension include the cranial head of the sartorius, tensor fasciae latae, rectus femoris, and the vastus group. Predominant stifle flexors include the semitendinosus, semimembranosus, biceps femoris, and gastrocnemius. Additionally, these muscles provide dynamic stabilization and the demand placed upon them may be increased due to the deficiency in static joint stabilization. Careful evaluation of these muscles for evidence of taut bands and MTPs should be performed in dogs with CCLD. MTPs can also be found in the gracilis and adductor due to their attempts to counter the slight pelvic limb abduction seen with CCLD as described by Tashman et al. (2004). Severity of MPS is directly related to the chronicity and severity of the CCLD.

Articular dysfunction of the coxofemoral joint related to hip dysplasia can also lead to MTP formation in its functional muscle units. The pectineus muscle in particular can become exquisitely painful and taut. Myalgia in this small muscle is almost always the result of articular disturbance and mechanical overload of the muscle due to its attempt to counter the subluxation of the femoral head. Other muscles that may show MTPs include the gluteal muscles and hip flexors including the iliopsoas, and iliocostalis lumborum near its origination.

Pelvic limb disorders, both orthopedic and neurologic, can result in increased distribution of body weight to the thoracic limbs. The formation of MTPs in the triceps, infraspinatus, supraspinatus, deltoids, latissimus dorsi, in the region of its fusion with the teres major, and/or serratus ventralis can be observed. The more chronic and severe the pelvic limb problem(s) are the more profound the MPS in the muscles described above.

MTPs can also be related to radiculopathy, such as thoracic limb lameness related to structural, compressive lesions of the C6–T2 region. Clinically MTPs can be observed in any of the muscles receiving innervation from an irritated spinal nerve(s). A pattern of increased development of MTPs in the triceps on the affected side in a C6–T2 radiculopathy is often observed.

6.6 Clinical Significance

MPS and MTPs in human healthcare are not without their skeptics and critics: A critical literature review published in 2014 dismissed MPS and MTP concepts and hypotheses (Quintner et al. 2015). However, in this author's opinion, Quintner et al. (2015) provided a biased review and failed to review current literature. In contrast, the rather lengthy published response of Dommerholt and Gerwin (2015) based on more current scientific advances supported the concepts of MPS and MTP.

This controversy is in part due to the reliance upon palpation and pain responses when diagnosing MPS. Further research is needed to clearly answer the clinical implications of MPS and MTP in people and dogs. However, the use of ultrasound and magnetic resonance elastography offers a method for more objective identification of MTPs (Gerwin 2016). For example, recent research utilizing MRI has confirmed the presence of taut bands in people but also showed that they are overestimated by clinicians (Chen et al. 2016).

Muscle pain and dysfunction resulting from the presence of MTPs should be considered in canine lameness as a potential cause (primary MPS) and/or a finding (secondary MPS) associated with a comorbid issue(s). In primary MPS, the localization of pain and dysfunction causing lameness will not be properly identified without a myofascial examination. As such, the diagnosis may be missed and appropriate treatment may not be initiated. Secondary MPS is highly prevalent in both people and dogs affected by any orthopedic condition or recovering from orthopedic and/or neurologic surgeries as described above.

Many treatment options for MPS have been described (Gerwin 2016). For example, treatment with dry needling has been shown to benefit patients with secondary MPS (Janssens 1991; Espejo-Antunez et al. 2017). It has also been successfully used to improve comfort after total knee arthroplasty in people (Mayoral et al. 2013). While there is still some controversy about the use in veterinary medicine, a better understanding of the patterns of myalgia and dysfunction associated secondary MPS may assist in localization of the primary issue as well as identification of additional areas for therapeutic intervention.

It is important to understand that common imaging modalities (radiography as well as standard ultrasound) are unable to diagnose MTPs. This in turn may place fault with a lesion that is not the real etiology (but can be identified with these diagnostic means).

References

Alvarez, D.J. and Rockwell, P.G. (2002). Trigger points diagnosis and management. *American Family Physician* 65 (4): 653–660.

Chen, Q., Wang, H.-J., Gay, R.E. et al. (2016). Quantification of myofascial taut bands. *Archives of Physical Medicine and Rehabilitation* 97 (1): 67–73.

Dommerholt, J. and Gerwin, R.D. (2015). A critical evaluation of Quintner et al.: missing the point. *Journal of Bodywork and Movement Therapies* 19 (2): 193–204.

Espejo-Antunez, L., Tejeda, J.F., Albornoz-Cabello, M. et al. (2017). Dry needling in the management of myofascial trigger points: a systematic review of randomized controlled trials. *Complementary Therapies in Medicine* 33: 46–57.

Frank, E.M. (1999). Myofascial trigger point diagnostic criteria in the dog. *Journal of Musculoskeletal Pain* 7 (1–2): 231–237.

Gerwin, R.D. (2010). Myofascial pain syndrome. In: *Muscle Pain: Diagnosis and Treatment* (eds. S. Mense and R.D. Gerwin), 15–83. Berlin: Springer.

Gerwin, R.D. (2016). Myofascial trigger point pain syndromes. *Seminars in Neurology* 36 (5): 469–473.

Janssens, L.A. (1991). Trigger points in 48 dogs with myofascial pain syndromes. *Veterinary Surgery* 20 (4): 274–278.

Janssens, L.A. (1992). Trigger point therapy. *Problems in Veterinary Medicine* 4 (1): 117–124.

Lavelle, E.D., Lavelle, W., and Smith, H.S. (2007). Myofascial trigger points. *Anesthesiology Clinics* 25 (4): 841–851. vii–viii.

Mayoral, O., Salvat, I., Martin, M.T. et al. (2013). Efficacy of myofascial trigger point dry needling in the prevention of pain after total knee arthroplasty: a randomized, double-blinded, placebo-controlled trial. *Evidence-based Complementary and Alternative Medicine* 2013: 694941.

Quintner, J.L., Bove, G.M., and Cohen, M.L. (2015). A critical evaluation of the trigger point phenomenon. *Rheumatology (Oxford)* 54 (3): 392–399.

Shah, J.P. and Gilliams, E.A. (2008). Uncovering the biochemical milieu of myofascial trigger points using in vivo microdialysis: an application of muscle pain concepts to myofascial pain syndrome. *Journal of Bodywork and Movement Therapies* 12 (4): 371–384.

Simons, D.G. and Stolov, W.C. (1976). Microscopic features and transient contraction of palpable bands in canine muscle. *American Journal of Physical Medicine* 55 (2): 65–88.

Stecco, A., Gesi, M., Stecco, C., and Stern, R. (2013). Fascial components of the myofascial pain syndrome. *Current Pain and Headache Reports* 17 (8): 352.

Tashman, S., Anderst, W., Kolowich, P. et al. (2004). Kinematics of the acl-deficient canine knee during gait: serial changes over two years. *Journal of Orthopaedic Research* 22 (5): 931–941.

Wall, R. (2014). Introduction to myofascial trigger points in dogs. *Topics in Companion Animal Medicine* 29 (2): 43–48.

Weller, J.L., Comeau, D., and Otis, J.A.D. (2018). Myofascial pain. *Seminars in Neurology* 38 (6): 640–643.

Part II

Diagnostic Techniques

7

Arthrocentesis Technique

Bryan T. Torres[1] and Felix Michael Duerr[2]

[1] Department of Veterinary Medicine and Surgery, College of Veterinary Medicine, University of Missouri, Columbia, MO, USA
[2] Department of Clinical Sciences, College of Veterinary Medicine and Biomedical Sciences, Colorado State University, Fort Collins, CO, USA

7.1   Introduction

Joints are complex structures that can allow varying degrees of motion. Fibrous joints (e.g. tibiofibular joint) and cartilaginous joints (e.g. pubic symphysis) offer little to no motion and have no joint cavity. However, synovial or diarthrodial (freely movable) joints (e.g. hip joint) allow wide degrees of motion and have fluid-filled joint cavities. This fluid, called synovial fluid, is a protein-rich ultrafiltrate of plasma and plays an important role in joint health. It contains hyaluronic acid, sugars, electrolytes, and enzymes that help provide nutrition to intra-articular structures, aid in joint lubrication, and act as a shock absorber during joint motion. By sampling it, clinicians can glean valuable information on the health of a joint or the presence and type of pathology (Chapter 9). Fluid evaluation is indicated for various clinical presentations (e.g. Box 7.1) and can also be used to gauge a patient's response to therapy. Despite the relative simplicity in obtaining synovial fluid samples by arthrocentesis (i.e. joint tap), this diagnostic tool remains underutilized in veterinary medicine.

Box 7.1   Principal Indications for Arthrocentesis

When to consider arthrocentesis?

- Joint effusion or swelling
- Joint pain
- Lameness (e.g. shifting leg and unexplained lameness)
- Altered gait or limb function
- Fever of unknown origin
- Generalized pain and weakness
- Suspected sepsis

7.2 Risks and Contraindications

Generally, there is little risk with appropriately performed arthrocentesis; however, iatrogenic damage to the joint and joint sepsis are possible complications. The overall incidence of joint sepsis after arthrocentesis and intra-articular administration of medications in horses has been reported to be less than 0.1% or 1 case per 1279 injections (Steel et al. 2013), but this has not been studied in dogs. To avoid the risk of contamination, arthrocentesis should not be performed when any evidence of infection/pyoderma is present in the area. Additionally, arthrocentesis should be performed under sterile conditions and with appropriate restraint/sedation.

7.3 Restraint

We recommend that sedation be used to ensure that the best synovial fluid samples are obtained in a pain-free manner that reduces patient stress during the procedure. There are anecdotal reports of performing canine joint taps without any or with only mild sedation using topical lidocaine–prilocaine cream (EMLA); however, these creams require 30–60 minutes of contact time (van Oostrom and Knowles 2018). Although joint taps are commonly performed without sedation in horses, canine joints are much smaller, and sedation helps reduce iatrogenic damage to the joint structures. Clinicians should choose a sedation method that they are comfortable with, provide adequate analgesia for the procedure, and minimize patient motion to ensure atraumatic aspiration of joint fluid. Please refer to Chapter 8 for specific sedation recommendation when joint fluid aspiration is combined with diagnostic joint anesthesia (e.g. joint block).

7.4 Site Preparation

All arthrocentesis sites should undergo a standard aseptic preparation process prior to acquiring a synovial sample. The goal of the aseptic skin preparation is to reduce gross contamination as well as the transient bacterial flora on the skin. Hair should be removed (clipped) from an area of approximately 5 cm × 5 cm (for a medium-sized dog) prior to cleaning and aseptic preparation. The size of the prepared site may vary by joint, size of dog, and/or clinician preference. The removal of hair helps reduce *tissue* contamination during arthrocentesis in horses; however, Wahl et al. (2012) found that angled insertion of the needle (at 45° to the skin) through unclipped hair results in the least amount of *hair* (not tissue) contamination. Additionally, the authors of this study suggested that hair debris is more likely to contain bacteria and cause sepsis and, therefore, recommended that (for horses) hair clipping may not be beneficial. However, since this has not yet been studied in dogs, when performing arthrocentesis on dogs, we recommend clipping hair prior to cleaning and aseptically preparing the insertion site.

7.5 Equipment

The equipment needed for arthrocentesis is readily available in most clinical environments. Sterile disposable syringes and hypodermic needles of varying sizes will be needed along with sterile gloves, glass slides for evaluation, culture medium (ideally pediatric blood culture flasks), hair clippers, and sterile preparation materials. General recommendations are listed in Table 7.1.

When selecting needles, clinicians should remember that joint fluid is viscous and smaller bore needles (e.g. 25 g) can make aspiration difficult. However, larger gauge needles appear to be associated with an increased risk of contamination (Waxman et al. 2015). Therefore, needle size should

Table 7.1 Supplies required for performing arthrocentesis.

	Arthrocentesis supplies
Sedation	• Sedation and monitoring supplies and equipment
Site preparation	• Hair clippers • Sterile scrub solution and alcohol • Sterile gauze • Sterile gloves
Needles	• Small dogs and cats = 25–22 g needles; 5/8″ to 1″ length • Medium to large dogs = 22–20 g needles; 1–1.5″ length • Giant-breed dogs = may require spinal needle; 2.5″ length

Syringes	• Sterile disposable syringes
	  ○ Small dogs and cats = 1–3 ml
	  ○ Medium- to Giant-breed dogs = 3–6 ml

Sample submission supplies	• Glass slides (and slide mailer) for
	  ○ submission of freshly prepared smears
	• Pediatric blood culture flasks for
	  ○ obtaining bacterial culture and sensitivity[a]
	• Ethylenediaminetetraacetic acid (EDTA) blood tubes (*purple or lavender top* tubes)[b] for
	  ○ total nucleated cell count
	  ○ cytology
	  ○ total protein (if not underfilled)
	• Sterile, no additive blood tubes (*red top* glass tubes)[c] for
	  ○ biochemical analytes (lactate, glucose, and total protein)
	  ○ mucin clot test (rarely indicated)
	  ○ obtaining bacterial culture and sensitivity[a]
	• Heparin blood tubes (*green top*)[b,c] for
	  ○ mucin clot test (rarely indicated)
	  ○ total nucleated cell count
	  ○ total protein (if not underfilled)

[a] Pediatric blood culture flasks are preferred (over culturette swabs or red top tubes) particularly if >0.5 ml of synovial fluid is available to increase the chances of obtaining a successful culture result. If large amounts of sample are available, cultures should be submitted in blood culture flasks and red top tubes (Chapter 9).
[b] Small volume (pediatric) heparin and EDTA tubes are recommended to reduce dilutional effects that may lead to testing errors.
[c] Unless EDTA blood tubes are unavailable, heparin blood tubes are generally not utilized. Please note that heparin tubes cannot be used for cytology.

not only be appropriate to the animal and joint, but also chosen with care to minimize the potential for iatrogenic trauma, to permit easy collection of joint fluid in as few attempts as necessary, and to ensure samples are free of blood contaminant.

The use of spinal needles with the stylet inserted is controversial (e.g. for hip and shoulder joint aspiration in large dogs), since some studies have suggested that it may result in increased contamination due to the hairs getting stuck in between the space of the stylet and needle (Adams et al. 2010; Wahl et al. 2012). To reduce the risk of contamination with arthrocentesis, Wahl et al. (2012) recommend using regular, disposable hypodermic needles. However, the tip of these needles is more oblique than the tip of a spinal needle (Wahl et al. 2012) and thus may not enter the lumen of the joint completely in smaller joints. For this reason, some authors recommend using a spinal needle for small joints (Degner 2014).

7.6 Approaches

The approach that clinicians use to perform arthrocentesis of different joints can vary and has been described by numerous authors (Clements 2006; Degner 2014). The following section/images describe some of the more common approaches as well as our preferred methods for obtaining joint fluid from appendicular joints. Recommended patient positioning, needle placement, and structures to avoid are summarized in Table 7.2.

Table 7.2 Summary of arthrocentesis recommendations and structures to avoid by region.

Area	Patient positioning	Needle placement	Structures to avoid	Figure
Carpus (radiocarpal joint)	Lateral recumbency with the target joint/limb up	From cranial, just below the palpable distal radius	Cephalic and accessory cephalic vein	Figure 7.1
Elbow		*Medial aspiration*		Figure 7.2
	Lateral recumbency with the target joint/limb down	From medial, distal, and caudal to the medial epicondyle	Ulnar nerve	
		Caudal aspiration		
	Lateral recumbency with the target joint/limb up	From lateral, in between the lateral epicondylar crest and anconeal process	None	
Shoulder	Lateral recumbency with the target joint/limb up	*Lateral aspiration*		Figure 7.3
		From lateral, just below (or slightly caudal to) the acromion process	Suprascapular nerve	
		Cranial aspiration		
		From cranial, just medial or lateral to the greater tubercle	Biceps tendon (if medial to greater tubercle)	
Tarsus (tibiotarsal joint)	Lateral recumbency with the target joint/limb up	*Cranial aspiration*		Figure 7.4
		From lateral, just medial and cranial to the lateral malleolus	Cranial branch of lateral saphenous vein	
		Caudal aspiration		
		From lateral, caudal to the lateral malleolus/distal tibia	Caudal branch of lateral saphenous vein	
Stifle	Lateral recumbency with the target joint/limb up or dorsal recumbency with the target joint/limb facing the clinician	From cranial, medial, or lateral to patellar tendon	Meniscus	Figure 7.5
Hip	Lateral recumbency with the target joint/limb up	From lateral, just proximal to greater trochanter	Sciatic nerve	Figure 7.6

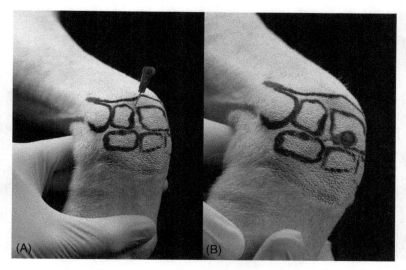

Figure 7.1   Carpus: (A) aspirate the radiocarpal joint by palpating the distal end of the radius and inserting the needle in a craniocaudal direction; (B) aspirate the middle carpal joint by inserting the needle in between either the second and third or third and fourth carpal bones.

7.6.1   Carpus

The antebrachiocarpal (radiocarpal) joint is one of the most frequently aspirated joints. Arthrocentesis can be performed by flexing the carpus to increase the joint space and improve needle access. The joint space can be palpated cranially at the distal end of the radius (a depression should reveal the landmark for the radiocarpal joint and will identify the site for needle insertion). The needle should be inserted from the cranial aspect of the joint and aligned perpendicular to the joint surface (Figure 7.1A and Video 7.1). Arthrocentesis of the middle carpal joint (Figure 7.1B) is performed between the second and third or third and fourth carpal bones. However, joint fluid may not always be obtained and therefore aspiration of this joint is less commonly performed. Clinicians should take care to palpate and avoid the cephalic and accessory cephalic vein when performing arthrocentesis of this joint.

Video 7.1:

Procedural details for aspiration of the carpal joint.

7.6.2   Elbow

It is the authors' preference to aspirate the elbow joint from a straight medial direction. If significant effusion is present, aspiration in a craniolateral direction at the caudal joint may also be performed. For *medial aspiration* (Figure 7.2A and Video 7.2), the patient should be placed in lateral recumbency with the affected limb down on the table. The elbow should be "opened" up by gently levering it over a towel while extending the joint. The ulnar nerve should be palpated prior to inserting the needle (which can easily be found just caudal to the epicondyle). The needle should be inserted at the level below the epicondyle and slightly caudal to this area – NOTE: in a medium-sized dog, the location will be a little less than 1 cm distal and caudal to the medial epicondyle.

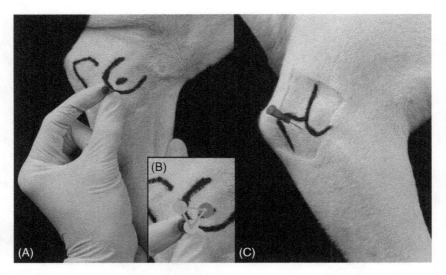

Figure 7.2 Elbow: (A) aspirate the elbow joint by inserting the needle in a straight medio-lateral direction at a location distal and caudal to the medial epicondyle (which can easily be palpated); (B) to identify the joint space location, imagine an equidistant triangle with the medial epicondyle (blue dot) and the caudal aspect of the epicondylar ridge (orange dot) as the two palpable landmarks, whereby the tip of the triangle then identifies the location of the arthrocentesis point (green dot); (C) for caudal aspiration, the needle is inserted in a distomedial direction along the long axis of the ulna.

Video 7.2:

Procedural details for aspiration of the elbow joint.

For *caudal aspiration* (Figure 7.2C), the joint is held in a flexed or neutral position and the needle is inserted alongside the olecranon and angled cranially. The needle is placed at the proximal level of the olecranon, medial to the lateral epicondyle (i.e. between the lateral epicondylar crest and anconeal process), and inserted in a distomedial direction along the long axis of the ulna.

7.6.3 Shoulder

The shoulder joint is most frequently aspirated laterally in an area below the acromion but can also be aspirated from a cranial and caudal location. Regardless of aspiration location, the patient should be placed in lateral recumbency with the affected shoulder up. It sometimes is helpful to distend the joint by pulling the distal limb away from the body; however, a neutral position typically provides good access.

For *lateral aspiration* (Figure 7.3A and Video 7.3), the needle should be inserted just below the acromion process in most dogs. In larger dogs, placement may be slightly caudal to the acromion process. The needle should be directed in a straight mediolateral direction, in a manner that is perpendicular to the skin. If the joint is not penetrated, a slightly more distoproximal angle should be attempted. Clinicians should be aware that acromion anatomy may differ in some dogs affecting its shape and position and making joint aspiration challenging. Radiographs of the joint and evalu-

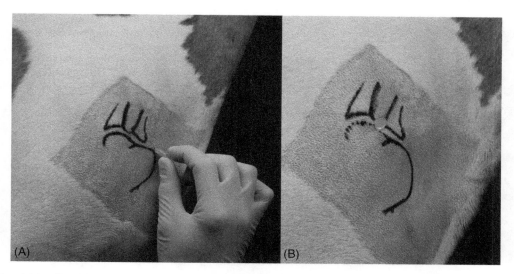

Figure 7.3 Shoulder: (A) aspirate the shoulder joint by inserting the needle just below the acromion process in a straight lateromedial direction; (B) alternatively, the joint can also be aspirated by inserting the needle laterally or medially to the greater tubercle in a caudal direction.

ation of the bony anatomy may be beneficial (to assess the location of the acromion process in relation to the joint space).

For *cranial aspiration* (Figure 7.3B), palpate the greater tubercle and insert the needle in a caudal direction either medial or lateral to this structure. If the needle is inserted medially to the greater tubercle, the biceps tendon should be palpated and avoided during insertion of the needle.

Video 7.3:

Procedural details for aspiration of the shoulder joint.

7.6.4 Tarsus

The tibiotarsal joint is the most frequently aspirated joint of the tarsus and is generally aspirated from the cranial or caudal aspect of the joint, approaching from either the medial or lateral side. The authors prefer the lateral aspect since it is easier to access. *Aspiration of the cranial aspect* of the joint (Figure 7.4A and Video 7.4) is done with the tarsus in slight extension and the needle is inserted into the joint space in a dorsomedial direction beginning at a point just medial and cranial to the lateral malleolus (distal fibula). *Aspiration of the caudal aspect* of the joint (Figure 7.4B) is done with the tarsus in slight flexion and the needle is inserted into the joint space by beginning needle insertion parallel to the calcaneus with insertion in a craniomedial direction. The tarsus is a small joint and often a smaller gauge needle may be more appropriate. It is also important to remember that the cranial and caudal branches of the saphenous vein are located laterally. If palpable, care should be taken to avoid the vein during aspiration. Thorough palpation of joint/landmarks, prior to aspiration, during range of motion is advised.

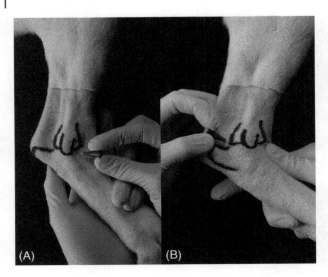

(A)   (B)

Figure 7.4 Tarsus: (A) aspirate the tarsal joint cranially by inserting the needle in a dorsomedial direction beginning at a point just medial and cranial to the lateral malleolus, or (B) caudally by inserting the needle in a craniomedial direction.

Video 7.4:

Procedural details for aspiration of the tarsal joint.

7.6.5 Stifle

The stifle is a large joint that can be aspirated in several ways, depending on clinician preference. It is aspirated either medially (Figure 7.5A and Video 7.5) or laterally (Figure 7.5B) to the patellar tendon. Some clinicians prefer to insert the needle through the central portion of the patellar ligament and one of the authors (BT) has not noticed any adverse events using this approach. In all cases, the joint is held in mild flexion. If aspiration is to occur medial or lateral to the patellar tendon, it may help to palpate the femoral condyle and the joint pouch and push fluid from the side opposite of where aspiration is to occur. Aspiration is performed by first locating the point for needle insertion, which is typically halfway between the patella and the tibial tuberosity. The needle is then inserted in a craniocaudal direction and angled toward the intercondylar space of the distal femur. A longer (1.5″) needle is ideal for the stifle. Due to the fat pad, joint fluid may be difficult to aspirate particularly in a normal joint because it contains little joint fluid.

Video 7.5:

Procedural details for aspiration of the stifle joint.

7.6.6 Hip

The coxofemoral joint is most commonly aspirated from the lateral side of the body. The limb is placed in slight abduction and the joint is identified by palpating the greater trochanter (illustrated in Figure 7.6). A long needle should be used and inserted just proximal to the greater trochanter at

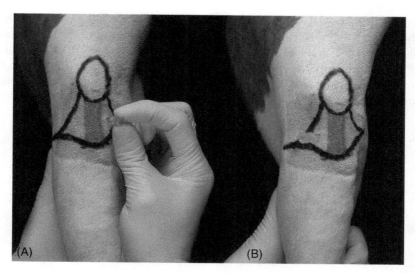

Figure 7.5   Stifle: aspirate the stifle joint by inserting the needle (A) medially or (B) laterally to the patellar tendon angled towards the intercondylar space of the distal femur.

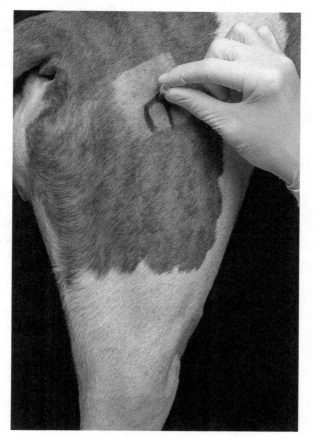

Figure 7.6   Hip: aspirate the hip joint by inserting the needle just proximal to the greater trochanter at an angle that is perpendicular to the long axis of the femur.

an angle that is perpendicular to the long axis of the femur (Video 7.6). If straight insertion does not allow for joint aspiration, the needle should be redirected slightly ventrally. Alternatively, the needle may be inserted cranially to the greater trochanter at ~45° angling caudomedially. Positioning the needle caudal to the greater trochanter or angling the needle toward the caudal aspect of the acetabulum should be avoided to prevent iatrogenic trauma to the sciatic nerve. Ventral aspiration has been described but is rarely performed.

Video 7.6:

Procedural details for aspiration of the hip joint.

References

Adams, S.B., Moore, G.E., Elrashidy, M. et al. (2010). Effect of needle size and type, reuse of needles, insertion speed, and removal of hair on contamination of joints with tissue debris and hair after arthrocentesis. *Veterinary Surgery* 39 (6): 667–673.

Clements, D. (2006). Arthrocentesis and synovial fluid analysis in dogs and cats. *In Practice* 28 (5): 256–262.

Degner, D.A. (2014). Arthrocentesis in dogs. Clinician's Brief. https://www.cliniciansbrief.com/article/arthrocentesis-dogs (accessed 31 January 2019).

Steel, C.M., Pannirselvam, R.R., and Anderson, G.A. (2013). Risk of septic arthritis after intra-articular medication: a study of 16,624 injections in Thoroughbred racehorses. *Australian Veterinary Journal* 91 (7): 268–273.

Van Oostrom, H. and Knowles, T.G. (2018). The clinical efficacy of EMLA cream for intravenous catheter placement in client-owned dogs. *Veterinary Anaesthesia and Analgesia* 45 (5): 604–608.

Wahl, K., Adams, S.B., and Moore, G.E. (2012). Contamination of joints with tissue debris and hair after arthrocentesis: the effect of needle insertion angle, spinal needle gauge, and insertion of spinal needles with and without a stylet. *Veterinary Surgery* 41 (3): 391–398.

Waxman, S.J., Adams, S.B., and Moore, G.E. (2015). Effect of needle brand, needle bevel grind, and silicone lubrication on contamination of joints with tissue and hair debris after arthrocentesis. *Veterinary Surgery* 44 (3): 373–378.

8

Diagnostic Joint Anesthesia

Bryan T. Torres[1] and Felix Michael Duerr[2]

[1] *Department of Veterinary Medicine and Surgery, College of Veterinary Medicine, University of Missouri, Columbia, MO, USA*
[2] *Department of Clinical Sciences, College of Veterinary Medicine and Biomedical Sciences, Colorado State University, Fort Collins, CO, USA*

8.1   Introduction

The use of intra-articular anesthetic agents to aid in the diagnosis of lameness has been long established in equine veterinary medicine (Dyson 1986). However, within the past few years, there has been an increased interest in employing diagnostic joint anesthesia (DJA) or "joint blocks" as a diagnostic tool in small animals to aid clinicians in pinpointing the source of lameness (Van Vynckt et al. 2012a). Principles of DJA are outlined in Box 8.1.

8.2   Patient Selection

In general, any dog with an unidentifiable source of lameness may benefit from DJA. Particularly if advanced diagnostics (such as CT/MRI) are not readily available, DJA may be helpful to justify that such diagnostics are indicated. If DJA results in a positive response, it allows the clinician to determine the injected joint as the most likely source of lameness. If DJA results in a negative response, it places other differential diagnoses higher on the list. As is true in horses, DJA aims to identify the joint responsible for a lameness rather than provide a specific diagnosis. This approach can be clinically useful in the following scenarios:

- Patients presenting with a lameness that is thought to be joint related, but the physical exam and available diagnostics are not definitive (e.g. a dog with suspected elbow dysplasia that shows no pain on examination and radiographs only show minor/no abnormalities). In this scenario, a positive DJA result (of the elbow joint) may aid to confirm the elbow as the source of lameness.
- Patients presenting with a lameness and multiple joints show abnormalities (e.g. a dog with shoulder and elbow osteoarthritis). In this scenario, a positive DJA result (of the elbow or shoulder joint) may aid to confirm the elbow or shoulder as the source of lameness.
- Patients presenting with a lameness and multiple detected abnormalities (e.g. a dog with shoulder osteoarthritis and possible axillary pain). In this scenario, a negative DJA result (of the shoulder joint) may aid to confirm that further diagnostics (such as MRI) investigating a possible neurologic reason (such as brachial plexus tumor) for the lameness is indicated. On the other hand, a positive result would confirm the shoulder as the source of lameness.

Box 8.1   Principals of Diagnostic Joint Anesthesia (DJA)

- Use only for patients with obvious lameness.
- Use sedation protocol A for stressed/anxious animals and A or B for calm animals.
- Use 2% mepivacaine (20 mg/ml Carbocaine®) at 1.5 mg/kg. A total dose of 5 mg/kg per dog and 4 ml/joint should not be exceeded.
- A 20% improvement in lameness is considered a positive response.
- Ideally objective gait analysis is used to evaluate response.
- False-negative and false-positive (due to diffusion of anesthetic or pain modulating effects of sedation) results are possible.

The most common joints where DJA has been applied to aid in lameness diagnosis have been in the thoracic limb (Van Vynckt et al. 2012b, 2013). This is understandable due to the frequent difficulty in isolating the location and cause of thoracic limb lameness (as compared to pelvic limb problems). However, DJA has also been used in all major canine pelvic limb joints (Van Vynckt et al. 2012a). The utility of DJA as a diagnostic aid should not be underestimated as the sensitivity and specificity of DJA has been shown to be up to 90 and 100%, respectively (Van Vynckt et al. 2012a). Therefore, the use of this technique can be a valuable clinical tool. However, as with many diagnostic tests, understanding the potential limitation is critical. Most importantly, false-negative results have been reported in approximately 10% of dogs. Furthermore, in dogs with more subtle lameness, the clinical interpretation of DJA is challenging due to the less significant degree of improvement seen and the potential effects of sedation on lameness. However, in dogs with more moderate-to-severe lameness, the degree of improvement after DJA is often more dramatic and this makes clinical interpretation easier. Clinicians should consider these factors when performing DJA as a diagnostic test and when evaluating the treatment response.

8.3   Sedation Protocols

While routinely performed in horses, we do not recommend performing DJA without sedation in dogs. Sedation ensures a pain-free, atraumatic joint injection, in a manner that reduces patient stress during the procedure (Chapter 7). General anesthesia should not be performed because this technique is employed as a diagnostic tool and patients are required to walk prior to and after injection to evaluate the efficacy of treatment.

Because DJA is a diagnostic test, unlike arthrocentesis, the choice of sedative agent(s) is a more important clinical consideration. Ideally, an effective sedative, that also allows quick ambulation and does not affect lameness interpretation, is used. Unfortunately, our understanding on how sedative agents affect lameness in dogs (positive or negative) and ultimately how they may influence our clinical interpretation of DJA is limited. Currently, only one study has evaluated the effect sedative agents have on lameness in dogs (Van Vynckt et al. 2011); it evaluated the two sedation protocols outlined below and found both to be suitable for use with DJA:

8.3.1   Sedation Protocol A: Sedation with an α_2-Adrenergic Receptor Agonist

This protocol is based on one of the most common and familiar methods of sedation in small animal medicine. The clinical benefits include rapid and effective sedation as well as sedation reversal

---

Box 8.2   DJA Protocol A

- *Step 1 – Sedative agent is administered intravenously –* dexmedetomidine (0.5 mg/ml) given IV at a dose of 250 mcg/m².
- *Step 2 – Intra-articular anesthetic is instilled in the target joint.*
- *Step 3 – Reversal agent is administered intramuscularly immediately after intra-articular anesthetic is administered –* atipamezole (5.0 mg/ml) is administered IM at a volume (ml) that is the same as the preceding dose volume of dexmedetomidine.
- *Step 4 – Lameness evaluation is performed seven minutes* after reversal agent (atipamezole) is administered.

---

with an antagonist agent. These aspects make it well suited for DJA. Available studies were performed with medetomidine; however, currently clinicians in North America are more likely to have access to dexmedetomidine. The recommended steps for DJA with an α_2-adrenergic receptor agonist are listed in Box 8.2.

8.3.2   Sedation Protocol B: Sedation with a Neuroleptanalgesic and Opiate

The use of acepromazine with an opiate has also been investigated and serves as a good option for use with DJA. This method of sedation is used for light-to-moderate sedation and analgesia while still allowing the patient to ambulate. Since sedation is less effective, more physical restraint was needed in one study (Van Vynckt et al. 2012b). Therefore, we prefer to use protocol A unless there are contraindications for the use of an α_2-adrenergic receptor agonist. Unlike sedation protocol A, there is no reversal agent administered. It is possible that stressed or anxious animals may require a higher sedative dose; however, Van Vynckt et al. (2012b) found the dose range in the steps listed in Box 8.3 suitable for DJA.

Currently, our understanding of how other sedatives affect lameness in dogs is limited to the protocols discussed above. It is possible that other protocols (such as use of Propofol or local anesthetics in addition to sedation) may be equally useful. However, the degree of effect and more importantly a means to account for that effect in our clinical interpretation is lacking. For example, if a local anesthetic is used, it could result in a change in lameness because of diffusion (and providing local anesthesia) into the extra-articular structures. This is not to say that other sedatives or combinations of sedatives are not appropriate for DJA, just that their effect on lameness interpretation is currently unknown. Therefore, it is recommended that clinicians use the tested and studied methods.

Box 8.3   DJA Protocol B

- *Step 1 – Sedative agent is administered intravenously –* acepromazine (0.01–0.02 mg/kg IV) and methadone (0.1–0.2 mg/kg IV).
- *Step 2 – Intra-articular anesthetic is instilled in the target joint.*
- *Step 3 – Lameness evaluation is performed two minutes* after intra-articular anesthetic is administered.

8.4 Intra-articular Anesthetic Instillation

The basic principles (including patient positing and preparation) used with arthrocentesis (Chapter 7) apply when using DJA. However, given the possibility of performing injections into normal joints, great attention to detail is required to avoid iatrogenic trauma to the joint. Ultrasound-guided injections may help improve the accuracy of injections and reduce trauma to the cartilage. A technique description for canine ultrasound-guided injection of the coxofemoral joint is available (Bergamino et al. 2015). Ultrasound guidance allows to place the needle more superficially in the joint, thereby causing less trauma. Furthermore, confirmation of placement of the anesthetic into the joint can be confirmed by observing distention of the joint capsule. If ultrasound guidance is not available, prior to instilling the anesthetic agent, joint fluid should be aspirated to confirm the location of the needle. In the case that joint fluid is unable to be aspirated, the needle should be slightly withdrawn, redirected, and aspiration attempted again. If joint fluid still cannot be aspirated, then careful instillation of the anesthetic agent can be performed. This should be done gradually and with great care to ensure that no resistance is met during instillation. If the needle is correctly located in the joint space, regardless of the aspiration of joint fluid, there should be no resistance met upon instillation of the anesthetic agent. Following instillation of the anesthetic agent, the joint flexion and extension should be performed to distribute the anesthetic throughout the joint (Van Vynckt et al. 2012a).

Because it is widely available and has a preferred safety profile for intra-articular use, 2% mepivacaine (i.e. 20 mg/ml Carbocaine®) is the recommended anesthetic agent for DJA in dogs. The use of lidocaine or bupivacaine for DJA is not recommended at this time as they may cause more local irritation when compared to mepivacaine (Van Vynckt et al. 2010). The recommended dose is 1.5 mg/kg instilled into a single joint (approximately 1–4 ml). A total dose of 5 mg/kg per dog and a total volume of 4 ml should not be exceeded (Van Vynckt et al. 2010, 2012a).

8.5 Lameness Evaluation and Interpreting the Effect of Diagnostic Joint Anesthesia

The localization of lameness to a specific joint with DJA is based on a change in lameness following instillation of the anesthetic. A *positive response* is when lameness improves, and a *negative response* is when the lameness is unchanged or worsens. Various grading scales are available, as described in Chapter 1. Currently available research used an 11-point numerical rating scale (with 0 = no lameness and 10 = non-weight-bearing) and a change of 2 scores was considered a positive response. As such, an approximately 20% improvement in degree of lameness should be used if other scoring systems are used. Ideally, objective gait analysis (Chapter 2) is used before and after DJA.

Lameness evaluation is recommended to begin seven minutes after the reversal agent is administered if an α_2-adrenergic receptor agonist is administered (Protocol A) for sedation (Figure 8.1). If a neuroleptanalgesia with an opioid is administered (Protocol B), then it is recommended that evaluation begins two minutes after the anesthetic agent is instilled. Regardless of sedation protocol, dogs should be evaluated at frequent intervals. The dogs should be walked continuously for the first five minutes after the initial evaluation. If an improvement in lameness is not seen during that time period, then repeat evaluations should be performed approximately every 5 minutes for a maximum of 30 minutes after injection (Van Vynckt et al. 2011, 2012a). An improvement in lameness at any time point during those 30 minutes is considered a positive response. The use of video recordings may aid in lameness evaluation by providing an ability to compare time points as well as providing material for secondary observers, if needed.

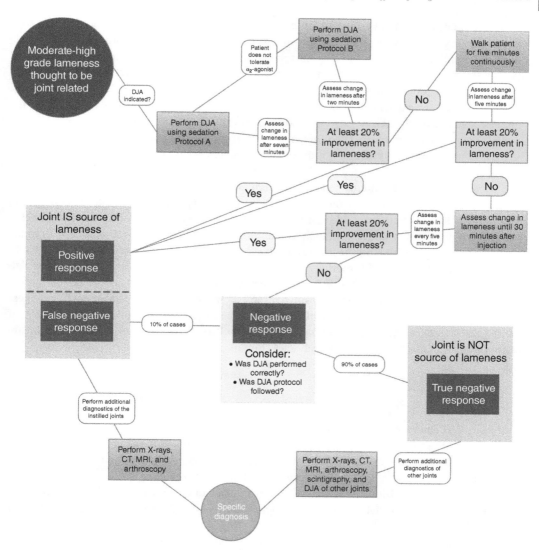

Figure 8.1 Decision tree for determining DJA protocol and interpretation of lameness assessment.

Both protocols outlined above were found to have the potential to influence lameness and thereby DJA interpretation. Van Vynckt et al. (2011) evaluated the influence of sedation on dogs with lameness (without performing DJA) and found that most dogs (72% for protocol A and 80% for protocol B) experienced no change in lameness due to sedation. However, sedation lead to a worsening of lameness by 1–2 grades in up to 20% of lame dogs (20% for protocol A and 12% for protocol B) and an improvement by 1 grade in 8% (for both groups). In general, lameness may become more obvious in anxious dogs (since the sedation results in them relaxing and being less distracted by the unfamiliar environment) while the pain modulation associated with the sedation may improve the lameness in less anxious dogs. Based on these findings, it is recommended that a positive response to DJA be interpreted only when lameness improves by two or more grades (using an 11-point scale).

DJA has been reported to be 100% specific and 90% sensitive for the identification of joint pain and lameness: Van Vynckt et al. (2012a) performed DJA in almost 200 dogs with thoracic or pelvic limb lameness that was thought to be joint related. In that study, all dogs who received DJA in a painful joint showed an improvement in lameness (100% specificity). Therefore, a positive response clearly indicates that the infused joint is painful and contributing to the observed lameness. However, 10% of lame dogs with a negative response to DJA (i.e. unchanged or worsening of the lameness) were actually false negatives, meaning that the joint was the source of lameness based on other diagnostics performed. Therefore, a negative response only indicates a 90% certainty that the joint infused is non-painful and not the source of lameness. As such, a negative response does not completely rule out the treated joint as the source of pain and lameness in all cases. Negative results should therefore be interpreted with caution and additional diagnostics should be utilized if the clinician is suspicious that the result may be a false-negative (rather than true negative) result (Figure 8.1). Alternatively, additional joints can be tested using DJA. It is also possible that specific joint disorders or pathology (such as pain originating from subchondral bone with intact cartilage or severe arthritis) may be less responsive to DJA (Dyson 1986; Van Vynckt et al. 2010).

As mentioned above, a slight improvement in lameness may be attributed to the pain-modulating effects of the sedation. While this response may be considered a false-positive response, Van Vynckt et al. (2012a) reported no false-positive responses when using an improvement in lameness by approximately 20% as the cutoff. While this has not been reported in dog studies, leakage of anesthetic to surrounding extra-articular structures as well as errors in lameness interpretation are other reasons for false-positive results in horses (Jordana et al. 2016).

References

Bergamino, C., Etienne, A.L., and Busoni, V. (2015). Developing a technique for ultrasound-guided injection of the adult canine hip. *Veterinary Radiology and Ultrasound* 56 (4): 456–461.

Dyson, S. (1986). Problems associated with the interpretation of the results of regional and intra-articular anaesthesia in the horse. *Veterinary Record* 118 (15): 419–422.

Jordana, M., Martens, A., Duchateau, L. et al. (2016). Diffusion of mepivacaine to adjacent synovial structures after intrasynovial analgesia of the digital flexor tendon sheath. *Equine Veterinary Journal* 48 (3): 326–330.

Van Vynckt, D., Polis, I., Verschooten, F., and Ryssen, V.B. (2010). A review of the human and veterinary literature on local anaesthetics and their intraarticular use. *Veterinary and Comparative Orthopaedics and Traumatology* 23 (04): 225–230.

Van Vynckt, D., Samoy, Y., Mosselmans, L. et al. (2012a). The use of intra-articular anesthesia as a diagnostic tool in canine lameness. *Vlaams Diergeneeskundig Tijdschrift* 81 (5): 290–297.

Van Vynckt, D., Samoy, Y., Polis, I. et al. (2011). Evaluation of two sedation protocols for use before diagnostic intra-articular anaesthesia in lame dogs. *Journal of Small Animal Practice* 52 (12): 638–644.

Van Vynckt, D., Verhoeven, G., Samoy, Y. et al. (2013). Anaesthetic arthrography of the shoulder joint in dogs. *Veterinary and Comparative Orthopaedics and Traumatology* 26 (04): 291–297.

Van Vynckt, D., Verhoeven, G., Saunders, J. et al. (2012b). Diagnostic intra-articular anaesthesia of the elbow in dogs with medial coronoid disease. *Veterinary and Comparative Orthopaedics and Traumatology* 25 (4): 307–313.

9

Joint Fluid Analysis and Collection Considerations

Adam Harris and Kelly Santangelo

Department of Microbiology, Immunology, and Pathology, College of Veterinary Medicine and Biomedical Sciences, Colorado State University, Fort Collins, CO, USA

9.1 Introduction

Synovial fluid is a viscous substance produced and contained within diarthrodial (i.e. freely movable) joints. Synovial fluid analysis is a valuable tool used to diagnose and monitor primary and secondary articular joint disorders. Information gained from cytological evaluation of synovial fluid is most helpful when combined with patient history, physical exam, imaging findings, and other laboratory data, such as bacterial culture and serology. For procedural details of arthrocentesis, please refer to Chapter 7.

9.2 Sample Submission and Prioritization of Diagnostic Tests

Pre-analytical errors involving sample collection and specimen handling can vastly alter results. In general, synovial fluid should be shipped at 4 °C and delivered within 24 hours. Fresh smears made at the time of collection are best for maintaining cellular morphology. If cytology is a primary outcome but adequate smears cannot be made by the referring clinician at the time of sample aspiration, smears should be made at the clinical pathology laboratory from samples stored in ethylenediaminetetraacetic acid (EDTA) tubes. Heparinized samples will not adequately preserve mammalian cell architecture.

Between 0.01 and 1 ml of synovial fluid may be aspirated from non-pathologic joints of dogs, with larger joints normally containing more fluid for sampling. As little as a single drop of joint fluid can be considered within normal limits, particularly in small-breed dogs. Joint pathology often increases joint fluid volume and clinicians should be suspicious of pathology in cases where the aspirated volume is >1 ml (Clements 2006). Given that aspiration of synovial fluid can yield variable amounts, allocation of the available sample for priority of diagnostic tests is important (Figure 9.1) and should be made considering the most likely differential diagnoses. If adequate joint fluid is retrieved, submission of the sample as direct smears, in EDTA tubes (purple or lavender tubes), sterile no-additive tubes (red top glass tubes), and blood culture flasks (if culture is indicated) are recommended.

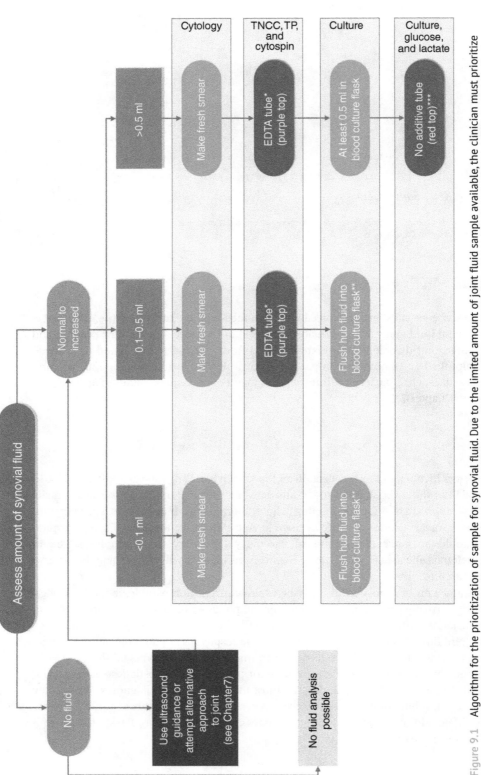

Figure 9.1 Algorithm for the prioritization of sample for synovial fluid. Due to the limited amount of joint fluid sample available, the clinician must prioritize allocation of the available sample. [*Most automated hematology analyzers require a minimum of 200 μl to process the sample submitted. If there is limited sample, the reader is encouraged to use the appropriate size EDTA tube, which generally requires submission in a pediatric/small tube. Submission in the appropriate size tube is critical because inappropriate anticoagulant to sample ratios can cause erroneous results. **If limited sample is available and an infectious etiology is suspected, some labs suggest submitting the capped needle directly to the diagnostic laboratory. Please contact the lab beforehand to ensure this is possible and provide instructions to flush the needle hub using sterile technique prior to processing cultures. Alternatively, the content of the syringe may be sterilely flushed into the culture media. ***If sufficient sample is available, red top tubes should be used to collect the additional sample. Further tests such as a secondary culture (in addition to the culture from the blood culture flask), mucin clot test, and biochemical analytes (such as lactate, glucose, and

9.3 Gross, Biochemical, and Cytologic Examination

Joint fluid analysis and evaluation typically involve assessment of gross appearance, protein concentration, total nucleated cell count (TNCC), and cytologic interpretation. Other biochemical parameters, such as glucose and lactate, can also be measured but the availability of these tests may vary from laboratory to laboratory. A summary of typical findings in non-affected canine joints and general interpretation guidelines are provided in Figure 9.2 and Table 9.1.

9.3.1 Gross Appearance

Gross appearance of synovial fluid assesses turbidity, color (particularly regarding the presence of blood), viscosity, and the amount of volume sampled from each joint. In healthy patients, joint fluid is typically clear and pale yellow, as well as thick and viscous. While these characteristics will be determined by the laboratory, it is also helpful to note such qualities at the time of sample collection. Viscosity can be evaluated empirically by forming a string of synovial fluid between the tips of the fingers, but this is only recommended to be performed in cases with ample amount of sample. A fingertip stretch distance of ~2–3 cm is generally considered appropriate viscosity. Recording the presence or absence of blood is particularly helpful to the clinical pathologist for distinguishing blood contamination due to sample collection from overt hemorrhage.

9.3.2 Protein Concentration

While protein concentrations are typically estimated using a refractometer, automated chemistry measurements and electrophoresis have also been used to determine and/or characterize such. However, some laboratories will not perform automated protein concentration analyses on joint fluids if the fluid is too viscous. When using a refractometer, it is important to note that the presence of other solutes in the fluid may affect the measurement of protein concentration, as does underfilling EDTA tubes or aspirating joints previously treated with intra-articular injections. Therefore, it is critical to use appropriately sized EDTA tubes due to the possibility of erroneous results secondary to EDTA dilution when tubes are underfilled. Alternatively, if sufficient sample is available, red top tubes can be used to measure protein concentrations.

Normal protein levels in synovial fluid are between 1.5 and 3.0 g/dl (MacWilliams and Friedrichs 2003). In disease states or when there is inadvertent sampling of blood, protein concentrations can begin to rise and approach levels similar to serum or plasma.

9.3.3 Total Nucleated Cell Counts

TNCCs are typically performed by an automated analyzer, most often on samples collected into EDTA. TNCCs within synovial fluid are predominately composed of white blood cells. However, other nucleated cells may also be included in the analyzer count as part of the TNCC (e.g. synoviocytes, nucleated red blood cells, neoplastic cells, etc.) making cytological analysis in addition to the TNCC imperative. If an analyzer is not available, or the amount of synovial fluid retrieved is insufficient to process through an analyzer, hemocytometers or direct smears can be used to assess cellularity. If a direct smear is used to estimate cellularity, the average number of cells per 40× objective high-power field over 10 fields can be multiplied by 1000 to yield an approximate number of cells per microliter. However, the evaluator should be aware that visual estimates are less accurate than automated methods. The viscosity of joint fluid can make estimation of cellularity

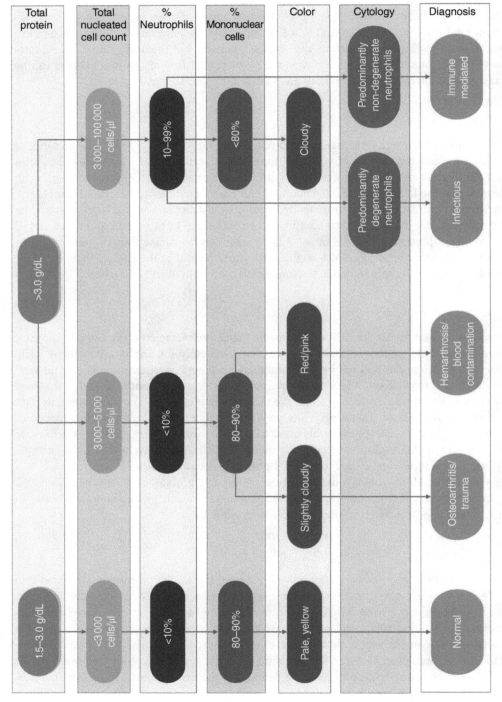

Figure 9.2 Guidelines for interpretation of synovial fluid samples. Please note that the provided interpretation is based on most commonly observed values for each disease and individual patients may not fit within these guidelines. Refer to Table 9.1 for further details on normal values and percentage of cell distribution.

Table 9.1 Typical joint fluid analysis findings associated with normal and diseased joints.

Category	Subtype	Appearance	Volume	Protein concentration (g/dl)	Mucin clot	TNCC	% Neutrophils	% Mononuclear cells
Normal	N/A	Clear, pale yellow	Normal	1.5–3.0	Good	<3000	<10	80–90
Nonsuppurative	Osteoarthritis and trauma	Slightly cloudy and red (trauma)	Reduced, normal, or increased	>3.0	Fair to poor	3000–5000	<10	80–90
Suppurative	Infectious and immune-mediated	Cloudy and turbid	Increased	>3.0	Fair to very poor	3000–100000	20–99	0–80
Neoplastic	Highly variable – cytology primarily used as the differentiating feature							

TNCC, total nucleated cell count (cells/μl).

difficult and, therefore, direct smears have been recommended to be assessed using broader categories such as normal, mild-moderately increased, or markedly increased (Dusick et al. 2014). Nevertheless, if an automated analyzer is not available, it is important to obtain or estimate a TNCC as this can be used to determine response to treatment.

Normal canine joints typically have a TNCC of less than 3000 cells/μl. TNCCs in pathologic joints will vary depending on the underlying pathological cause. Suppurative arthropathies often yield the highest cell counts, which have been reported to range from >3000 to >100000 cells/μl (MacWilliams and Friedrichs 2003). Nonsuppurative arthropathies typically do not exceed 10000 cells/μl and most often range from 3000 to 5000 cells/μl.

9.3.4 Cytological Analysis

Cytologic analysis of joint fluid is typically performed by evaluating direct smears. If smears prepared by the clinician at the time of collection are adequate, these will be utilized for interpretation. Many laboratories will often also prepare their own direct smears and cytospin preparations using sample from the EDTA tubes; the latter slides can be helpful for distinguishing cellular morphology or characteristics not obvious on direct smears. Slides are generally evaluated microscopically using 10× and 100× objectives to confirm automated TNCCs, provide a differential cell count, and assess cell morphology and/or inclusions. Direct smear preparations of synovial fluid in healthy patients typically have a dense eosinophilic stippled background (Figure 9.3). Cells may align in a linear fashion, commonly referred to as "windrowing," due to the viscosity of joint fluid (Figure 9.4A, B). High protein content can also result in dense preparations, which make it challenging to determine cellular morphology, cellularity, and the presence of infectious agents. The thinnest portions of the slide and/or cytospin slides are best for cellular evaluation. The number of red blood cells and the presence of platelets/platelet clumps should be noted as this can indicate increases of WBC proportions due to blood contamination.

Cells frequently seen on cytologic evaluation of normal joints include large and small mononuclear cells, synovial lining cells (i.e. synoviocytes), and rare-to-occasional neutrophils (Figure 9.3). Large mononuclear cells are the predominate cell population identified in healthy joints and compose approximately 90% of cells identified. On cytological evaluation, it can be difficult to differentiate synovial macrophages from synoviocytes, which is why the term "large mononuclear cells" is used. Large mononuclear cells are typically identified by their amount of blue grey to deeply basophilic cytoplasm, vacuolization, cytoplasmic inclusions, and the size of their nucleus (approximately 1.0×–1.5× the size of a neutrophil). Synoviocytes can have a similar morphology as macrophages and have a round to spindle shape, with round-to-ovoid nuclei, and a moderate amount of basophilic cytoplasm. Small mononuclear cells are usually representative of the lymphocyte population present. They are identified by a thin rim of cytoplasm, an absence of cytoplasmic vacuolization, and a nucleus that is round and approximately 0.5–1.0× the size of a neutrophil (Figure 9.3B). Nondegenerate neutrophils are readily identified by their segmented nucleus and clear, granular cytoplasm (Figure 9.5E). Of note, in the absence of blood contamination, neutrophil numbers will be low; however, if blood contamination is present, the number will increase. As mentioned above, it can be challenging to differentiate cell types in dense cytological preparations, so in some cases, cytospin preparations or dilution of the sample might be required to fully assess cellular morphology.

9.3.5 Mucin Clot Test

The mucin clot test is a semiquantitative assessment of the hyaluronic acid content in synovial fluid. The test estimates the ability of the synovial fluid to form a clot after the addition of acetic

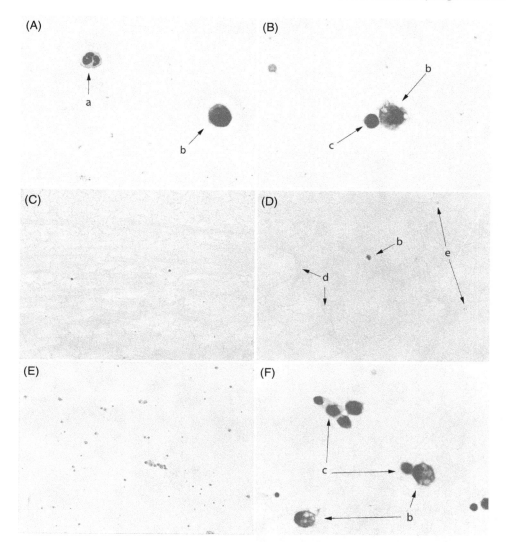

Figure 9.3 Representative examples of the appearance of the cells found in (A–D) normal joint fluid versus (E, F) mononuclear inflammation in joint fluid from a dog with osteoarthritis. Predominantly (b) large and (c) small mononuclear cells and occasional blood cells, such as (a) neutrophils and (e) red blood cells are present; (d) protein crescents are artifactual folds in the background material indicating a normal content of protein and other solutes (e.g. hyaluronic acid) found within synovial fluid. Note the stippled eosinophilic background, which is typical of proteinaceous samples such as synovial fluid, as well as the increased number of large (b) mononuclear cells, in a (E) low-power versus a (F) high-power field of view. Magnification: (A, B, F): 100×; (C, E): 10×; (D): 20× objective.

acid. It should be performed on samples that have been collected in no additive (red top glass tubes) or heparin tubes, as EDTA can hinder clot formation. Fluid from non-pathologic joints forms a clot rapidly after the addition of the acetic acid. In contrast, pathologic or inflamed joints typically have delayed or poor clot formation. However, because quantitative data for interpretation of the mucin clot test is lacking, the results should be interpreted together with other clinical findings (Clements 2006).

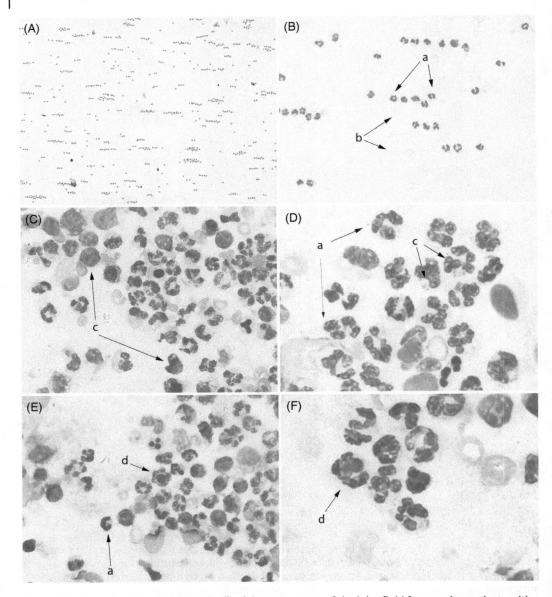

Figure 9.4 Representative examples (A–F) of the appearance of the joint fluid from canine patients with immune-mediated polyarthritis (IMPA): (A, B) note the increased number of (a) nondegenerate neutrophils relative to (b) red blood cells and the non-pathologic windrowing pattern that can occur with viscous fluid samples such as joint fluid; (C, D) samples showing (c) ragocytes seen with IMPA; care should be taken to distinguish ragocytes from neutrophils containing phagocytized bacteria (see also Figure 9.3C); (D, E) cytoprep samples clearly illustrating the high number of (a) nondegenerate neutrophils typically seen with IMPA; (E, F) samples showing (d) lupus erythematous cells seen with IMPA. Magnification: (A): 10×; (B): 50×; (E): 100× objective; (C, D, F): 100× objective digitally magnified.

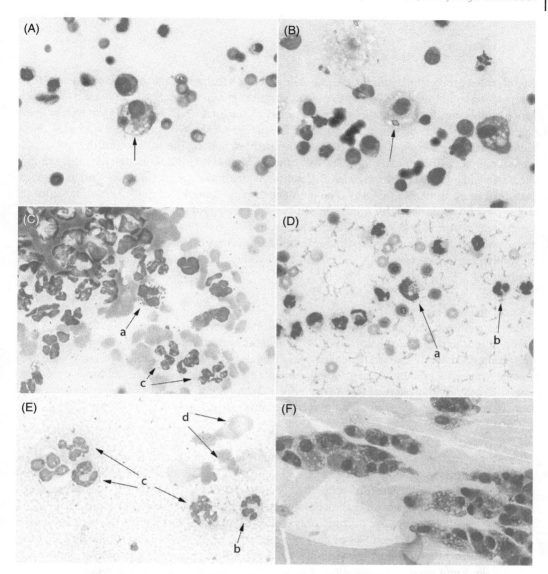

Figure 9.5   Representative examples of the appearance of the joint fluid from canine patients with (A, B) hemarthrosis, (C–E) septic arthritis, and (F) synovial sarcoma: (A) erythrophagia and (B) hematoidin crystals (both indicated by black arrows) in large mononuclear cells seen in joint fluid of dogs with hemarthrosis; (C, D) samples showing representative images of intracytoplasmic bacteria in (a) neutrophils present in a synovial fluid sample from a dog with septic arthritis. Note the high number of (b) nondegenerate to (c) degenerate neutrophils present; (E) sample collage illustrating the difference between (c) degenerate and (b) nondegenerate neutrophils: nondegenerate neutrophils maintain their shape and segmented nuclei while degenerate neutrophils lose their segmented nucleus and display cellular swelling. The glycosaminoglycan background of this image is diluted and a few (d) ruptured cells are present; (F) sample showing cell features consistent with a diagnosis of synovial sarcoma: wispy cytoplasmic borders, cells are loosely aggregated together or individualized, moderate anisocytosis and anisokaryosis and multiple prominent nucleoli. The bright eosinophilic cytoplasmic granules are compatible with a secretory product. Magnification: (A, B, C, D): 100× objective; (E, F): 100× objective digitally magnified.

9.4 Canine Arthropathies

9.4.1 Suppurative Arthropathies

An increased proportion of nondegenerate to degenerate neutrophils above what is suspected to be due to blood contamination is indicative of suppurative inflammation. Specifically, neutrophil percentages are considered increased when above 10% of the total nucleated cells. However, in many cases, they are even higher, often between 20 and 99% (MacWilliams and Friedrichs 2003). Hemorrhage may accompany suppurative arthropathies, making the source contributing to neutrophil numbers difficult to discern. The two forms of suppurative inflammation include immune-mediated and infectious arthropathies. Differentiating these two forms can be difficult as cytologic features can be similar (Table 9.1). The presence of degenerate neutrophils is suspicious for an underlying infectious etiology. However, caution should be used when relying on the presence of degenerate neutrophils in synovial fluid since neutrophils can deteriorate rapidly once in fluid or tissue due to their short life span. As neutrophils decline, they can acquire cytologic features, such as swollen nuclei and basophilic cytoplasm, that overlap with the appearance of true degenerate neutrophils.

9.4.1.1 Immune-mediated

Immune-mediated joint disease is a common cause for suppurative polyarthritis in canine patients. Since immune-mediated polyarthritis (IMPA) generally affects multiple joints, samples from several joints, particularly the carpi and tarsi, should be collected and evaluated. Cytologic evaluation typically reveals a predominance of nondegenerate neutrophils. Ragocytes and lupus erythematous (LE) cells are indicative of IMPA (Figure 9.4) but are not commonly observed and should not be relied on for diagnosis of an immune-mediated process.

9.4.1.2 Infectious

Microscopic interpretation of infected joints reveals mildly to markedly increased TNCCs that are primarily composed of nondegenerate and degenerate neutrophils. While degenerate neutrophils are one feature of septic arthritis, some patients may not display many of these cells and septic arthritis should not be ruled out in these instances (Marchevsky and Read 1999; Mielke et al. 2018). Similarly, infectious agents are uncommonly identified on cytology (Figure 9.5C, D) and cultures are also only positive in about 50% of the cases (Scharf et al. 2015; Mielke et al. 2018). Therefore, infectious arthritis can mimic immune-mediated polyarthritis on cytology and correlation with clinical signs and careful classification of neutrophils as degenerate or nondegenerate is recommended before initiating treatment.

Obtaining a culture in cases of suspected infection is crucial for establishing a diagnosis and enabling selection of appropriate antibiotics. Therefore, every attempt should be made to facilitate a successful culture result in these scenarios. The use of blood culture media is recommended to increase sensitivity and the likelihood of obtaining a positive result (Montgomery et al. 1989; Miller et al. 2018). Unfortunately, the smallest blood culture medium flasks available (pediatric blood culture flasks, which are generally used in veterinary medicine) still require at least 0.5 ml of fluid. If too little synovial fluid is available for culture via direct ejection into the blood culture flask, yield can be maximized by sterilely flushing the culture media back and forth between the collection needle and culture bottle to remove as much of the sample from the needle/hub as possible. Alternatively, the hub of a capped needle can be submitted to some diagnostic laboratories, with instructions to flush the sample. However, submission in the blood culture bottle is preferred due to the potential for desiccation when submitted in the syringe/needle. It is important to note that the sensitivity for a true positive result can decrease with small sample volumes (i.e. if less than 0.5 ml are used in a blood culture flask). On the other hand, use of a culturette swab as the single method of culture is least likely to produce a positive culture result and therefore should be avoided (Font-Vizcarra et al. 2010).

Blood culture flasks are available with and without antibiotic-binding resin. In general, and particularly in situations where an animal is receiving antibiotics, use of resin-containing media is advised to reduce the activity of antibiotics previously administered to the patient (Lorenzo-Figueras et al. 2006). If excessive amounts of fluid are available (such as frequently seen in septic arthritis), culture from a red top tube in addition to the blood culture flask is ideal since blood culture flasks have a higher propensity for contamination. As such, matching culture results from both the red top and blood culture flask cultures provides greater confidence in the diagnosis. Culturing of the synovial membrane has not been shown to be superior to synovial fluid and, therefore, likely does not justify the additional cost and potential morbidity associated with the sample collection procedure (Montgomery et al. 1989).

Infectious agents (bacteria, rickettsial, fungal, protozoal, or viral) typically require additional specific tests (i.e. culture or genetic isolation) to diagnose. Many agents can infect joints either via direct penetration or the hematogenous route (Martinez and Santangelo 2017). Some organisms, such as *Borrelia burgdorferi,* may not necessarily cause synovial infections, but disease is typically thought to be due to immune complex deposition, resulting in polyarthritis (Littman et al. 2018).

Additional diagnostics, such as the measurement of lactate and glucose in synovial fluid, as well as serum C-reactive protein, have shown promise for including or excluding septic arthritis if cytology, culture, and clinical signs are not conclusive (Proot et al. 2015; Hillström et al. 2016). Further work is warranted to validate use of these tests for diagnosing septic arthritis, particularly given a lack of knowledge regarding how other musculoskeletal and non-musculoskeletal conditions may affect the test results. It should be noted that, prior to adopting these or any other novel assays clinically, each individual diagnostic laboratory will need to confirm assay sensitivity and specificity for synovial fluid on the designated high-throughput or point-of-care instrument, determine in-house reference intervals, and validate their own diagnostic cutoffs.

9.4.2 Nonsuppurative Arthropathies

9.4.2.1 Mononuclear Inflammation
Mild to moderately increased TNCCs with predominantly large mononuclear cells are typically due to either degenerate joint disease, such as osteoarthritis, or trauma. Both conditions can result in increased populations of large mononuclear cells, typically both synoviocytes and macrophages, within the synovial fluid. Investigation into clinical history and additional diagnostic information is crucial for interpreting synovial fluid that shows increased nuclear cellularity due to large mononuclear cells. If trauma is suspected, evidence of previous or acute hemorrhage and/or other fragments of surrounding structures such as cartilage or bone might also be visualized on cytological examination.

Foreign body reactions can induce mononuclear-to-mixed inflammation, the latter of which may contain neutrophils, lymphocytes, and/or plasma cells. Pseudogout (deposition of calcium pyrophosphate crystals in articular cartilage), while very rare in dogs, can cause acute arthritic clinical signs and is associated with a mixed inflammatory response composed of mononuclear cells and neutrophilic inflammation. A distinguishing feature of pseudogout is the presence of variably sized square-to-rhomboid-shaped crystals (Forsyth et al. 2007).

9.4.2.2 Hemarthrosis

True hemarthrosis, defined as hemorrhage within the synovial space, can be difficult to differentiate from inadvertent blood contamination. Therefore, the clinician should communicate any difficulties encountered during sample collection or irregular amounts of blood seen during aspiration to the laboratory. Joint fluid associated with true hemarthrosis is typically homogeneously pink/orange/red. Cytological evaluation reveals an increased density of red blood cells, a dilute glycosaminoglycan background, increased hemosiderin laden and erythrophagocytic macrophages, and, if chronic, hematoidin crystals (Figure 9.5). Erythrophagocytic macrophages are macrophages with erythrocytes in their cytoplasm. Hemosiderin is an iron storage complex that forms within macrophages as erythrocytes are being broken down. The pigment granules on Wrights–Giemsa staining appear dark blue green to almost black and can vary between very fine to globular within the cytoplasm. Special stains to identify iron (i.e. Prussian blue) can be performed to identify hemosiderin from other pigment granules. Hematoidin crystals are breakdown products of bilirubin that crystalize to form diamond-to-rectangular-shaped light brown-gold refractile crystals. Of note, macrophages are capable of phagocytizing erythrocytes post-collection and within collection tubes. Therefore, it is crucial to make fresh smears at the time of collection to discern *in vivo* from *in vitro* erythrophagia. The presence of hemosiderin and hematoidin is more definitive for true hemorrhage because they take longer to form and suggest chronicity. Possible differentials for patients with hemarthrosis include trauma, coagulation disorders (hemophiliacs versus anticoagulants), or any condition that disrupts blood supply and causes hemorrhage (i.e. neoplasia).

9.4.3 Neoplasia

All cell populations within the joint organ have the potential to become neoplastic. Diagnosis of a neoplastic disorder can be reached by combining the clinical picture with the cytological findings. Establishing a diagnosis based on synovial fluid analysis can be difficult; neoplastic synovial fluid is highly variable in cellular and protein composition and can appear similar to any of the other categories described above. It is the presence of cells that display atypia and criteria of malignancy that should alert the evaluator to consider neoplastic differentials (e.g. synovial cell sarcoma in Figure 9.5F). Ancillary diagnostics, such as biopsy, immunocytochemistry or immunohistochemistry, and/or flow cytometry, are typically required to reach a definitive diagnosis, as multiple types of sarcomas have similar morphological feature. Additionally, other tumor tissue types, such as carcinomas and lymphomas, have been reported to metastasize or localize to synovial tissue and fluid.

References

Clements, D. (2006). Arthrocentesis and synovial fluid analysis in dogs and cats. *In Practice* 28 (5): 256–262.

Dusick, A., Young, K.M., and Muir, P. (2014). Relationship between automated total nucleated cell count and enumeration of cells on direct smears of canine synovial fluid. *Vet. J.* 202 (3): 550–554.

Font-Vizcarra, L., Garcia, S., Martinez-Pastor, J.C. et al. (2010). Blood culture flasks for culturing synovial fluid in prosthetic joint infections. *Clin. Orthop. Relat. Res.* 468 (8): 2238–2243.

Forsyth, S.F., Thompson, K.G., and Donald, J.J. (2007). Possible pseudogout in two dogs. *J. Small Anim. Pract.* 48 (3): 174–176.

Hillström, A., Bylin, J., Hagman, R. et al. (2016). Measurement of serum C-reactive protein concentration for discriminating between suppurative arthritis and osteoarthritis in dogs. *BMC Vet. Res.* 12 (1): 240.

Littman, M.P., Gerber, B., Goldstein, R.E. et al. (2018). ACVIM consensus update on Lyme borreliosis in dogs and cats. *J. Vet. Intern. Med.* 32 (3): 887–903.

Lorenzo-Figueras, M., Pusterla, N., Byrne, B.A., and Samitz, E.M. (2006). In vitro evaluation of three bacterial culture systems for the recovery of *Escherichia coli* from equine blood. *Am. J. Vet. Res.* 67 (12): 2025–2029.

Macwilliams, P.S. and Friedrichs, K.R. (2003). Laboratory evaluation and interpretation of synovial fluid. *Vet. Clin. North Am. Small Anim. Pract.* 33 (1): 153–178.

Marchevsky, A.M. and Read, R.A. (1999). Bacterial septic arthritis in 19 dogs. *Aust. Vet. J.* 77 (4): 233–237.

Martinez, C.R. and Santangelo, K.S. (2017). Preanalytical considerations for joint fluid evaluation. *Vet. Clin. North Am. Small Anim. Pract.* 47 (1): 111–122.

Mielke, B., Comerford, E., English, K., and Meeson, R. (2018). Spontaneous septic arthritis of canine elbows: twenty-one cases. *Vet. Comp. Orthop. Traumatol.* 31 (6): 488–493.

Miller, J.M., Binnicker, M.J., Campbell, S. et al. (2018). A guide to utilization of the microbiology laboratory for diagnosis of infectious diseases: 2018 update by the infectious diseases society of America and the American society for microbiology. *Clin. Infect. Dis.* 67 (6): e1–e94.

Montgomery, R., Long, I., Milton, J., and Dipinto, M. (1989). Comparison of aerobic culturette, synovial membrane biopsy, and blood culture medium in detection of canine bacterial arthritis. *Vet. Surg.* 18 (4): 300–303.

Proot, J.L., De Vicente, F., and Sheahan, D.E. (2015). Analysis of lactate concentrations in canine synovial fluid. *Vet. Comp. Orthop. Traumatol.* 28 (5): 301–305.

Scharf, V., Lewis, S., Wellehan, J. et al. (2015). Retrospective evaluation of the efficacy of isolating bacteria from synovial fluid in dogs with suspected septic arthritis. *Aust. Vet. J.* 93 (6): 200–203.

10

Diagnostic Imaging Techniques in Lameness Evaluation

Angela J. Marolf

Department of Environmental and Radiological Health Sciences, College of Veterinary Medicine and Biomedical Sciences, Colorado State University, Fort Collins, CO, USA

10.1   Introduction

Diagnostic imaging is usually necessary in the assessment of patients presenting with lameness and can often provide definitive diagnosis. Radiography and ultrasound have been performed in dogs for evaluation of musculoskeletal conditions for many years in veterinary medicine, with newer imaging techniques such as magnetic resonance imaging (MR or MRI), computed tomography (CT), and positron emission tomography (PET)/CT being utilized increasingly for diagnosis of musculoskeletal disease in animal patients. Ideally, the diagnosis is made using the least costly and most readily available imaging modality. This chapter will provide a brief overview of imaging modalities used in the diagnosis of musculoskeletal conditions and discuss which are better selected for identification of certain clinical conditions. Imaging indications and findings for individual regions are discussed in greater detail in Section 2, as they apply to the thoracic limb and pelvic limb specifically. Table 10.1 provides an overview of current imaging modalities.

10.2   Radiography

Long the mainstay of imaging of the musculoskeletal system, radiography (Figure 10.1) continues to be the frontline imaging choice in many disease processes because it is readily available, obtained quickly, and relatively inexpensive. Moreover, it is excellent at identifying osseous changes including fractures, advanced osteoarthritis, and certain congenital diseases. Many soft tissue changes can be noted as well on radiographs, including joint effusion/hypertrophy and calcifying tendinopathies (Lafuente et al. 2009). Additional views, such as special oblique (Figures 12.3 and 18.2), skyline (Figure 15.12), and stress radiographs (Figure 13.8), are particularly useful in determining location and extent of disease. However, disadvantages of radiography include ionizing radiation and the possibility of underdiagnosis of certain disease processes. It is important for the clinician to remember that normal radiographs of a limb or body part do not exclude disease, and additional advanced imaging may be required for diagnosis.

Table 10.1 Imaging modality comparisons.

Imaging modality	Advantages	Disadvantages	Common uses
Radiography	Readily available Detects osseous disease and soft tissue calcification	Underdiagnoses soft tissue disease Superimposition of structures	First-line diagnosis
Ultrasonography	More available Detects periarticular soft tissue, muscle, and meniscal injury in larger joints	Highly operator dependent Underdiagnoses smaller joints and medial shoulder structures	Soft tissue injuries of the shoulder Achilles tendinopathy Detection of meniscal tears Evaluation of specific muscles (such as iliopsoas)
Computed tomography	Excellent osseous detail Good soft tissue detail Can use intravenous contrast Multi-plane reconstruction	Less availability Cost May need general anesthesia Multiple regions scanned quickly	Elbow dysplasia Detection of OCD-lesions Complex fractures Angular limb deformities
Magnetic resonance imaging	Excellent soft tissue detail Can use intravenous contrast Multiple sequences/planes	Limited availability Cost General anesthesia Limited to specific region	Soft tissue injuries of the shoulder Evaluation of specific muscles (such as iliopsoas) Detection of meniscal tears
Nuclear medicine	Physiologic/metabolic activity detection Lesion localization and diagnosis (PET/CT)	Very limited availability Cost General anesthesia (PET/CT) Long scan times (PET/CT)	Obscure lameness

10.3 Ultrasonography

Ultrasonography (Figure 10.2) is used often to evaluate soft tissue changes and can differentiate fluid and soft tissue thickening, as well as muscle fiber pattern changes; whereas, radiographs cannot. Ultrasonography is often complementary to radiographs when obvious osseous disease is not present and muscular injury is suspected. Dynamic evaluation of muscle and joint movement with ultrasound is beneficial, and ultrasound imaging has become common in musculoskeletal diagnosis. Regions commonly evaluated with ultrasound include the shoulder, calcaneal tendon and tarsus, and stifle (Long and Nyland 1999; Lamb and Duvernois 2005; Caine et al. 2009; Cook 2016). Advantages to ultrasonography include the ability to perform the study on either awake or sedate patients and the use of nonionizing sound waves. However, ultrasound is highly operator dependent, and thorough and accurate evaluation can be limited due to a sonographer's level of experience.

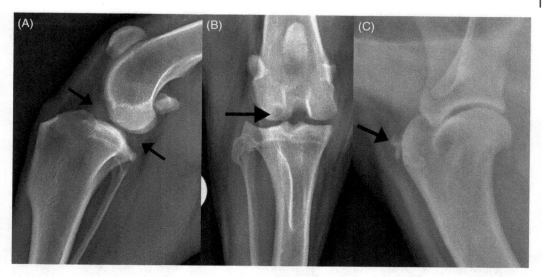

Figure 10.1 Radiographic images – diagnostic examples: (A) lateral view of the stifle. Note the increased intra-articular soft tissue opacity within the cranial and caudal aspects of the joint (arrows). This is likely either effusion or synovial hypertrophy; (B) craniocaudal view of the stifle. Note the subchondral articular lucency with surrounding sclerosis in the lateral femoral condyle (arrow). This is consistent with an osteochondrosis lesion; (C) lateral view of the shoulder. Note the smoothly marginated soft tissue mineralization adjacent to the greater tubercle of the humerus (arrow). This is likely mineralization within the supraspinatus tendon.

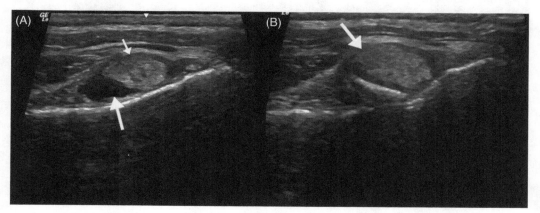

Figure 10.2 Ultrasound images – diagnostic examples: (A) transverse ultrasound image of the proximal biceps tendon. Note the heterogeneity of the tendon (small arrow) and increased fluid within the sheath (large arrow); (B) transverse ultrasound image of the more distal biceps tendon. Note the enlargement and heterogeneity of the tendon at this level (arrow). Sonographic diagnosis was biceps tenosynovitis and tendinopathy.

10.4 Computed Tomography

CT (Figure 10.3) has been performed for years to assess the musculoskeletal system in people; however, the increased availability of CT scanners in veterinary hospitals in recent years has led to this imaging modality becoming readily accessible for use in dogs as well. Further, with the advent and greater availability of multi-slice CT scanners (i.e. a CT with multiple rows of detectors), the

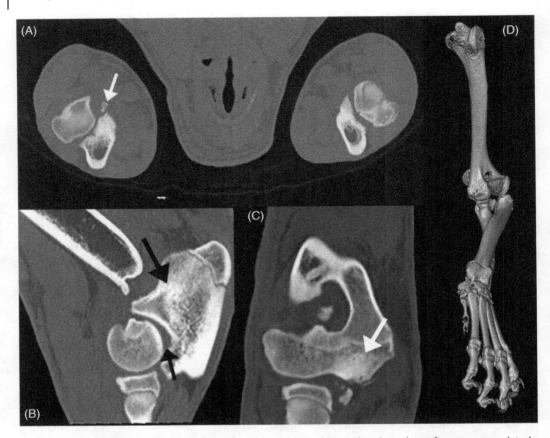

Figure 10.3 CT images – diagnostic examples: (A) transverse image showing a large fragment associated with the medial coronoid process of the right elbow (arrow). The adjacent coronoid process is sclerotic and abnormally shaped; (B) sagittal plane reconstruction of the right elbow. A widening of the humero-ulnar joint (small arrow) occurs with mild sclerosis of the anconeal process (large arrow). Humero-ulnar incongruity is present; (C) dorsal plane reconstruction of the right elbow. Note the sclerosis of the humeral trochlea (arrow) with irregular articular margin and small fragments; (D) 3D reconstruction of a dog with congenital elbow luxation.

speed at which CT studies can be performed has increased, thus allowing for musculoskeletal CT imaging to be performed with light sedation only. CT provides excellent contrast resolution of soft tissues and bones, is relatively fast, and can cover multiple regions in one study. It can be combined with intravenous iodinated contrast to better evaluate the blood flow to tissues (i.e. contrast-enhanced CT). The speed of CT, combined with its ability to image regions without superimposition of overlying structures, offers distinct advantages over other imaging methods. Disadvantages to CT imaging include ionizing radiation, added expense, need for anesthesia or sedation, and limited availability in comparison to the ubiquity of ultrasound and radiography.

CT imaging is an excellent diagnostic choice to identify osseous disease or osteochondrosis dissecans and to evaluate regions with complex osseous anatomy. The shoulder, elbow, and tarsus joints are some of the most common regions evaluated with CT (Reichle et al. 2000; De Rycke et al. 2002; Gielen et al. 2005). Bones, muscles, and joints can be evaluated in dorsal and sagittal imaging planes (Figure 10.4) in unlimited angles for thorough assessment via

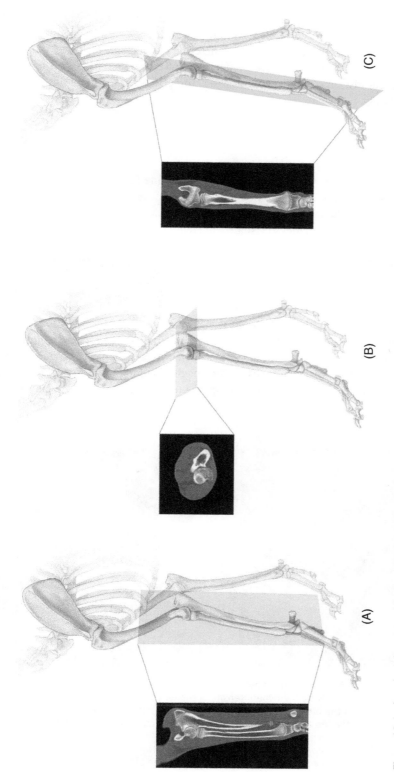

Figure 10.4 Imaging planes used for lower limb multi-planar imaging modalities: (A) sagittal plane; (B) transverse plane; and (C) dorsal plane.

multi-planar reconstructions (using a commercially available software imaging tool), thus permitting complete visualization of all anatomic structures.

CT terminology uses the term "attenuation" to describe tissue characteristics in relation to each other: tissues presenting as bright are described as hyperattenuating, dark tissues are described as hypoattenuating, and tissues of similar brightness are described as isoattenuating. Fluids are typically hypoattenuating.

10.5 Magnetic Resonance Imaging

MR (Figure 10.5) is a newer modality in veterinary medicine for evaluation of musculoskeletal conditions. Soft tissue injuries of the shoulder are often diagnosed with MR imaging (Agnello et al. 2008; Murphy et al. 2008; Schaefer et al. 2010). It provides excellent contrast resolution of the soft tissues and multiple anatomic planes to visualize the region of interest. Although CT and MR both offer excellent contrast resolution, MR is considered the gold-standard imaging modality for evaluation of soft tissue injuries. CT uses X-rays and attenuation differences in tissues, whereas MR uses electromagnetic radiation to evaluate the hydrogen nuclei (protons) composition in tissues. Because different tissues have different amounts of protons, MR imaging can characterize tissues more sensitively than CT.

However, MR is not without its limitations. Detection of subtle bone changes is more difficult with MR imaging, and in contrast to CT imaging, MR is usually limited to one region and is often more time-consuming due to the multiple sequences in different planes that need to be acquired for a complete study. Other disadvantages to MR imaging include the need for general anesthesia, added expense, and decreased availability compared to radiography, ultrasonography, and CT imaging.

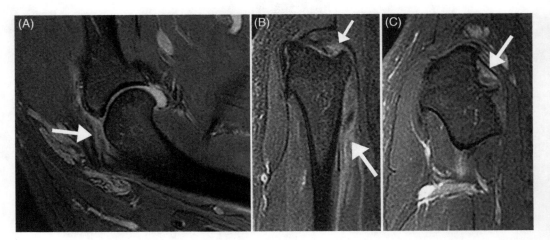

Figure 10.5 MR images of the shoulder showing proton density fat-saturated images: (A) sagittal plane at the level of the biceps tendon. Note the hyperintensity of the tendon and surrounding bursa (arrow); (B) dorsal plane at the level of the biceps tendon within the intertubercular groove of the humerus. Note the hyperintensity within the tendon and surrounding bursa (small arrow) and the hyperintensity within the muscle belly distally (large arrow); (C) transverse plane at the level of the biceps tendon within the intertubercular groove of the humerus. Note the hyperintensity within the biceps tendon and adjacent bursa (arrow). Diagnosis was biceps tenosynovitis and with possible biceps tendon tear.

Intravenous contrast media are frequently used with MR and CT imaging to improve contrast resolution and to evaluate the blood flow (i.e. perfusion and vascularity) of tissues. This can help differentiate different pathologic processes (e.g. neoplastic versus degenerative). The type of intravenous contrast agents differs between MR and CT. Specifically, MR utilizes gadolinium based while CT utilizes iodinated contrast media.

Standard imaging sequences obtained in MR include T1, T2, and proton density (PD)-weighted sequences, which demonstrate the molecular differences in various tissues and can detect abnormalities due to differences in tissue appearance in the sequences. MR terminology uses the term "intensity" to describe tissue characteristics and appearance on various sequences, whereby tissues that are bright are described as hyperintense; dark tissues as hypointense; and tissues of a similar intensity as isointense. Fluids are typically hypointense on T1-weighted images, hyperintense on T2-weighted images, and of intermediate signal intensity on PD-weighted images. An additional technique often used in MR imaging is called "fat saturation." This technique makes fat appear hypointense on T1-, T2-, and PD-weighted images and can highlight inflammation and edema in tissues.

10.6 Nuclear Medicine

In the past, nuclear medicine imaging in small animals was limited to an imaging modality described as bone scan or bone scintigraphy. This technology uses a gamma camera that captures gamma radiation emitted by specific radiopharmaceuticals (typically ^{99m}Technetium methylene diphosphonate) after intravenous administration, thereby highlighting areas of increased uptake. It has been found to be helpful in dogs with obscure lameness by several authors (Schwarz et al. 2004; Samoy et al. 2008). Scintigraphy localizes areas of increased radiopharmaceutical uptake due to inflammation or neoplasia; however, it does not provide a specific diagnosis. Therefore, further structural imaging of the identified areas is always needed to establish a diagnosis.

Currently, the newest imaging modality for evaluation of the musculoskeletal system is PET imaging combined with a conventional CT, termed PET/CT (Figure 10.6). PET is a form of nuclear medicine that uses radiopharmaceuticals that are positron emitters. Positrons are positively charged particles, also called beta + particles, or β^+. These particles travel a short distance (1–2 mm) before colliding with a negatively charged electron. When the two collide, two annihilation gamma photons are created and travel 180° from each other. The special detectors in a PET scanner detect and register these coincident photons – photons that are emitted 180° from each other and arrive within a few nanoseconds of each other. Fluorine-18-fluorodeoxyglucose (FDG), an analog of glucose, is widely used for PET imaging in human medicine and veterinary oncology. FDG is characterized by uptake and retention by hypermetabolic cells, hence it is frequently used for diagnosis of cancer and metastatic disease; however, it can also be used to evaluate muscle activity. The most common way to quantify PET tracer accumulation is by standardized uptake values (SUVs), and the tissue activity concentration is normalized by the fraction of the injected dose/unit weight (Kinehan and Fletcher 2010).

When this technology was first developed, PET/CT acquired a PET scan and CT scan on separate machines at different times. However, advances in machine technology now provide the ability to acquire images using a dual PET/CT scanner as part of one imaging exam. The CT images offer excellent anatomic depiction of normal and abnormal structures, while PET with FDG identifies areas of high glucose metabolism. Once obtained, CT and PET images are compared, side by side and fused, to determine if areas of noticeably high metabolic activity are normal or abnormal on

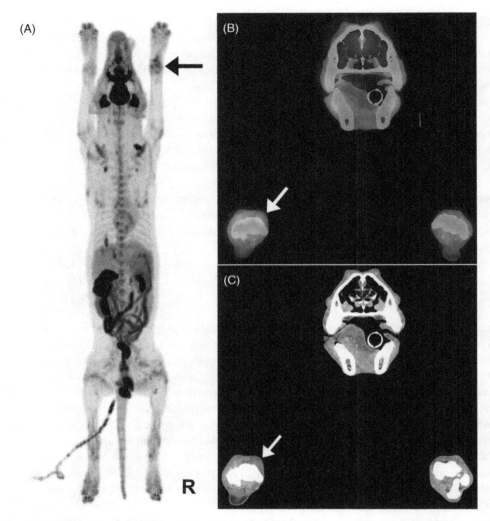

Figure 10.6   PET/CT images of a dog with subtle right thoracic limb lameness: whole body PET scan fused PET/CT and CT images of the right and left carpus (left included for comparison): (A) whole body PET scan showing areas of uptake throughout the body. Salivary gland, brain, gastrointestinal, and urinary tract uptake is normal. Note the right carpus with increased metabolic activity (arrow) compared to left carpus (right is on right side in this image [R]); (B) fused PET/CT transverse image at level of right and left carpus. Note the increased metabolic activity of the right carpus with mild soft tissue thickening (arrow) compared to left carpus; (C) CT post-contrast study in soft tissue window at the level of the right and left carpus. Note the soft tissue thickening of the right carpus (arrow). Right carpal arthrocentesis revealed chronic synovial inflammation.

CT. PET alone is substantially limited by low spatial resolution and its inability to provide anatomical detail. Combining PET with structural imaging techniques such as CT (or even MRI) provides useful physiologic information to detect abnormalities while allowing exact anatomic localization of pathology.

PET/CT imaging can be used to localize lameness and identify areas of abnormality due to higher metabolic activity compared to normal (Mann et al. 2016; Grobman et al. 2018). These changes may guide further diagnostics to determine the cause of the increased metabolic activity (if the CT imaging is not sufficient to establish a diagnosis). Such diagnostics may include ultrasound (for muscle pathology), fine-needle aspirate, biopsy, or arthrocentesis to differentiate specific disease processes causing increased SUV, such as infection, inflammation, or cancer.

All nuclear medicine studies require special imaging equipment and appropriate nuclear medicine facilities. Disadvantages of PET/CT imaging include extremely limited availability, long scan times, ionizing radiation, need for general anesthesia, and cost. Currently, this imaging modality is mostly limited to university and tertiary referral hospitals.

References

Agnello, K.A., Puchalski, S.M., Wisner, E.R. et al. (2008). Effect of positioning, scan plane, and arthrography on visibility of periarticular canine shoulder soft tissue structures on magnetic resonance images. *Vet Radiol Ultrasound* 49 (6): 529–539.

Caine, A., Agthe, P., Posch, B., and Herrtage, M. (2009). Sonography of the soft tissue structures of the canine tarsus. *Vet Radiol Ultrasound* 50 (3): 304–308.

Cook, C.R. (2016). Ultrasound imaging of the musculoskeletal system. *Vet Clin North Am Small Anim Pract* 46 (3): 355–371.

De Rycke, L.M., Gielen, I.M., Van Bree, H., and Simoens, P.J. (2002). Computed tomography of the elbow joint in clinically normal dogs. *Am J Vet Res* 63 (10): 1400–1407.

Gielen, I., Van Ryssen, B., and Van Bree, H. (2005). Computerized tomography compared with radiography in the diagnosis of lateral trochlear ridge talar osteochondritis dissecans in dogs. *Vet Comp Orthop Traumatol* 18 (2): 77–82.

Grobman, M., Cohn, L., Knapp, S. et al. (2018). (18) F-FDG-PET/CT as adjunctive diagnostic modalities in canine fever of unknown origin. *Vet Radiol Ultrasound* 59 (1): 107–115.

Kinehan, P. and Fletcher, J. (2010). PET/CT standardized uptake values (SUVs) in clinical practice and assessing response to therapy. *Semin Ultrasound CT MR* 31 (6): 496–505.

Lafuente, M.P., Fransson, B.A., Lincoln, J.D. et al. (2009). Surgical treatment of mineralized and nonmineralized supraspinatus tendinopathy in twenty-four dogs. *Vet Surg* 38 (3): 380–387.

Lamb, C.R. and Duvernois, A. (2005). Ultrasonographic anatomy of the normal canine calcaneal tendon. *Vet Radiol Ultrasound* 46 (4): 326–330.

Long, C.D. and Nyland, T.G. (1999). Ultrasonographic evaluation of the canine shoulder. *Vet Radiol Ultrasound* 40 (4): 372–379.

Mann, K., Hart, J., and Duerr, F. (2016). 18F-FDG positron emission tomography: an innovative technique for the diagnosis of a canine lameness. *Front Vet Sci* 3: 45.

Murphy, S.E., Ballegeer, E.A., Forrest, L.J., and Schaefer, S.L. (2008). Magnetic resonance imaging findings in dogs with confirmed shoulder pathology. *Vet Surg* 37 (7): 631–638.

Reichle, J.K., Park, R.D., and Bahr, A.M. (2000). Computed tomographic findings of dogs with cubital joint lameness. *Vet Radiol Ultrasound* 41 (2): 125–130.

Samoy, Y., Van Ryssen, B., Van Caelenberg, A. et al. (2008). Single-phase bone scintigraphy in dogs with obscure lameness. *J Small Anim Pract* 49 (9): 444–450.

Schaefer, S.L., Baumel, C.A., Gerbig, J.R., and Forrest, L.J. (2010). Direct magnetic resonance arthrography of the canine shoulder. *Vet Radiol Ultrasound* 51 (4): 391–396.

Schwarz, T., Johnson, V.S., Voute, L., and Sullivan, M. (2004). Bone scintigraphy in the investigation of occult lameness in the dog. *J Small Anim Pract* 45 (5): 232–237.

11

Diagnostic Approach to Neoplastic Conditions Causing Lameness

Bernard Séguin

Department of Clinical Sciences, College of Veterinary Medicine and Biomedical Sciences, Flint Animal Cancer Center, Colorado State University, Fort Collins, CO, USA

11.1   Introduction

Neoplasia is a frequent cause of lameness and therefore must be considered as a differential diagnosis for most patients. Signalment, history, and physical exam may raise suspicion of a neoplastic condition. Neoplasia is a common differential diagnosis in certain breeds and older patients, although osteosarcoma can affect any breed and is known to affect younger animals as well (Liptak et al. 2004). Certain histories can raise the suspicion of a neoplastic condition, such as one that indicates a pathologic fracture (e.g. progressive thoracic limb lameness followed by a nontraumatic event that causes acute non-weight-bearing lameness). A general approach to the patient with neoplasia causing lameness is outlined in Figure 11.1.

11.2   Diagnostic Methods

11.2.1   Physical Examination

Lameness is a common finding with tumors but it may not always be present. Given the paucity of soft tissues around the lower limb, it is common to visualize a "swelling" or mass effect if tumors affect these regions. Soft tissue masses should be assessed for their ability to be freely movable, to determine their origin (skin versus subcutaneous tissue versus deeper soft tissues or bone) and adherence to the underlying bone. Palpation of the soft tissues or bones affected by cancer generally is painful, and frequently a mass effect may be observed (Figure 13.13). With osseous neoplasia, pain can be elicited when direct pressure is placed on the bone, while arthropathies cause pain during end range of motion. Tendinopathies can be diagnosed by isolating the muscle and stretching it (Chapter 5). Physical exam findings should always be confirmed with diagnostic imaging.

11.2.2   Fine-needle Aspirate and Biopsy

In order to diagnose neoplasm, a fine-needle aspirate (FNA; which leads to cytology) or biopsy (which leads to histopathology) is required. If a nondiagnostic sample or reactive tissue is obtained

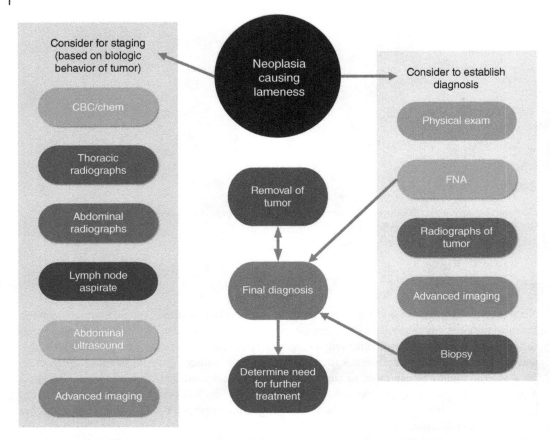

Figure 11.1 Schematic representation of the clinical approach to a patient exhibiting lameness caused by neoplasia. The veterinarian should attempt to establish a diagnosis for the primary tumor and determine the extent of distant disease (staging). The biologic behavior of the tumor influences the appropriate diagnostic methods (for example, advanced imaging may not be necessary for all tumor types).

with cytology, this does not rule out the possibility of neoplasm and another attempt at FNA or a biopsy is necessary. In one study, Ghisleni et al. (2006) reported that the cytology of cutaneous and subcutaneous masses agreed with the histologic diagnosis in 90% of the diagnostic samples obtained. Similarly, in a retrospective study that compared the accuracy of using cytology and histological biopsies to diagnose destructive bone lesions, Sabattini et al. (2017) observed non-accurate results in about 20% of the cases for each technique, thus suggesting that cytology is a valid alternative to histology. When results suggest a false negative (e.g. reactive bone; which has been reported to occur in up to 17% of biopsies of malignant bone tumors), it is recommended to repeat the biopsy (Powers et al. 1988; Sabattini et al. 2017). Yet, even this may be nondiagnostic in some cases, and a final diagnosis can only be obtained once the entire lesion is removed (e.g. via amputation or limb sparing). Ultrasound guidance can be helpful to increase the likelihood of acquiring a diagnostic sample with an FNA for bone lesions (Britt et al. 2007). With ultrasound, breaks in the cortex can be found and used to guide the needle into the intramedullary component of the tumor. Tumors that have a significant soft tissue component may be successfully aspirated without ultrasound guidance. If cytology of a bone lesion is obtained, alkaline phosphatase (ALP) staining can be performed. ALP staining is highly sensitive but not entirely specific for osteosarcoma

(Barger et al. 2005; Ryseff and Bohn 2012). Other bone tumors that can stain positive for ALP include chondrosarcoma and multilobular osteochondrosarcoma (MLO), but MLO typically affects the axial skeleton. Bone biopsies are best performed with a Jamshidi needle (Powers et al. 1988; Sabattini et al. 2017). For bone lesions that are small, using fluoroscopy or performing radiographs throughout the procedure is helpful to ensure the biopsies were indeed taken from the lesion. It is best to sample the middle of a bone lesion for a biopsy and not the periphery (Powers et al. 1988; Liptak et al. 2004).

11.2.3   Diagnostic Imaging

Radiographs of the affected region of the limb are indicated when neoplasia is suspected, particularly for tumors that are fixed and poorly movable on palpation. Soft tissue tumors may show bone invasion on radiographs and as such this technique is still indicated. Primary tumors of bone typically display lytic and proliferative changes but only one dominant feature may be present. Particularly for the proximal humerus, it can be difficult to differentiate subtle lytic lesions from underlying tissues, making orthogonal views mandatory for these cases (Figure 17.1). Tumors of the synovium typically display lytic changes in the bones on "both sides" (i.e. proximal and distal) of the joint. It can sometimes be difficult to differentiate between severe osteoarthritis, septic arthritis, and a neoplasm of the synovium on radiographs (Figure 14.12C). Computed tomography (CT) can be used to image the area and is more sensitive to show both soft tissue and bone changes. Magnetic resonance is another useful imaging modality and is superior to CT for imaging soft tissue tumors. It can also be used to image bone tumors, particularly when assessing the extent of the tumor is important (Davis et al. 2002).

11.2.4   Staging

Once a diagnosis of neoplasia is suspected or confirmed, staging should be performed for any neoplasia with metastatic potential. A complete blood count and chemistry panel are indicated to assess overall health of the patient and can be helpful for diagnostic or prognostic purposes in certain cases (e.g. hyperglobulinemia with multiple myeloma or alkaline phosphatase for osteosarcoma, respectively). In general, thoracic radiograph (or CT) is recommended for all malignant neoplasms to evaluate for pulmonary metastases. Abdominal radiographs and ultrasound should be considered for tumors known to metastasize to intra-abdominal lymph nodes, spleen, or liver. Similar to the approach for diagnosing the primary tumor, FNA of these structures is generally the next step to confirm metastatic disease. If nondiagnostic samples are obtained, biopsy samples may need to be obtained via exploratory laparotomy/laparoscopy.

Some tumors, such as mast cell tumors and histiocytic sarcomas, are more likely to metastasize to lymph nodes. For these tumors, any palpable lymph node draining the area from which the tumor is arising from, even when not enlarged, should be aspirated. But even in the presence of tumors that uncommonly metastasize to lymph nodes, aspirating the lymph nodes is still recommended. A metastatic lymph node can provide a diagnosis and also have a significant impact on the prognosis. A good example is osteosarcoma: lymph node metastasis is seen in only about 5% of cases, but when present the median survival is only about two months (Hillers et al. 2005).

Other staging tests such as bone scintigraphy, or positron emission tomography (PET-CT), may be utilized based on the tumor and availability. PET-CT is a sensitive test to diagnose metastatic foci in both soft tissue and bone and is therefore an excellent staging modality to evaluate the entire body with a single test (Selmic et al. 2017). However, availability of this modality is limited.

11.3   Specific Tumors

Many histologic types of neoplasm cause lameness in dogs. Both skin and subcutaneous tumors may occur in the thoracic and pelvic limbs. Tumors can also originate from muscles, bones, or the joint capsule.

11.3.1   Skin and Subcutaneous Neoplasia

Tumors of the skin and subcutaneous tissues can affect any aspect of the limbs. Common tumors of the skin and subcutaneous tissues are mast cell tumors, soft tissue sarcomas, and lipomas. Both skin and subcutaneous tumors can cause lameness if they are painful. Furthermore, subcutaneous tumors can interfere with the tendons, muscles, and joint motion or irritate adjacent nerves and thereby result in lameness. Infiltrative tumors into a muscle, such as infiltrative lipoma or soft tissue sarcoma, are examples of a tumor that can interfere with muscle function.

11.3.2   Muscle Neoplasia

Tumors of the muscles are not well described in the canine literature, and primary tumors of the muscles, such as rhabdomyosarcomas, appear to be quite rare. Anecdotally, other tumors arising within a muscle, such as hemangiosarcoma, histiocytic sarcoma, and soft tissue sarcoma, are more common than primary muscle tumors. Other differentials for mass effects in muscles include infection and muscle tears. Tumors of the muscle should be considered as a differential diagnosis, particularly if swelling and muscle tears are observed without a history of trauma.

11.3.3   Bone Neoplasia

Tumors of the bones and synovium frequently cause severe lameness because of their intimate association with the tissues involved in motion. Tumors of the bone can be either primary or metastatic. Primary bone tumors can be osteosarcoma, chondrosarcoma, fibrosarcoma, and hemangiosarcoma. By far the most common (98% in one study) tumor of the appendicular skeleton is osteosarcoma with large and giant breeds being predisposed. Osteosarcoma is most commonly diagnosed in 7–9 year old dogs, however, even dogs of 1–2 years of age may be affected (Liptak et al. 2004). Osteosarcoma most commonly occurs in the metaphyseal regions of bones, most frequently in the distal radius and proximal humerus. Diaphyseal lesions have been reported but are uncommon. Chondrosarcoma is the second most common bone tumor.

As a rule, any carcinoma of a bone should be considered metastatic. As such, once a bone carcinoma is diagnosed, the primary tumor should be identified. In general, a thorough physical exam (including a rectal exam), radiographs of the chest and abdomen, and abdominal ultrasound are appropriate first steps.

Other tumors affecting the bones include lymphoma and plasma cell tumor/multiple myeloma. Multiple myeloma can be associated with hyperglobulinemia. A chemistry panel and protein electrophoresis may be used to detect a monoclonal gammopathy.

11.3.4   Joint Capsule Neoplasia

The most common tumors arising from the joint capsule are histiocytic sarcoma, synovial myxomas, and synovial cell sarcoma (Craig et al. 2002). The most common breeds affected are the

Golden Retriever, Labrador Retriever, and Rottweiler (Schultz et al. 2007; Klahn et al. 2011; Manor et al. 2018). Prior joint disease is associated with increased risk of developing periarticular histiocytic sarcoma in dogs (Manor et al. 2018). Whereas myxomas are identified by their unique histologic appearance, immunohistochemistry with CD 18 or CD204 is required to distinguish histiocytic sarcoma from synovial cell sarcoma (Craig et al. 2002). Other types of sarcomas (malignant fibrous histiocytoma, fibrosarcoma, and undifferentiated sarcoma) have also been rarely reported from the synovium in dogs (Craig et al. 2002). Although neoplastic cells can at times be identified with joint fluid analysis, this is not a reliable method to diagnose tumors that involve the joint capsule in the author's experience. FNAs and biopsies are preferred to make a definitive diagnosis.

Villonodular synovitis (also called pigmented villonodular synovitis; PVNS) has been described in all of the major joints, including the carpus (Hanson 1998). PVNS is considered a benign neoplasia (Dempsey et al. 2018); however, the etiology is still not fully understood. The condition causes proliferation of synovial tissues resulting in lameness and pain (Akerblom and Sjostrom 2006). PVNS has most commonly been described as a monoarticular condition; however, a dog with bilateral stifle PVNS has been reported (Marti 1997). Diagnostic imaging is generally nonspecific, requiring histopathology to establish the diagnosis. Even though PVNS is extremely rare, it should be considered as a differential diagnosis when diagnostics are inconsistent with more commonly observed conditions.

References

Akerblom, S. and Sjostrom, L. (2006). Villonodular synovitis in the dog: a report of four cases. *Vet Comp Orthop Traumatol* 19 (2): 87–92.

Barger, A., Graca, R., Bailey, K. et al. (2005). Use of alkaline phosphatase staining to differentiate canine osteosarcoma from other vimentin-positive tumors. *Vet Pathol* 42 (2): 161–165.

Britt, T., Clifford, C., Barger, A. et al. (2007). Diagnosing appendicular osteosarcoma with ultrasound-guided fine-needle aspiration: 36 cases. *J Small Anim Pract* 48 (3): 145–150.

Craig, L.E., Julian, M.E., and Ferracone, J.D. (2002). The diagnosis and prognosis of synovial tumors in dogs: 35 cases. *Vet Pathol* 39 (1): 66–73.

Davis, G.J., Kapatkin, A.S., Craig, L.E. et al. (2002). Comparison of radiography, computed tomography, and magnetic resonance imaging for evaluation of appendicular osteosarcoma in dogs. *J Am Vet Med Assoc* 220 (8): 1171–1176.

Dempsey, L.M., Maddox, T.W., Meiring, T. et al. (2018). Computed tomography findings of pigmented villonodular synovitis in a dog. *Vet Comp Orthop Traumatol* 31 (4): 304–310.

Ghisleni, G., Roccabianca, P., Ceruti, R. et al. (2006). Correlation between fine-needle aspiration cytology and histopathology in the evaluation of cutaneous and subcutaneous masses from dogs and cats. *Vet Clin Pathol* 35 (1): 24–30.

Hanson, J.A. (1998). Radiographic diagnosis-canine carpal villonodular synovitis. *Vet Radiol Ultrasound* 39 (1): 15–17.

Hillers, K.R., Dernell, W.S., Lafferty, M.H. et al. (2005). Incidence and prognostic importance of lymph node metastases in dogs with appendicular osteosarcoma: 228 cases (1986–2003). *J Am Vet Med Assoc* 226 (8): 1364–1367.

Klahn, S.L., Kitchell, B.E., and Dervisis, N.G. (2011). Evaluation and comparison of outcomes in dogs with periarticular and nonperiarticular histiocytic sarcoma. *J Am Vet Med Assoc* 239 (1): 90–96.

Liptak, J.M., Dernell, W.S., Ehrhart, N., and Withrow, S. (2004). Canine appendicular osteosarcoma: diagnosis and palliative treatment. *Compend Contin Educ Vet* 26 (3): 172–182.

Manor, E.K., Craig, L.E., Sun, X., and Cannon, C.M. (2018). Prior joint disease is associated with increased risk of periarticular histiocytic sarcoma in dogs. *Vet Comp Oncol* 16 (1): E83–E88.

Marti, J.M. (1997). Bilateral pigmented villonodular synovitis in a dog. *J Small Anim Pract* 38 (6): 256–260.

Powers, B.E., Larue, S.M., Withrow, S.J. et al. (1988). Jamshidi needle biopsy for diagnosis of bone lesions in small animals. *J Am Vet Med Assoc* 193 (2): 205–210.

Ryseff, J.K. and Bohn, A.A. (2012). Detection of alkaline phosphatase in canine cells previously stained with Wright-Giemsa and its utility in differentiating osteosarcoma from other mesenchymal tumors. *Vet Clin Pathol* 41 (3): 391–395.

Sabattini, S., Renzi, A., Buracco, P. et al. (2017). Comparative assessment of the accuracy of cytological and histologic biopsies in the diagnosis of canine bone lesions. *J Vet Intern Med* 31 (3): 864–871.

Schultz, R.M., Puchalski, S.M., Kent, M., and Moore, P.F. (2007). Skeletal lesions of histiocytic sarcoma in nineteen dogs. *Vet Radiol Ultrasound* 48 (6): 539–543.

Selmic, L.E., Griffin, L.R., Nolan, M.W. et al. (2017). Use of PET/CT and stereotactic radiation therapy for the diagnosis and treatment of osteosarcoma metastases. *J Am Anim Hosp Assoc* 53 (1): 52–58.

Section 2

Regional Diagnosis

Part III

Distal Limb Lameness

12

Distal Limb Region

Metacarpals, Metatarsals, Digits, Sesamoids, and Associated Structures

Nicolaas E. Lambrechts

Department of Clinical Sciences, College of Veterinary Medicine and Biomedical Sciences, Colorado State University, Fort Collins, CO, USA

12.1 Introduction

Although often overlooked because of the small size and complexity of their component anatomic structures, minor clinical findings, and paucity of available information regarding disease manifestation and methods of clinical examination for this region, injuries and diseases of the distal limb are a frequent and important source of lameness. This chapter describes many conditions that may subtly or profoundly affect a dog's normal gait and ambulatory performance. Figure 12.1 and Table 12.1 outline common differential diagnoses and diagnostic steps for the distal limb region.

12.2 Normal Anatomy

12.2.1 Thoracic Limb

The five metacarpals, numbered from medial to lateral, have a cylindrically shaped *body* articulating proximally with the distal row of carpal bones at their *base* and distally with the similarly numbered phalanges at their *head* (Figure 12.2). Metacarpal I, the smallest, only has a proximal epiphysis, does not bear weight, and may be supernumerary in some individuals or breeds (e.g. Saint Bernards). Metacarpals II–V all bear weight, although the longer III and IV are believed to bear greater loads. They all have a single distal physis and diverge from each other as they course distally. At each of the metacarpophalangeal joints II–V, there are also articulations with a single dorsal sesamoid (Figure 12.3), which lies within the common digital extensor tendons and two (single in metacarpal I) elongated, inwardly curved sesamoids within the ligamentous insertion of the interosseous muscles. These palmar sesamoids are also numbered from medial to lateral; however, only the paired sesamoids are numbered (Cake and Read 1995; Figure 12.2).

The metacarpal bones are attached to the distal row of carpal bones by synovial membranes and numerous straight and oblique ligaments. Distal to the synovial reflections, the individual bones are held to each other by interosseous metacarpal ligaments. There is very little movement at the carpometacarpal joint. At the transversely oriented metacarpophalangeal joints, movement is mainly flexion

Table 12.1 Key features for selected diseases affecting the distal limb region.

Disease	Common signalment	Exam findings	Diagnostic test of choice	Treatment	Clinical pearls	Terminology
Fractures/ luxations	Any breed or age – racing Greyhounds develop stress/ fatigue fractures	Pain, swelling, crepitus, and possibly instability or deviations	Survey radiographs, rarely CT for complex fractures	External coaptation or surgical fixation	The choice between surgical vs. nonsurgical treatment is controversial and depends on severity/ digits involved	
Other trauma	Any breed or age	Laceration, stabs, and foreign body penetrations and splits	Clinical appearance, radiographs, and ultrasound to detect involvement of underlying structures or potential foreign bodies	When appropriate, suturing and surgical exploration	Trauma to the distal limb is common and frequently missed	
Osteoarthritis	More commonly seen in adult animals. Metacarpophalangeal joints IV and V more common than II and III	Initial pain with later thickening and stiffening of the joint, variable lameness, can be associated with "flat digits"	Survey radiographs	Nonsurgical, rarely arthrodesis or amputation	May be overuse injury	
Sesamoid disease	Mainly racing Greyhounds and young Rottweilers. Sesamoids II and VII of either thoracic limb most commonly affected – others can be involved if traumatic origin	Focal pain and swelling. Reduced flexion of adjacent joint(s)	Survey radiographs or CT	Nonsurgical or surgical excision	Can be differentiated from bipartite sesamoids via imaging and lack of pain	Sesamoiditis and sesamoid fracture
Digital flexor muscle and tendon injury	Any breed, more likely athletic individuals	Digit(s) flattened with isolated SDF injury; last phalanx and claw angled dorsally with combined DDF and SDF injury	Radiographs to detect bony changes; ultrasound to localize site, extent, and stage of the disease	Appositional suturing of acutely transected muscle and tendons. For less severe or chronic strains and nonsurgical management	Injury can occur anywhere along the length of the muscle	"Dropped toe" (SDF); "Kicked up toe" or "knocked up toe" (DDF)

	Signalment	Clinical findings	Diagnosis	Treatment	Comments	Other terms
Corns	Sight hounds, especially Greyhounds	Well-circumscribed hyperkeratotic lesions with central keratin core	Biopsy and histopathology	Symptomatic or with surgical excision if unresponsive	90% affect digital pads of digits 3 and 4 of the thoracic limbs and consider other DD if located in other digits	Sweet corns: "wart-like lesion" or "Porokeratosis plantaris discreta"
Dermatologic conditions causing lameness	Multiple etiologies. Predisposed breeds for specific conditions, any breed and age for infectious conditions	Visually identifiable changes to paw pads, claws, and nail bed	Clinical appearance, skin scraping, exudate cytology, FNA, bacterial and fungal culture. Radiographs to detect potential underlying bone involvement	Depending on cause. Pharmacologic and surgical treatment (amputation if extensive bone involvement)	Important differential for lameness – careful evaluation of the paws/pad necessary to establish diagnosis	
Hypertrophic osteopathy	Any breed or age, older animals more common since most commonly associated with thoracic neoplasia	Limb thickening and pain	Radiographs of limbs and thoracic and abdominal imaging	Treat underlying thoracic and/or abdominal cause	Periosteal reaction and pain in all four limbs	Marie's disease of the dog, hypertrophic osteoarthropathy/ osteopathy
Digit neoplasia	Older animals	Swelling or mass effect of the digits – third phalanx most commonly affected	Fine-needle aspirate or biopsy, and radiographs (malignant melanoma frequently does not cause lytic changes)	Digit amputation, partial foot amputation; rarely requires partial or full-limb amputation	Squamous cell carcinoma and malignant melanoma most common rarely can affect multiple digits	

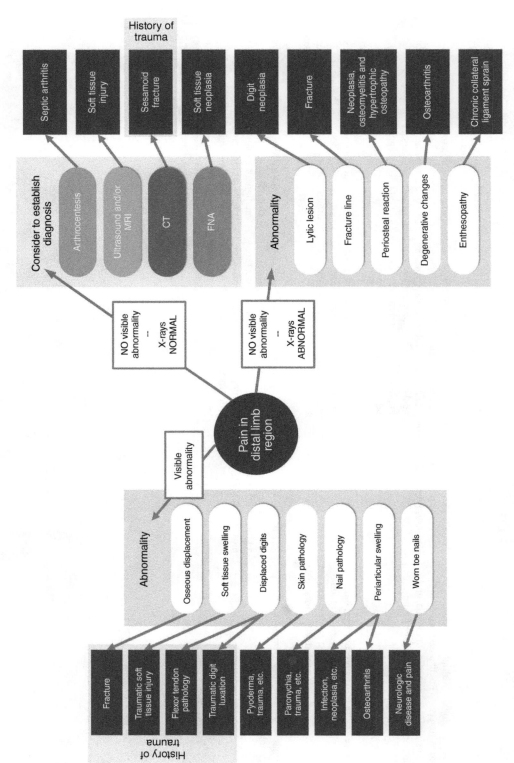

Figure 12.1   Schematic of common diseases affecting the distal limb region and the steps necessary to establish a diagnosis.

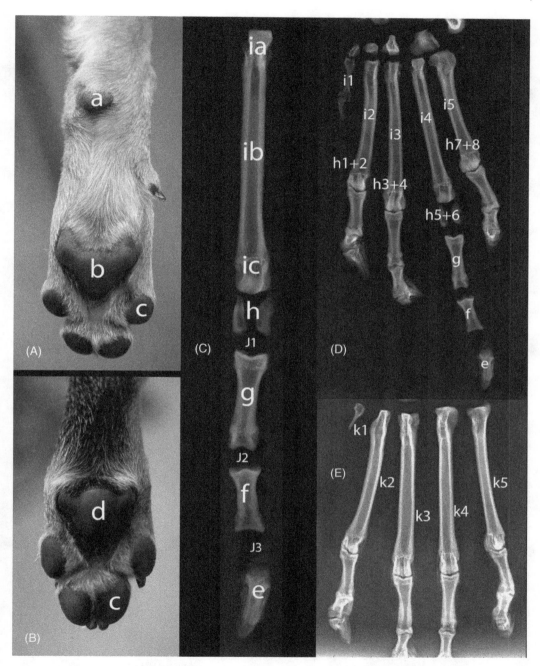

Figure 12.2 Normal anatomy of the paws: pads of the (A) thoracic limb and (B) pelvic limb; (C) fourth digit of the thoracic limb; (D) forepaw; and (E) hindpaw. (a) Carpal pad; (b) metacarpal pad; (c) digital pads; (d) metatarsal pad; (e) distal (third) phalanx with claw; (f) middle (second) phalanx; (g) proximal (first) phalanx; (h) proximal sesamoid bones (paired sesamoids are labeled from medial to lateral; i.e. the sesamoids of digit II are labeled number 1 + 2); (i) metacarpi (numbered from medial to lateral), (ia) base, (ib) body, (ic) head; (j1) metacarpophalangeal joint; (j2) proximal interphalangeal joint; (j3) distal interphalangeal joint; and (k) metatarsi (numbered from medial to lateral).

with lateral and medial movement restrained by the joint morphology, the bilateral collateral ligaments, and the lateral and medial collateral sesamoidean ligaments. Extension is limited by the short sesamoidean ligaments and the cruciate ligaments (located between the distal pole of the sesamoid bones and the proximal palmar surface of the first phalanges). The paired sesamoids are connected to each other by short palmar ligaments, and the four bones of each joint share a single joint capsule.

The powerful interosseous muscles originate from the palmar side of the bases of metacarpals II–V. They split into two tendons which each receive a sesamoid bone before inserting on the bases of the adjacent first phalanx. The muscle bellies run between the bifurcating tendons of the deep and superficial digital flexors and flex the metacarpophalangeal joints. The flexor carpi radialis muscle inserts on the proximal palmar surfaces of metacarpals II and III body. The two heads of the flexor carpi ulnaris muscle both insert on the accessory carpal bone. The two accessory carpal ligaments anchor the accessory carpal bone to the base of metacarpals IV and V. Together, they serve to flex the carpus and may also provide antigravity support in dogs. There are numerous small muscles which lie deep to the deep digital flexor in this area. The extensor carpi radialis muscles insert on the dorsal surface of the base of metacarpals II and III.

There are three phalanges for each of digits II–V, whereas the underdeveloped digit I has no second phalanx (Figure 12.3). The first phalanx is a short cylinder with a concave proximal joint and a distal joint which is sagittally convex, is transversely concave, and extends further on the palmar than the dorsal surface. This arrangement provides for more flexion than extension and limited lateral movement. The second phalanx, similarly cylindrical but shorter, forms a flexion angle of 135° with first phalanx. The four tendons of the superficial digital flexor, which bifurcate from the primary tendon at the proximal third of the metacarpus and are surrounded by a long synovial sheath, insert on their proximal bases. They serve to flex both the metacarpophalangeal

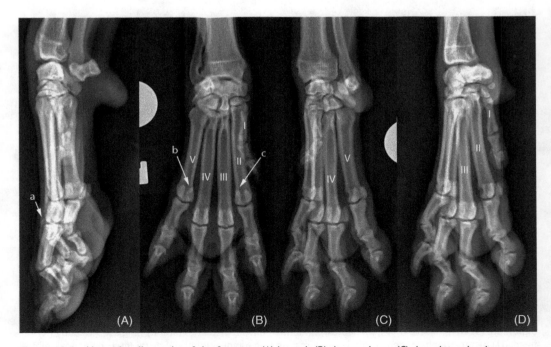

Figure 12.3 Normal radiographs of the forepaw: (A) lateral; (B) dorsopalmar; (C) dorsolateral palmaro-medial oblique (DLPMO); and (D) dorsomedial palmaro-lateral oblique (DMPLO) view: (a) dorsal sesamoid; (b) sesamoid 2; and (c) sesamoid 7 (these are the sesamoids most commonly affected by "sesamoid disease"); metacarpals 1–5 are labeled with roman numerals (I–V).

and proximal interphalangeal joints of digits II–V. The transversely and dorsally oriented base of the third phalanx results in it forming an almost 90° dorsal angle with the second phalanx. On their palmar surfaces, broad, low tubercles receive one of the five branches of the deep digital flexor tendons. The tendon of this muscle first sends a small medial branch to the first phalanx at the level of the proximal metacarpus before splitting into its four main branches. The principle tendon is surrounded by a synovial sheath from the level of the distal radius to proximal metacarpus, and the individual branches are similar enveloped. On the dorsal surface just distal to the joint, the extensor processes of digits II–V receive one of the four tendons of the common digital extensor muscle. Distal to this, the conical, ventrally curved, and tapered ungula process receives the claw (nail). The ungula crest surrounds the process dorsally and laterally.

The proximal interphalangeal joints, formed between the first and second phalanx in digits II–V, are stabilized laterally and medially by stout collateral ligaments. The extensor tendons dorsally and the flexor tendons on the palmar aspect are attached to the joint capsule. The joint capsule of the distal interphalangeal joint is thickened to form collateral ligaments. Each of digits II–V has two dorsal ligaments which extend from the base of the second phalanx to the ungula crest. These passive extensors keep the claws elevated off the ground and counter the tension of the deep digital flexors. The digital flexor tendons are held in place by annular ligaments at each phalanx. In the metacarpophalangeal region, the fascia forms the transverse metacarpal ligament which holds the digits together and anchors the metacarpal footpad.

Five of the six palmar paw pads occur in this region; whereas the sixth, the carpal pad, is located adjacent to the accessory carpal bone (Figure 12.2). Palmar pads include the heart-shaped metacarpal pad as well as four digital pads which lie under the distal interphalangeal joints of digits II–V. The digital pads are anchored in place by fibroelastic strands from the digital fascia. Deep to the dermis and heavily keratinized epidermis, the pad is composed of fat, laced with reticular, collagenous, and elastic fibers, along with a scattering of eccrine sweat glands. This arrangement allows the pads to deform under load yet return to their original shape and size. Pads also provide traction, load transfer, shock absorption, sensory perception, insulation, plus an additional cooling mechanism.

12.2.2 Pelvic Limb

Metatarsals II–V are similar to the corresponding metacarpals although they are longer (Figure 12.4), and their bases are flattened and compressed transversely, resulting in them being more crowded together and having smaller intermetatarsal spaces compared to the thoracic limb. Metatarsal I is significantly reduced in size (Figure 12.4) and sometimes fused to the first tarsal bone (Figure 18.2). Although not always present, the associated phalanx, the dewclaw, is often vestigial and supernumerary in some breeds. Phalanges II–V are very similar to those of the thoracic limb, as are the joints and ligaments.

The superficial digital flexor muscle divides into four branches at the level of the distal row of tarsal bones. These branches insert on the plantar surface of the proximal base of phalanges II–V. The lateral and medial heads of the deep digital flexor muscle converge and at the level of the proximal metatarsus, the common tendon splits into four branches which insert on the plantar flexor tubercles of the third phalanx of digits II–V. The synovial and ligamentous structures of both these muscles are similar to the flexor muscles of the thoracic limb. The tendon of cranial tibial extensor muscle runs obliquely across the tarsus and inserts on the palmer base of metatarsals I and II. The long digital extensor tendon branches into four at the proximal metatarsus; these synovial-sheathed tendons run along the dorsal surfaces to phalanges II–V and receive a single sesamoid at the proximal interphalangeal joint, before inserting on the dorsal surface of the ungula process.

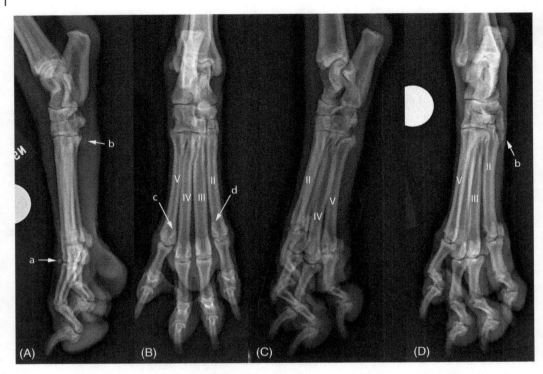

Figure 12.4 Normal radiographs of the hindpaw: (A) lateral; (B) dorsoplantar; and (C) dorsolateral plantaro-medial oblique (DLPMO); and (D) dorsomedial plantaro-lateral oblique (DMPLO) view. (a) Dorsal sesamoid; (b) metatarsal I; (c) sesamoid 2, and (d) sesamoid 7; metatarsals 2–5 are labeled with roman numerals (II–V).

12.2.3 Function, Posture, and Carriage

The metacarpal and digital pads should all touch the contact surface. Additionally, the digits should be slightly splayed, dorsally angled relative to the metacarpals, with digits III and IV elevated above and extending forward relative to digits II and V. The dorsal surface between the distal interphalangeal joint and the nail bed should be slightly concave. The claws (nails) should curve downwards, but if appropriately worn or trimmed, the tips should not touch the contact surface while standing, but rather be suspended slightly above it, ending square as well as caudally beveled. The metacarpophalangeal and metatarsophalangeal joint angles have been measured using three-dimensional videography (Nielsen et al. 2003); however, they are infrequently measured objectively in the clinical setting. With increasing velocity, the digits splay slightly more, the pads expand, and the claws rotate distally into the contact surface. Reported normal range of motion angles for the carpus and tarsus are described in Chapter 5.

12.3 Arthritis

Osteoarthritis of the lower limb region is poorly described. The condition can involve any joint, although the metacarpophalangeal joints IV and V have a higher incidence than those of II and III as well as the metatarsophalangeal joints (Franklin et al. 2009). Individual or multiple joints may be involved. The condition may be secondary to trauma or associated with strain injuries of the collateral ligaments and is sometimes seen with flexor tendon injuries or, as observed by the author, in dogs with excessively long nails and apparent rotary angulation of the digits and their joints. Clinical signs may be absent or mild. However, dogs with visible swelling are more likely to have clinical lameness (Franklin et al. 2009) and affected joints may be painful during the early stages of the disease. In chronic cases, there is thickening of the joint and loss of range of motion. Severe joint thickening may cause cutaneous impingement of the adjacent digit(s), with ensuing abrasion and pain. Radiographic imaging may reveal soft tissue proliferation, osteophytosis and enthesopathy, as well as extensive periosteal reaction, which may give the appearance of a neoplastic process (Franklin 2009). In the author's experience, the condition may also be accompanied (and potentially related) to the clinical syndrome of the hyperextension of multiple digits frequently seen in geriatric dogs (Figure 12.5).

Infective and immune-mediated arthritis are uncommon conditions for this region. The former may occur from bacterial introduction through local wounding or from adjacent infected tissues, or spontaneously through hematogenous bacterial extension (see Section 14.12). Typical signs include acute onset lameness with a warm, swollen, and painful joint (usually single). Immune-mediated arthritis usually involves multiple joints and may be erosive or nonerosive (Chapter 13). Erosive forms show bone erosions, subluxation, or luxation of the joints with periarticular bone proliferation and mineralization of the periarticular soft tissue possible. Joint fluid analysis and culture is required for diagnosis of both conditions.

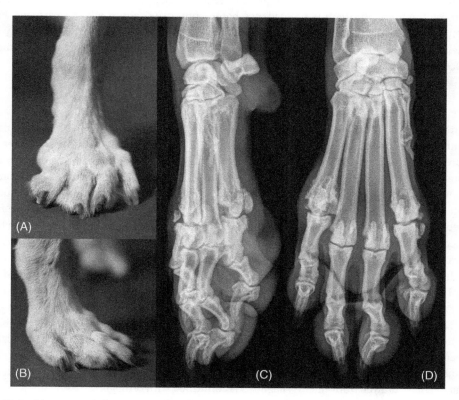

Figure 12.5 Metacarpophalangeal osteoarthritis: (A, B) this dog presented with hyperextension of all digits; (C, D) note the severe degenerative changes of the metacarpophalangeal joints of the second and fourth digits with soft tissue proliferation, osteophytosis, and enthesopathy, as well a periosteal reaction.

12.4 Fractures of the Distal Limb Region

12.4.1 Metacarpal and Metatarsal Fractures

Fractures of these bones usually occur following a traumatic event. In racing Greyhounds, they are considered stress/fatigue fractures and most commonly involve metacarpal II of the right limb and metacarpal V of the left. In these dogs (and possibly other working dogs where the bones are exposed to cyclical injury and have not had enough time to adaptively remodel), bone injury is common and manifests as an ill-defined continuum of periostitis, stress fracture, and finally, complete fracture. In racing Greyhounds, a single bone is most commonly fractured (Boemo 1998). In contrast, traumatic fractures in pets frequently involve multiple bones (Kornmayer et al. 2014).

Clinical signs can range in severity depending on the extent of the force, number of bones affected, degree of injury, and the size of the animal. There is usually some adjacent swelling and there may be associated cutaneous injuries. Palpation will reveal pain, swelling, crepitus, and possibly topographical deformity of the region.

Diagnostic confirmation and fracture details are generally provided through orthogonal radiographs. Lateral views give confusing superimposition of the bones, which may be resolved through oblique projections and/or gentle elevation or depression of an individual bone to assist with orientation. CT can be useful to elucidate comminuted fractures, especially those that involve the joints.

Numerous surgical and nonsurgical treatments (e.g. external coaptation) have been described to treat these fractures but there is no evidence-based consensus as to the best treatment. Factors influencing the choice of treatment include the age and mass of the dog, intended activity of the dog, which bones are fractured, number of bone fractures, site of the fractures, extent of fragment displacement, and concurrent local and distant injuries.

12.4.2 Digit Fractures and Luxations

Digit fractures most commonly occur as a result of trauma and frequently involve only a single digit. The clinical signs and diagnostic approach are similar to those described for metacarpal/metatarsal fractures. Due to the complexity of this region, careful evaluation of radiographs is necessary for the diagnosis of minimally displaced fractures (Figure 12.6). There is also no clear consensus on treatment, with both surgical and nonsurgical treatment described. Most frequently these fractures are managed nonsurgically; however, because of the difficulty in adequately immobilizing the region, delayed unions and exuberant callus are common. Surgical repair of shaft fractures has been recommended in performance dogs, although there are no studies to support this (Eaton-Wells 1998).

Luxations or subluxations can occur at any level but are reportedly more common at the distal interphalangeal joints, especially in athletic dogs (DeCamp et al. 2016). These injuries are due to a strain injury of the associated collateral and/or sesamoid ligaments and usually involve a single joint. Dogs with this injury are often not lame at the walk but may show lameness during faster gaits. There is often no, or minimal pain (luxations of the metacarpophalangeal joints are reported to be more painful than those of the distal joints), swelling, nor crepitation (Blythe et al. 2007). With complete luxation, the phalanx is displaced laterally or medially (Figure 12.6).

Instability is palpated by gently opening the joints laterally or medially and performing a dorso-palmar/plantar "drawer" movement. Diagnosis is confirmed with orthogonal radiographs, but stress radiographs may be necessary to establish the diagnosis. Small avulsion fractures associated with the collateral ligaments are often seen. Ultrasound may be useful to identify ligamentous injuries or concurrent tendon injury, in larger dogs. Although reduction and nonsurgical treatments are frequently successful in the author's experience, surgical treatment is described for athletic dogs (Guilliard 2003).

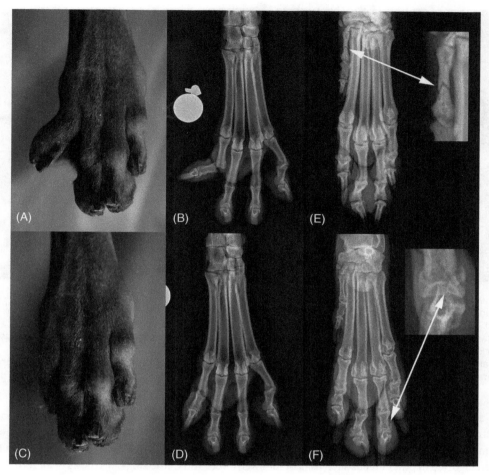

Figure 12.6   Digit luxation and fractures: the dog depicted in images (A–D) presented with acute lameness due to a luxation of the proximal interphalangeal joint of the fifth digit of the pelvic limb; (A, B) the luxation was (C, D) reduced and managed conservatively; (E) mid-diaphyseal fracture of the first phalanx of digit I, and (F) articular fracture of the second phalanx of digit IV illustrate the difficulty of diagnosing minimally displaced digit fractures in dogs.

12.4.3   Sesamoid Disease

Sesamoid disease refers to a group of diseases which include traumatic fractures, sesamoid inflammation (sesamoiditis), degeneration, and fragmentation (Read et al. 1992; Cake and Read 1995; Mathews et al. 2001; Daniel et al. 2008). The pathogenesis is unclear, and it is unknown whether these conditions are manifestations of a single disease or different diseases. The condition generally affects the thoracic limbs; however, it may occasionally occur in the pelvic limb as well. Sesamoids II and VII in Greyhounds and Rottweilers are most commonly affected (Figures 12.3 and 12.7).

Sesamoiditis is reported in Greyhounds as an inflammation of the sesamoid ligaments secondary to a strain injury (Blythe et al. 2007). Traumatic sesamoid fractures of sesamoids II and VII have also been described in racing Greyhounds and other large-breed dogs and are believed to be caused by excessive tension of the digital flexor tendons across the sesamoid bones (Eaton-Wells 1998).

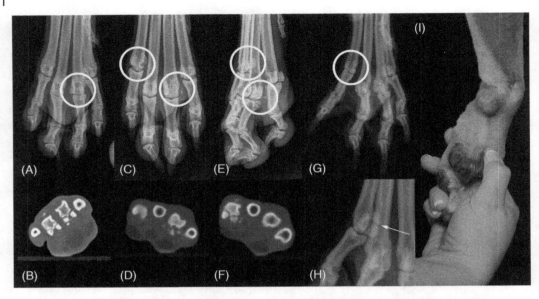

Figure 12.7 Sesamoid disease (white circles are used to outline the affected sesamoid bones in all images): (A) radiograph and (B) CT of traumatic sesamoid fracture of the fourth proximal sesamoid; note that establishing a diagnosis on radiographs is difficult, but fracture is clearly revealed on CT. (C–F) Sesamoid disease of sesamoids 3 and 7; note that radiographs (C, E) permitted to establish the diagnosis in this case, but (D, F) CT was used to determine the extent of the disease. (G, H) Radiographs of bipartite sesamoid (sesamoid 7, white arrow) permitted to establish the diagnosis. (I) Typical location for palpation of thoracic limb sesamoid 7.

Sesamoid fragmentation is a condition mainly occurring in young Rottweilers. It is not associated with trauma or specific athletic pursuits but, like traumatic fractures, usually also involves sesamoids II and VII of either of the thoracic limbs (Read et al. 1992; Mathews et al. 2001). Fragmentation has been reported in other breeds such as Labrador Retrievers and Cattle Dogs (Mathews et al. 2001), and clinical signs may vary greatly. Traumatic fractures are generally associated with an acute, severe lameness; whereas chronic conditions may present with mild or no lameness. Pain on deep, direct palpation and during flexion may be elicited, and local swelling may be palpable. Sesamoids II and VII are easily palpable adjacent to the metacarpal pad, while sesamoids III–VI may be covered by the pad (however, as noted above, these are rarely affected). Over time, a thickening of the area may develop and a reduction of flexion of the adjacent metacarpophalangeal joints may also occur. In normal animals, this joint should be able to flex to at least 90°.

Diagnosis is generally confirmed with dorsopalmar and oblique radiographs (Figure 12.7) but CT can also be used and simplifies the diagnosis. Tape traction and/or separation of the digits with cotton wool may allow better radiographic visualization. Imaging may reveal fragmentation (cluster of ossicles with sharp or rounded margins depending on chronicity) of the affected sesamoids. Enthesophytosis, soft tissue swelling, or calcification (Cake and Read 1995) and other secondary arthritic changes may also be observed. Since radiographic evidence of sesamoid disease can be an incidental finding (Vaughan and France 1986), it is imperative to rule out other causes of thoracic limb lameness. Further complicating the diagnosis is the fact that bipartite or multipartite sesamoids, a congenital abnormality where the sesamoid presents as multiple instead of a single bony structure, may be present. These are minimally displaced, usually have rounded margins, and are not accompanied by soft tissue swelling. Scintigraphy or CT can be used to differentiate this condition from pathological conditions of the sesamoids. Local analgesic blocks may also be used to evaluate whether sesamoid pathology contributes to a lameness. There is no consensus on treatment; however, sesamoidectomy (removal of the affected sesamoid) is possible in cases that are refractory to nonsurgical treatment (Mathews et al. 2001).

12.5 Conditions of Muscles, Tendon, and Ligaments

Numerous major muscles that insert in this region have their origins and muscle bellies well proximal on the limb. This allows for the muscle mass to be centralized towards the trunk rather than add to the distal "pendulum" weight and inertia of the limb. This means that many of these muscles cross multiple joints, which makes them more vulnerable to injury compared to those that only cross a single joint. Any of these muscles may be injured and probably are. The manifestation of these injuries might be obvious, for example an abnormally elevated digit (i.e. injury of the digital flexor muscles). Many, however, are insidious, as the impact of their injury may be muted by muscles with similar function taking over their roles. These injuries may be detectable but require familiarity with the regional anatomy upon a meticulous clinical examination. Treatment of these conditions may involve surgical (such as apposition of the injured structures) and nonsurgical (external coaptation, rest, and pain management) strategies.

12.5.1 Dorsal Digital Ligament Sprain

Dorsal digital ligament sprains occur when the distal phalanx is forcefully and excessively flexed and has been described in active Greyhounds (Blythe et al. 2007). It may be associated with injury of the adjacent digital extensor tendon. Animals might be slightly lame and on inspection of the affected paw, the dorsal (cutaneous) concavity between the proximal interphalangeal joint and claw is lost. This is caused by swelling of the area, which is accompanied by pain on palpation. Radiographs to investigate any concurrent fractures, for example avulsion fractures, and ultrasonographic examination are warranted to confirm the ligamentous injury.

12.5.2 Digital Flexor Muscle and Tendon Injuries

12.5.2.1 Superficial Digital Flexor Muscle

The superficial digital flexor muscle may be damaged through overexertion (causing overstretching or strain injury), or through external trauma, including contusion and laceration. The damage may occur in both the muscle or in the long tendon and its synovial sheath. The entire paw may be involved if the muscle is torn and elongates or if the main tendon or multiple branches are ruptured, for example following a deep laceration to the palmar/plantar aspect of the paw (usually in the region of the metacarpal or metatarsal footpad). Animals may or may not be lame, depending on the extent and chronicity of the condition. The clinical appearance is of one or more digits that appear to lie parallel to the contact surface (Figure 12.8); the proximal interphalangeal joint loses its normally flexed angle, referred to as "dropped toe" in dog racing circles. If the deep digital flexor tendon is intact, the claw elevates and points forward (but is not cocked dorsally, see Section 12.5.2.2).

Clinical diagnosis involves palpating for pain and swelling along the entire length of the affected muscle, since the injury may not be located at the site of obvious abnormality (i.e. the "dropped toe"). The affected digit(s) may be extended to a greater degree than their unaffected

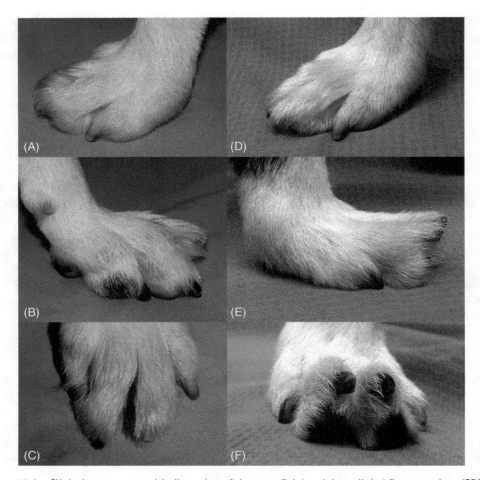

Figure 12.8 Clinical appearance with disruption of the superficial and deep digital flexor tendons (SDF/DDF) in two patients. *Patient I* (A–C): (A) normal leg for comparison; (B, C) disruption of the SDF only of the fourth digit; note the loss of the flexed angle of the proximal interphalangeal joint and that the digit appears to lie parallel to the contact surface (i.e. the claw is elevated and approximately parallel to the ground). *Patient II* (D–F): (D) normal leg for comparison; (E, F) disruption of the SDF and DDF of the third and fourth digit; note that compared to *Patient I* (B, C) the claw is elevated beyond parallel due to the complete loss of the flexor mechanism.

opposite number; however, resistance from the deep digital flexor is still palpable (i.e. inability to elevate the toe dorsally completely). The muscle of the opposite limb should be similarly palpated for comparison and to detect similar disease. Bear in mind that this muscle crosses multiple joints, so that stretching of the muscle (i.e. elbow, carpal, and digit extension) may result in a more pronounced pain response (Chapter 5), particularly if the level of injury is proximal. Establishing a diagnosis generally involves palpation, and confirmation can be accomplished by ultrasonographic examination of the muscle and tendons if the tendons are accessible. This may confirm the diagnosis and can be helpful to describe the extent of the disease, potentially directing treatment strategies. Radiographs are used to detect associated bony changes like avulsions, enthesiophytes, or dystrophic mineralization in chronically damaged tissues. Magnetic resonance imaging, although seldom used for this condition, may provide more detailed information.

12.5.2.2 Deep Digital Flexor Muscle

Mechanisms of injury are similar to those of the superficial tendon. Both muscles and/or their tendons may be affected concurrently. The deep digital flexor tendon is more commonly lacerated than the superficial tendon, as it lies superficial to the latter, and so is more vulnerable to injury. The clinical appearance is of the claw of one or more digits being elevated off the contact surface, colloquially referred to as "kicked up" or "knocked up" toe. If there is concurrent superficial flexor muscle injury, the digit becomes flattened as described above, but the claw is cocked dorsally. Clinical assessment and diagnostic options are similar for those of the superficial digital muscle.

12.5.2.3 Flexor Tendon Strain: *Bowed Tendon*

A condition termed "bowed tendon" has been described in racing Greyhounds (Blythe et al. 2007). This is a strain injury of one or more of the tendons of mainly the superficial and occasionally deep digital flexors of the thoracic limbs. The condition manifests clinically as a swelling on the palmar surface of the foot extending from the level of the accessory carpal bone to the level of the metacarpal footpad. Palpation of the affected tendon evokes pain and the tendon may feel thickened and more prominent than the adjacent, unaffected tendons.

12.6 Conditions of the Digital and Paw Pads

12.6.1 Trauma

Laceration of the metacarpal pad has been ascribed to be the most common traumatic injury in working dogs and pets. In one study, concurrent injuries were uncommon, and the prognosis remained favorable even for full-thickness injuries, regardless of treatment (Hansen et al. 2015). Diagnosis can generally be established by careful visual inspection and palpation. Concurrent damage to underlying structures, such as the flexor tendons, needs to be investigated; this can be accomplished by blunt probing through the laceration while extending the toes or through use of ultrasound. Radiographs may be required to detect radiopaque foreign bodies and to investigate the underlying osseous structures for osteomyelitis.

Aside from laceration, other traumatic injuries to the digital and paw pads include foreign bodies, blistering from hot surfaces, chemical damage (e.g. walking through wet cement or undiluted surface disinfectants), maceration when pads remain wet for extended periods, abrasions, and ulcerations. Specifically, ulcerations (Figure 12.9F) often occur when dogs are exposed to hard surfaces that they are not conditioned to, or through overuse in runs with cement floors such as found in communities of highly active and driven dogs (e.g. police and military work dogs). In such cases, the keratinized epidermis is worn away, leaving the sensitive dermis exposed ("hot spots") and can cause dogs to show a more pronounced lameness when walking on paved surfaces. Therefore, establishing a diagnosis may require walking affected animals on soft surfaces or donning paw covers to determine if the lameness disappears.

12.6.2 Corns

Corns are well-circumscribed hyperkeratotic lesions with a central, often conical core of keratin. The validity of the term "corn" has been questioned since in people, corns are generally non-painful. Other terminology suggested includes "wart-like lesion" or "Porokeratosis plantaris discreta" (Balara et al. 2009). The lesions appear as white, flat, and circular thickened areas

DISTAL LIMB REGION

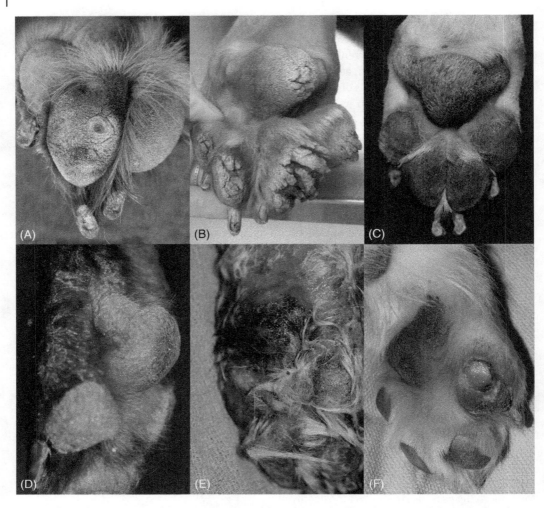

Figure 12.9 Pad conditions: (A) corns; (B) paw pad hyperkeratosis; (C) pad overgrowth from abnormal weight-bearing; (D) pemphigus foliaceus; (E) superficial necrolytic dermatitis; and (F) digital pad ulceration.

on the pads (Figure 12.9A). Sight hounds, especially Greyhounds, are prone to developing these lesions, perhaps because of the anatomical differences of these dogs compared to other breeds (i.e. long narrow feet with little distance separating the digital pads). The lesions may be incidental findings or may be painful and cause lameness. They occur most often (90%) on the digital pads of digits 3 and 4 of the thoracic limbs but can appear on the metacarpal and metatarsal pads as well (Guilliard et al. 2010). Their etiology is not known but hypothesized to be caused by scar tissue related to trauma or foreign bodies, or hypertrophy of the eccrine sweat glands due to pressure (Balara et al. 2009). Controversy exists as to whether they may be a result of a papilloma virus infection (Balara et al. 2009; Anis et al. 2016).

Clinical signs of corns frequently include lameness when walking on hard surfaces and excessively long nails due to the animal shifting its weight proximally onto its metacarpal/metatarsal pads to mitigate discomfort. Radiographs are used to rule out radiopaque foreign bodies. The diagnosis is made by visual inspection and pain response during palpation, however, confirmation requires biopsy and histopathology. Treatment is controversial. Nonsurgical treatment, digital ostectomy, and surgical excision have been reported; notably, surgical excision may be curative in some breeds, but recurrence is greater than 50% in Greyhounds (Guilliard 2003; Balara et al. 2009).

12.6.3 Abnormal Wear and Migration

Although not a primary cause of lameness, some conditions associated with abnormal weight-bearing on the paw (e.g. angular limb deformities, muscle and ligamentous conditions described above, and joint conditions that limit limb mobility) may cause eccentric loading or abrasion of the pads through abnormal motion, such as rotary movements. This may manifest as abnormal pad wear, ulceration, and/or migration. Pads that do not bear weight may also appear overgrown (Figure 12.9) or hyperkeratotic. The pads may then become secondary sources of pain and lameness. The attending clinician needs to distinguish between a primary paw problem and a paw manifestation of a distant condition of that limb.

12.6.4 Dermatologic Conditions Causing Lameness

Many dermatologic conditions can be associated with lameness or altered ambulation if they affect the distal limb region (Figure 12.10). A few select conditions are presented below; the reader is encouraged to refer to comprehensive texts for more detailed information (Duclos 2013; Outerbridge 2013).

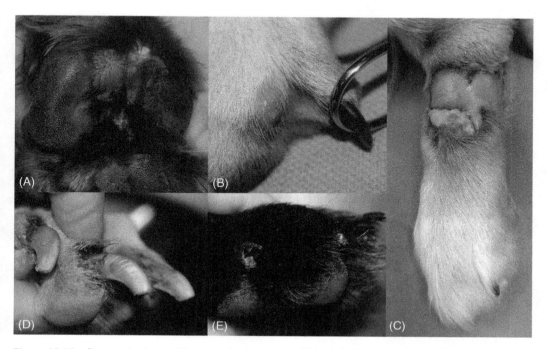

Figure 12.10   Dermatologic conditions causing lameness: (A) interdigital dermatitis (pododermatitis); (B) foreign body with draining sinus; (C) acral lick dermatitis; (D) paronychia; and (E) symmetrical lupoid onychodystrophy/onychitis.

12.6.4.1 Pemphigus Foliaceus

Pemphigus foliaceus is one of the most commonly reported immune-mediated dermatoses in dogs and is known to affect multiple sites, but in rare cases the footpad may be the only site affected. When it occurs on the footpads, it may cause lameness, because of changes to the pad that include thickening due to swelling and hyperkeratosis with scaling, crusting, hardening, and fissuring (Mueller et al. 2006). Severe cases may exhibit purulent exudate from beneath hyperkeratotic foot-pad crusts. Cytology of purulent exudate may demonstrate acantholytic keratinocytes. Diagnosis is generally confirmed by histopathology.

12.6.4.2 Superficial Necrolytic Dermatitis

Superficial necrolytic dermatitis, also called "necrolytic migratory erythema" and "metabolic epidermal necrosis," is an uncommon skin disorder associated with a systemic disease. Although most commonly ascribed to a hepatic disease (hepatocutaneous syndrome), it is also associated with pancreatic glucagonoma, phenobarbital use, and intestinal conditions. Hypoaminoacidemia appears to be the common pathophysiological pathway. Shetland Sheepdogs, West Highland White Terriers, Cocker Spaniels, and Scottish Terriers may be predisposed. Older animals are most commonly affected. Lameness and licking of the footpads are often the first signs of the condition. Typically affecting all the feet, superficial necrolytic dermatitis may also cause the pads to become hyperkeratotic, crusted, and fissured with secondary bacterial infections. Occasionally the skin of the muzzle, perineum, elbows, or hocks is also affected. Diagnosis is confirmed with skin biopsy. Elevated liver chemistry values and ultrasound confirming hepatopathy when accompanied by pad and skin lesion are highly suggestive of the syndrome (Outerbridge 2013).

12.6.4.3 Paw Pad Hyperkeratosis

Hyperkeratosis of the footpads is familial in Irish Setters, Kerry Blue Terriers, Dogue de Bourdeaux, and Golden Retrievers, but may also be associated with canine distemper virus (Duclos 2013). The condition affects all pads and generally presents in 4- to 6-month-old puppies. It is characterized by a defect of keratinization, causing excessive keratin of the paw pads (Figure 12.9B). The paw pad keratin presents as hard vegetative, feathered, and fissured projections of horny tissue. Some affected individuals may be very lame. A tentative diagnosis can be made based on the signalment and clinical appearance, but confirmation requires histopathology. An idiopathic nasodigital form which also involves the nasal planum is described in Labrador Retrievers.

12.6.4.4 Zinc-responsive Dermatoses

Zinc-responsive dermatosis is a systemic keratosis that may result in thickening, scaling, and crusting of the pads in approximately one-third of affected dogs (White et al. 2001). Similar changes are seen on other areas of skin, particularly the facial skin. The condition is described in genetically predisposed breeds such as Siberian Huskies and Alaskan Malamutes, as well as in rapid growing large- and giant-breed puppies fed zinc (Zn)-deficient diets. The disease may require biopsies to confirm the diagnosis (Outerbridge 2013). In genetically predisposed animals, supplementation with elemental Zn is often curative. In the dietary deficient cases, correcting the diet is curative.

12.7 Conditions of the Digit/Paw Skin

12.7.1 Interdigital Web Injuries

Interdigital web injuries have been most clearly described in racing Greyhounds (Blythe et al. 2007) but can occur in any breed of dog. Injuries include laceration, stabs, foreign body penetrations, and splits between adjacent digits. Such injuries often heal slowly and are vulnerable to reinjury because the healed tissue lacks the pliability and durability of the uninjured tissue. Unattended lesions that produce excessive granulation tissue leading to large fibrous scars and exaggerated cicatricial contraction may deform the interdigital skin, making it less distensible and interfere with individual digit movement. This interdigital deformation may itself result in lameness. Radiographs and ultrasound might be helpful to detect underlying bone involvement and to locate foreign bodies.

12.7.2 Pododermatitis

Pododermatitis (Figure 12.10a) is a nonspecific term to describe several inflammatory conditions that affect the skin of the paws (Breathnach et al. 2008; Duclos 2013). There are multiple causes for the condition: allergic dermatitis, foreign bodies, mechanical or chemical trauma, fungal and parasitic infections, in addition to psychogenic or idiopathic sterile pyogranulomas. Bacterial infection is usually secondary. Tissues that may be affected include the interdigital skin, paw pads, nails, and nail folds. Clinical signs include pruritus, edema, swelling, erythema, alopecia, paronychia, detaching or detached claws, and serous, hemorrhagic, or purulent discharge. A single, or multiple, digits or feet may be affected, and the degree of lameness varies.

12.7.3 Acral Lick Dermatitis

Acral lick dermatitis (or acral lick furunculosis/granuloma) is a condition characterized by excessive licking of the distal limb region of the front limbs, although the pelvic limbs may be affected occasionally (Shumaker 2019). The condition has multiple causes and may be precipitated by allergies, behavioral, or underlying orthopedic conditions that cause pruritus or pain. Occasionally a tumor, foreign body (Figure 12.10b), injury, or opportunistic fungal infection may be the inciting cause. The condition is often associated with a deep staphylococcal and/or mixed bacterial infection, either primarily, or through secondary invasion. The Doberman Pinscher, German Shepherd Dog, Golden and Labrador Retrievers, Great Dane, Weimaraner, and Irish setters are reported to be predisposed. Incessant licking produces lesions which appear as firm, raised, erythematous, and erosive plaques initially. With chronicity, these become more extensive, thickened, hairless, hyperpigmented, and ulcerated with scattered furuncles which erode and weep exudate. Diagnosis is generally confirmed by clinical appearance (Figure 12.10c). Radiography is indicated to identify underlying bone reaction and involvement, as well as to establish an underlying cause for the licking (e.g. joint disease). Tissue culture is recommended in severe cases for assessment and treatment of deep bacterial, or rarely, fungal infection. Treatment is aimed at identifying the underlying disease, treating the primary disease (if possible) as well as the secondary infection (if present), and stopping the licking behavior (Shumaker 2019).

12.8 Conditions of the Claws

Conditions of the claws are easily overlooked and often subtle, but they can be the primary cause of lameness (Mueller 1999). Excessively long claws may predispose animals to claw, digital, and musculotendinous injury as well as pododermatitis, all of which may lead to lameness. In addition, abnormal nail wear may indicate other conditions causing a lameness. For example, causes of excessively short nails due to abnormal wear include neurological conditions causing loss of conscious proprioception, conditions which cause abnormal foot carriage (e.g. dorsal curvature of the radius due to premature closure of the distal ulna growth plate), and conditions which cause the animal to "drag" its feet during the swing phase (e.g. severe bilateral, painful osteoarthritis of the stifles). Excessively long nails may be due to reduced wear, for example after injury to the digital flexor tendons resulting in diminished downward rotation of the digit.

12.8.1 Trauma

Trauma (such as traumatic split, cracked, bruised, and avulsed claws) is a frequent cause of claw injury and associated lameness. It usually affects a single, or only a small number of claws. To establish a diagnosis, the claw should be carefully observed for integrity and color abnormalities, palpated for pain, and pulled away from the nail bed to determine the firmness of its attachment.

12.8.2 Paronychia

Paronychia describes a nonspecific inflammation of the claw fold (Mueller 1999) whereby the nail bed becomes swollen, red, and painful, with possible purulent discharge (Figure 12.10d). The area is usually very sensitive to palpation. There are numerous causes for this condition; trauma is considered the most common primary cause, while bacterial infections are usually secondary. An allergic or immune-mediated cause is also common. In addition to the examination, skin scrapings for Demodex, exudate cytology, bacterial and fungal culture, and fine-needle aspirates (FNAs) may be indicated. Radiographs of the affected digit are useful to identify any underlying bone involvement. Paronychia may lead to deformity and accelerated growth of the claw.

12.8.3 Deformed Claws

Deformed claws usually indicate previous, unappreciated physical injury to, infection, or immune insult of the nail bed. They may also cause lameness via various mechanisms. For example, although claws may not be painful themselves, they may impinge on adjacent skin causing abrasion and pain. Accelerated growth of the claw may lead to ingrown claws, where the apex curves back and impinges on the adjacent digital footpad or skin.

12.8.4 Symmetrical Lupoid Onychodystrophy

Symmetrical lupoid onychodystrophy/onychitis, also called symmetrical onychomadesis (Ziener and Nødtvedt 2014), is a claw-specific disease of mainly young to middle-aged dogs. Gordon Setters and German Shepherd Dogs appear to be predisposed. The usual presentation is licking of the paws, lameness, and sloughing of the affected claw(s). Inspection of the claw reveals paronychia and separation or sloughing of the claw. Claws may be dry, roughened, short, and misshapen as they regrow (Figure 12.10E). The condition usually progresses until all claws are affected. A purulent discharge may be present due to secondary bacterial infection. Diagnosis is based on signalment, clinical appearance, and the absence of clinical manifestation elsewhere. Diagnosis can be confirmed histopathologically. Treatment is difficult but involves removal of damaged claw plates, treatment of secondary infections, as well as pharmacologic therapy to allow for regrowth of normal claws (Ziener and Nødtvedt 2014).

12.9 Other Conditions Affecting the Distal Limb Region

12.9.1 Neurological Conditions

Neurological conditions causing lameness and proprioceptive deficits (Chapters 16 and 21) may cause abnormal claw (Figure 4.4) and footpad wear or result in abrasive damage to the dorsal aspect of the digital skin. Neurological conditions may also manifest in hyper- or paresthesia, with resultant foot mutilation, poor or nonhealing wounds, and profound atrophy of the soft tissues including muscles and tendons, with resultant osteopenia of the underlying bones of the affected region. It is important that the attending clinician performs a careful neurological examination to identify such conditions.

12.9.2 Dysostoses

Dysostoses are constitutional bone diseases characterized by abnormal development of individual bones, or parts of bones. Examples of dysostoses include hemimelia (the congenital absence of a part or all of one or more bones), dimelia (the duplication of the whole or part of limb), ectrodactyly (congenital split formation or separation between metacarpal bones, also called "split-hand deformity"), polydactyly (the occurrence of one or more extra digits), and syndactyly (the partial or complete lack of separation between adjacent digits). Each of these conditions can cause lameness. Diagnosis is made through clinical examination and confirmed with radiographs. Treatment of these conditions depends on the severity of the disease and the clinical symptoms and may include surgical correction (Towle-Millard and Breur 2018).

12.9.3 Hypertrophic Osteopathy

Hypertrophic osteopathy, also called Marie's disease or hypertrophic pulmonary osteoarthropathy, is characterized by the proliferation of periosteal new bone of especially the distal extremities (Figure 12.11). These distinct osseous changes are generally bilaterally symmetrical and involve all four limbs. They occur secondary to a separate disease process within the thorax or

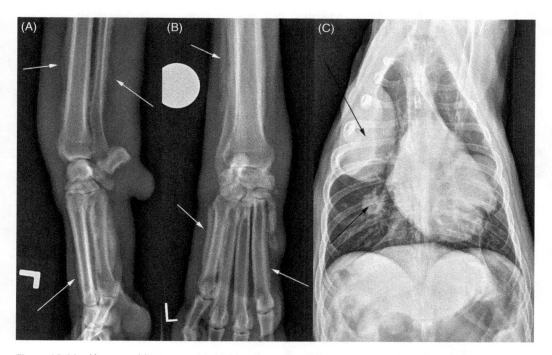

Figure 12.11 Hypertrophic osteopathy: (A, B) radiographs of the thoracic limb show smooth and irregular palisading periosteal reaction along the cortices of the long bones (white arrows) with associated soft tissue swelling; (C) chest radiographs reveal an extrapleural thoracic wall mass (black arrow) and pulmonary nodules. The dog had previously received a thoracic limb amputation for treatment of appendicular osteosarcoma.

abdomen. The pathophysiology is still unknown; however, it may be due to a neurally or growth factor-mediated increase in peripheral blood flow. Hypertrophic osteopathy is typically a paraneoplastic condition, secondary to pulmonary neoplasia (Withers et al. 2015). However, various other conditions have been described as causes for hypertrophic osteopathy including extrapulmonary causes, such as esophageal granuloma formation secondary to *Spirocerca lupi*, right–left shunting, esophageal foreign bodies, and various abdominal neoplasia. The bony proliferation is associated with pain during early stages of the disease, such that this together with the thickening of the tissues, frequently causes lameness or difficulty ambulating. Other clinical signs may include coughing, hyperthermia, weight loss, and depression. These signs often precede signs associated with the primary disease. In a recent retrospective study, more than half of the dogs with hypertrophic osteopathy displayed bilateral ocular discharge (Withers et al. 2015).

Diagnostic investigation should include thoracic and abdominal radiographs in addition to ultrasound for identification of the primary cause. Radiographs of affected limbs show periosteal bone formation in a circumferential and columnar ("palisade-like") appearance. Initially, new bone formation will be absent or minimal. Treatment requires management of the primary condition. The osseous lesions resolve spontaneous if successful treatment of the primary disease can be accomplished.

12.9.4 Metabolic Bone Diseases

Metabolic bone diseases are rare conditions which affect calcium, phosphorus, and vitamin D metabolism. These can occur as a result of inappropriate nutrition, including deficiencies in calcium and/or phosphorous, hypo- or hypervitaminosis A and D, and hypovitaminosis E. They may also involve abnormal metabolism or production of these mineral and vitamins, such as primary and secondary (renal) hyperparathyroidism, chronic renal failure, and intestinal malabsorption conditions. These diseases tend to result in generalized bone conditions that may result in lameness, such as osteopenia, osteomalacia, pathological (spontaneous) fractures, fragile ("brittle") bones, deformed limbs, and excessive new bone production.

12.9.5 Distal Limb Region Neoplasia

Digit neoplasia is the most common tumor encountered in the distal limb region. Digital squamous cell carcinomas frequently cause bone lysis, whereas melanoma does not. Further details about digit tumors and other neoplastic conditions affecting the region are described in Chapter 11.

References

Anis, E.A., Frank, L.A., Francisco, R., and Kania, S.A. (2016). Identification of canine papillomavirus by PCR in Greyhound dogs. *Peer J* 4: e2744.

Balara, J.M., Mccarthy, R.J., Kiupel, M. et al. (2009). Clinical, histologic, and immunohistochemical characterization of wart-like lesions on the paw pads of dogs: 24 cases (2000–2007). *J Am Vet Med Assoc* 234 (12): 1555–1558.

Boemo, C.M. (1998). Injuries of the metacarpus and metatarsus. In: *Canine Sports Medicine and Surgery* (eds. M.S. Bloomberg, J.F. Dee and R.A. Taylor), 150–165. Philadelphia: Saunders.

Blythe, L.L., Gannon, J.R., Craig, A.M. and Fegan, D.F., 2007. "Break-in" or "schooling". In: *Care of the Racing and Retired Greyhound*, 1, 231–278. Abilene, KS: American Greyhound Council.

Breathnach, R.M., Fanning, S., Mulcahy, G. et al. (2008). Canine pododermatitis and idiopathic disease. *Vet J* 176 (2): 146–157.

Cake, M. and Read, R. (1995). Canine and human sesamoid disease. A review of conditions affecting the palmar metacarpal/metatarsal sesamoid bones. *Vet Comp Orthop Traumatol* 8 (2): 70–75.

Daniel, A., Read, R.A., and Cake, M.A. (2008). Vascular foramina of the metacarpophalangeal sesamoid bones of Greyhounds and their relationship to sesamoid disease. *Am J Vet Res* 69 (6): 716–721.

DeCamp, C.E., Johnston, S.A., Déjardin, L.M., and Schaefer, S.L. (2016). Fractures and other orthopedic conditions of the carpus, metacarpus, and phalanges. In: *Brinker, Piermattei, and Flo's Handbook of Small Animal Orthopedics and Fracture Repair*, 5e (eds. C.E. DeCamp, S.A. Johnston, L.M. Déjardin and S.L. Schaefer), 389–433. St. Louis: Elsevier.

Duclos, D. (2013). Canine pododermatitis. *Vet Clin North Am Small Anim Pract* 43 (1): 57–87.

Eaton-Wells, R. (1998). Injuries of the digits and pads. In: *Canine Sports Medicine and Surgery* (eds. M.S. Bloomberg, J.F. Dee and R.A. Taylor), 165–173. Philadelphia: Saunders.

Franklin, S.P., Park, R.D., and Egger, E.L. (2009). Metacarpophalangeal and metatarsophalangeal osteoarthritis in 49 dogs. *J Am Anim Hosp Assoc* 45 (3): 112–117.

Guilliard, M.J. (2003). Proximal interphalangeal joint instability in the dog. *J Small Anim Pract* 44 (9): 399–403.

Guilliard, M.J., Segboer, I., and Shearer, D.H. (2010). Corns in dogs; signalment, possible aetiology and response to surgical treatment. *J Small Anim Pract* 51 (3): 162–168.

Hansen, L.A., Hazenfield, K.M., Olea-Popelka, F., and Smeak, D.D. (2015). Distribution, complications, and outcome of footpad injuries in pet and military working dogs. *J Am Anim Hosp Assoc* 51 (4): 222–230.

Kornmayer, M., Failing, K., and Matis, U. (2014). Long-term prognosis of metacarpal and metatarsal fractures in dogs. A retrospective analysis of medical histories in 100 re-evaluated patients. *Vet Comp Orthop Traumatol* 27 (1): 45–53.

Mathews, K.G., Koblik, P.D., Whitehair, J.G. et al. (2001). Fragmented palmar metacarpophalangeal sesamoids in dogs: a long-term evaluation. *Vet Comp Orthop Traumatol* 14 (1): 7–14.

Mueller, R.S. (1999). Diagnosis and management of canine claw diseases. *Vet Clin North Am Small Anim Pract* 29 (6): 1357–1371.

Mueller, R.S., Krebs, I., Power, H.T., and Fieseler, K.V. (2006). Pemphigus foliaceus in 91 dogs. *J Am Anim Hosp Assoc* 42 (3): 189–196.

Nielsen, C., Stover, S.M., Schulz, K.S. et al. (2003). Two-dimensional link-segment model of the thoracic limb of dogs at a walk. *Am J Vet Res* 64 (5): 609–617.

Outerbridge, C.A. (2013). Cutaneous manifestations of internal diseases. *Vet Clin North Am Small Anim Pract* 43 (1): 135–152.

Read, R.A., Black, A.P., Armstrong, S.J. et al. (1992). Incidence and clinical significance of sesamoid disease in Rottweilers. *Vet Rec* 130 (24): 533–535.

Shumaker, A.K. (2019). Diagnosis and treatment of canine acral lick dermatitis. *Vet Clin North Am Small Anim Pract* 49 (1): 105–123.

Towle Millard, H.A. and Breur, G.J. (2018). Miscellaneous orthopedic conditions. In: *Veterinary Surgery: Small Animal*, 2e (eds. S.A. Johnston and K.M. Tobias), 1299–1315. St. Louis: Elsevier.

Vaughan, L.C. and France, C. (1986). Abnormalities of the volar and plantar sesamoid bones in Rottweilers. *J Small Anim Pract* 27 (9): 551–558.

White, S.D., Bourdeau, P., Rosychuk, R.A. et al. (2001). Zinc-responsive dermatosis in dogs: 41 cases and literature review. *Vet Dermatol* 12 (2): 101–109.

Withers, S.S., Johnson, E.G., Culp, W.T.N. et al. (2015). Paraneoplastic hypertrophic osteopathy in 30 dogs. *Vet Comp Oncol* 13 (3): 157–165.

Ziener, M.L. and Nødtvedt, A. (2014). A treatment study of canine symmetrical onychomadesis (symmetrical lupoid onychodystrophy) comparing fish oil and cyclosporine supplementation in addition. *Acta Vet Scand* 56 (1): 66.

Part IV

Thoracic Limb Lameness

13

Carpal Region

Denis J. Marcellin-Little[1] and Dirsko J.F. von Pfeil[2,3]

[1] Department of Veterinary Surgical and Radiological Sciences, School of Veterinary Medicine, University of California, Davis, CA, USA
[2] Small Animal Surgery Locum PLLC, Dallas, TX, USA
[3] Sirius Veterinary Orthopedic Center, Omaha, NE, USA

13.1   Introduction and Common Differential Diagnoses

The carpus connects the antebrachium to the manus. Overall in dogs, carpal region pathology is less common than elbow or shoulder pathology. The carpus is prone to instability, particularly excessive extension secondary to damage to the palmar ligaments. The carpus is also a common site of inflammation (e.g. immune-mediated polyarthritis [IMPA]). Carpal osteoarthritis is common and may occur as primary osteoarthritis (i.e. without an underlying disease) or secondary osteoarthritis (e.g. secondary to carpal hyperextension or other primary conditions). The identification of carpal problems most commonly relies on palpation, radiographs, and computed tomography (CT); MRI and ultrasound are helpful if soft tissue pathology is suspected. Figure 13.1 and Table 13.1 outline common differential diagnoses and diagnostic steps for this region.

13.2   Normal Anatomy and Osteoarthritis

The carpus is a complex joint that allows motion at three levels: antebrachiocarpal, middle carpal, and carpometacarpal (Figure 13.2). The carpus includes 14 bones: the distal aspect of the radius and ulna, proximal carpal row (intermedioradial carpal bone, ulnar carpal bone, and accessory carpal bone), distal carpal row (first, second, third, and fourth carpal bones), and the proximal aspect of the five metacarpal bones. The intermedioradial carpal bone (frequently referred to as radial carpal bone) is the largest of the carpal bones. The carpus functions mostly in flexion and extension, with approximately 170° of sagittal plane motion. The carpus is the only limb joint that functions past a straight line (i.e. 180°). All other joints extend to approximately 165° and stop short of a straight line. By comparison, the carpus extends 15–20° past a straight line to almost 200° (Jaegger et al. 2002). Extension is limited by the palmar fibrocartilage, by the radiocarpal and ulnocarpal ligaments, and, to a lesser extent, by the medial and the lateral collateral ligaments (Slocum and Devine 1982; Milgram et al. 2012). Approximately 70% of carpal motion occurs at the antebrachiocarpal joint level, 25% at the middle carpal joint level, and 5% at the carpometacarpal joint level (Yalden 1970).

Table 13.1 Key features for selected diseases affecting the carpal region.

Disease	Common signalment	Diagnostic test of choice	Exam findings	Treatment	Clinical pearls	Terminology
Hyperextension injury	All breeds	Stress radiographs	Increased carpal extension	Mild injuries are protected with a brace or splint. Arthrodesis for severe injuries	Conservative management most often fails	
Carpal bone fractures	Racing and sporting dogs	Computed tomography	Swelling and loss of carpal flexion	Bone screws placed with precision	Use intraoperative fluoroscopy to enhance precision of screw placement	
Distal R/U fractures	Toy-breed dogs	Radiographs	Swelling, pain, and obvious instability	Surgical Fixation	Frequently happen without substantial trauma	
Antebrachial deformities	Chondrodystrophic dogs and physeal injuries	Palpation, radiography, and computed tomography	Varus or valgus, length deficit, and elbow joint subluxation	External fixation or bone plate	Deformities should be treated promptly, before the onset of joint subluxation	Valgus = lateral deviation Varus = medial deviation
Lack or loss of carpal extension	Large-breed growing dogs	Gait observation and goniometry	Lack of extension	Conservative, coaptation, and exercise	Optimize growth in growing dogs by decreasing food intake	Flexural deformity and carpal laxity syndrome
Immune-mediated polyarthritis	Large-breed (nonerosive) and small-breed (erosive)	Radiographs and arthrocentesis	Effusion, pain, and hyperextension	Immunosuppressive drugs and pancarpal arthrodesis	Severe carpal effusion suggests polyarthritis Instability suggests that polyarthritis is erosive	
Hypertrophic osteodystrophy (HOD)	Large-breed puppies	Clinical signs and radiographs	Metaphyseal pain and swelling and hyperthermia	Supportive care	Most patients will recover Antebrachial deformities can occur as a consequence of HOD	

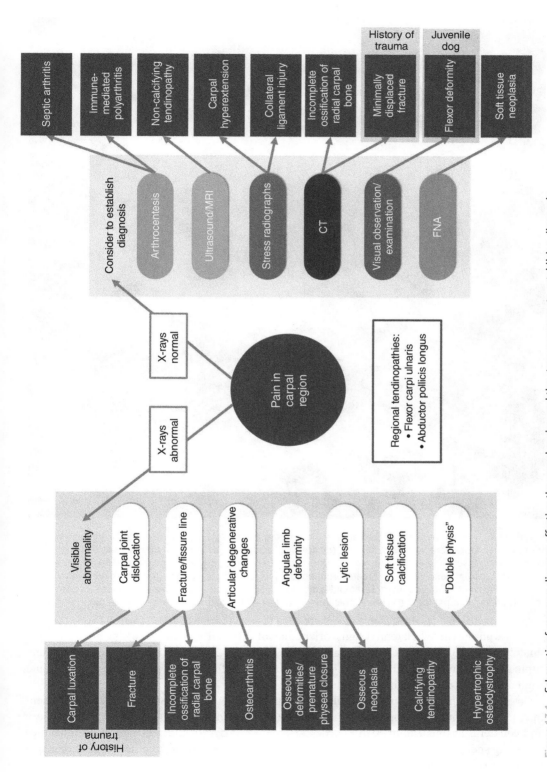

Figure 13.1 Schematic of common diseases affecting the carpal region and the steps necessary to establish a diagnosis.

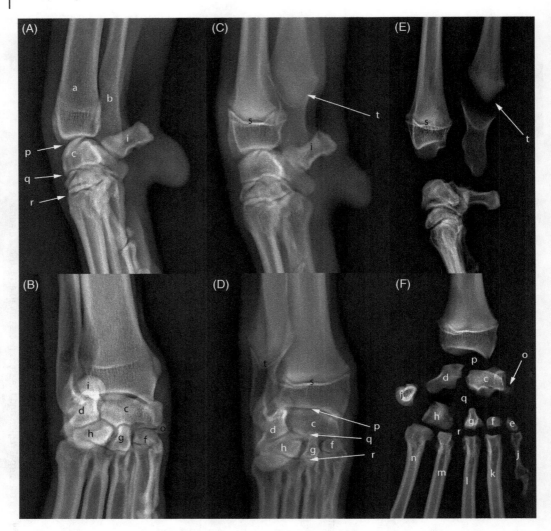

Figure 13.2 Normal anatomy of the carpal joint depicted by radiographs of (A, B) an adult dog and of (C–F) an immature dog: (a) radius; (b) ulna; (c) intermedioradial carpal bone; (d) ulnar carpal bone; (e) first carpal bone; (f) second carpal bone; (g) third carpal bone; (h) fourth carpal bone; (i) accessory carpal bone; (j) first metacarpal bone; (k) second metacarpal bone; (l) third metacarpal bone; (m) fourth metacarpal bone; (n) fifth metacarpal bone; (o) sesamoid bone of abductor pollicis longus muscle; (p) antebrachiocarpal joint; (q) middle carpal joint; (r) carpometacarpal joint; (s) distal radial physis; and (t) distal ulnar physis.

The carpus has a slight lateral (valgus) orientation of 5° (Goodrich et al. 2014) and allows approximately 20° of motion in the frontal plane (Jaegger et al. 2002). A small amount of pronation and supination occurs within the carpus but has not been differentiated from the pronation and supination that occurs within the antebrachium.

Osteoarthritis of the carpus can result from a variety of causes such as the subluxation present in dogs with chondrodystrophy (Theyse et al. 2005), joint instability (e.g. hyperextension injury and collateral ligament injury), intra-articular fracture, IMPA, or the presence of deep wounds including shearing injuries. Treatment of carpal osteoarthritis ranges from nonsurgical management to carpal arthrodesis.

13.2.1 Immune-Mediated Polyarthritis

The carpus is a common site of IMPA including erosive (i.e. radiographic evidence of bone lysis) and nonerosive (i.e. lack of erosive radiographic changes) forms of the disease. In contrast to other differential diagnoses (e.g. septic arthritis, neoplasia, and degenerative joint disease), immune-mediated diseases generally affect multiple joints, most frequently the distal joints (i.e. carpi and tarsi). Treatment consists of immunosuppressive drug therapy or carpal arthrodesis, if pain is severe.

Non-erosive polyarthritis can occur in all breeds but tends to affect middle-aged large-breed dogs (Johnson and Mackin 2012). It can be idiopathic (Type I), which is the most common form, or secondary to amyloidosis (Shar-Peis), to receiving sulfa drugs (Doberman Pinschers), or to the presence of neoplasia (Type IV), enterohepatic disease (Type III), or other chronic diseases, particularly infectious diseases (Type II). The clinical signs of polyarthritis vary but may include reluctance to walk, stiffness, vocalizing, exercise intolerance, and systemic signs such as inappetence and pyrexia. In one study, 40% of dogs with fever of unknown origin were diagnosed with polyarthritis (Lunn 2001). Lameness may be mild to severe and shift from one leg to another but frequently affects both thoracic limbs. Loss of carpal joint flexion secondary to carpal effusion, and pain response may be present; however, in one study, only 40% of dogs showed joint pain (Jacques et al. 2002). Besides joint effusion, the diagnosis of nonerosive polyarthritis relies on the lack of radiographic changes (Figure 13.3) and arthrocentesis showing suppurative inflammation without evidence of infection (Chapter 9). The most commonly affected joints are the tarsi, carpi, and the stifle. Aspiration of these joints is generally recommended (Johnson and Mackin 2012) since some dogs with polyarthritis do not have palpable carpal effusion or show signs of pain, so it is important to collect joint fluid when polyarthritis is suspected, even if effusion is not detected. It is also important to collect joint fluid to evaluate the response to therapy regardless of the presence or absence of effusion.

Erosive polyarthritis, also termed rheumatoid arthritis, tends to occur in smaller dogs and is rare. In one study, all dogs with erosive polyarthritis had erosive lesions of the carpal joint (Shaughnessy et al. 2016). The diagnosis of erosive polyarthritis relies on radiographs (to diagnose erosive lesions) in combination with joint fluid analysis. Carpal joint instability and hyperextension may occur secondarily. A *juvenile* form of polyarthritis has been reported in Akitas (Dougherty et al. 1991).

13.3 Fractures of the Carpal Region

Fractures of the carpal region (Figure 13.4) include fractures of the distal aspect of the radius and ulna, particularly Salter-Harris (SH) fractures of the distal radial and ulnar physes, as well as fractures of the carpal bones. Physeal fractures of the distal radial and ulnar physes appear to be the most common physeal fractures in dogs (Marretta and Schrader 1983). These fractures are generally classified using the SH classification system (Figure 13.5). In the radius, fractures across the distal radial physis without (*SH Type I*) or with a metaphyseal bone fragment (*SH Type II*) and asymmetric compressive lesions leading to premature physeal closure (described as *SH Type VI*) are most common. Physeal distal radial fractures that involve the articular surface without (*SH Type III*) or with a metaphyseal bone fragment (*SH Type IV*) rarely occur. In the ulna, the distal physis is cone-shaped and excessive bending leads to a compressive injury on one side of the cone and secondary premature closure (*SH Type V*). Since these distal ulna fractures frequently lead to angular limb deformity due to premature growth plate closure, their identification prior to the development of deformities

CARPAL REGION

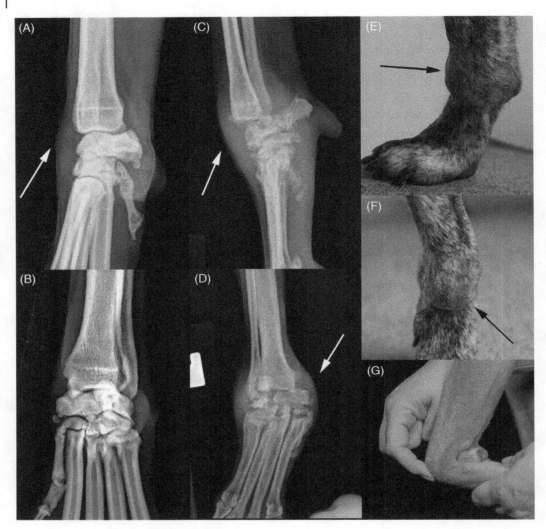

Figure 13.3 Immune-mediated polyarthritis: (A, B) dog with nonerosive polyarthritis; (C–F) dog with erosive polyarthritis: (A) lateral view of the carpus with (white arrow) soft tissue opacity; (B) no lytic osseous changes are seen; (C, D) note the (white arrow) soft tissue opacity and lytic osseous changes; (E, F) visible, severe carpal joint effusion; (G) joint effusion is best palpated dorsally by identifying the extent of the distal radius during flexion, identifying the joint space.

is crucial. In dogs with unilateral problems, comparing the length and geometry of the ulna and radius from both thoracic limbs greatly facilitates the assessment. Surgical treatment options that may prevent the development or limit the severity of deformities (e.g. distal ulnar ostectomy) are available, although they are only effective if performed while growth potential remains.

Carpal bone fractures are rare overall and most commonly occur in sporting dogs. Among these, accessory carpal bone fractures are among the most common fractures seen in racing Greyhounds. Accessory carpal bone fractures have been classified into Type I–V based on the avulsed or crushed portion of the bone (Johnson 1987; Johnson et al. 1989). To detect damage to the accessory carpal bone, digital pressure is applied to the bone while slowly extending the carpus. Radial carpal bone fractures have been seldom reported (Li et al. 2000; Tomlin et al. 2001). Incomplete ossification of the

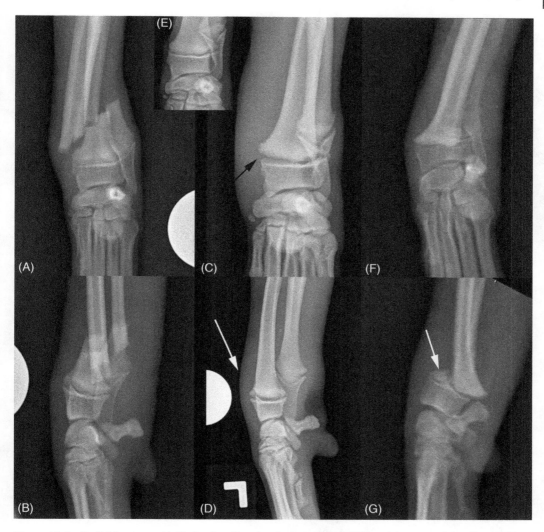

Figure 13.4 Radial fractures: (A, B) distal radius ulna fracture; (C, D) SH Type I fracture of the distal radius, note the widening of the physis (black arrow) and soft tissue swelling (white arrow), (E) is the contralateral normal limb for comparison; (F, G) SH Type II fracture of the distal radius: the white arrow indicates the metaphyseal portion.

radial carpal bone has been suggested as an underlying etiology (Gnudi et al. 2003; Perry et al. 2010). An ulnar carpal bone fracture has been reported in a Labrador Retriever (Vedrine 2013). A slab fracture of the fourth carpal bone has been reported in a racing Greyhound (Rutherford and Ness 2012).

13.3.1 Signalment and History

Traumatic fractures may be observed in any breed or age of dog. Distal radius/ulna fractures are frequently observed in Toy-breed dogs without a history of trauma. Commonly, these fractures or observed after falling or minor jumping (e.g. off the couch). This is related to the proportionally reduced cross-sectional diameter of the distal radius in these dogs (Brianza et al. 2006) compared to large-breed dogs, who more frequently sustain carpal hyperextension injuries instead.

(A) (B)

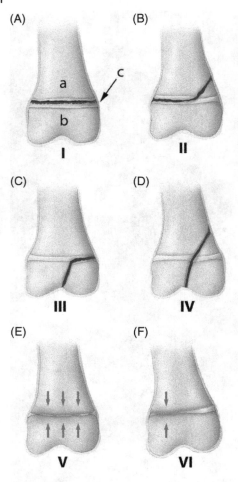

(C) (D)

(E) (F)

Figure 13.5 Salter-Harris (SH) fracture classification: the SH classification is intended for fractures in juveniles that are involving variable components of the (a) metaphysis, (b) epiphysis, and (c) physis. (A) SH Type I fractures describe a fracture directly though the physis without a fracture component of the metaphysis or epiphysis. (B) A Type II fracture, which is the most common physeal fracture type in dogs, involves the physis and a portion of the metaphysis. (C) Type III fractures involve a portion of the physis and epiphysis and, therefore, are articular fractures. (D) Type IV fractures involve all three components and, therefore, are also a type of articular fracture. (E) Type V fractures are symmetric, and (F) Type VI are asymmetric compressive fractures of the physis, both of which cannot initially be identified radiographically since no displacement is present.

13.3.2 Physical Examination

Carpal fractures can lead to varying degrees of lameness from a mild, weight-bearing lameness to a severe, toe-touching or non-weight-bearing lameness based on the potential loss of carpal stability. Slab fractures, chip fractures, and non-displaced carpal bone fractures often lead to mild lameness that may be more severe after a period of rest (dogs "warm out of the lameness") or after a period of heavy exercise. Fractures with ligamentous disruptions and loss of carpal stability are incompatible with weight-bearing and lead to a toe-touching stance and severe lameness. On palpation, carpal fractures are associated with mild and focal swelling to severe and diffuse swelling, based on carpal disruption. Swelling is generally most severe on the dorsal aspect of the joint. Carpal flexion is decreased and range of motion generally elicits a pain response. To flex and extend the carpus, the leg is held with one hand proximal to the carpus, and the other hand is placed distal to it. Motion of the elbow and shoulder joints should be avoided when performing the evaluation of the carpus to reduce a possible response from a painful source in these areas. A normal carpus can be flexed to a point where the metacarpal pad contacts the caudal surface of the antebrachium.

13.3.3 Diagnostics

Suspected carpal fractures are investigated using orthogonal radiographs. Soft tissue swelling over the carpus may be visible on radiographs. SH Type I fractures may be difficult to identify radiographically if they are minimally displaced (Figure 13.4). Early after injury, SH Type V and VI fractures are generally not visible radiographically, although soft tissue swelling may be present. If the history and physical exam suggests that these fractures are present, serial radiographs (e.g. every two weeks) should be performed since a few weeks later premature closure of the physis will be visible. Ideally radiographs of both limbs are performed allowing to monitor for a length deficit compared to the contralateral bone. The goal is to monitor for the development of secondary angular limb deformities and institute treatment early during the progression of the disease.

If the problem is chronic, focal periosteal reaction over the fracture site may be visible and the joint may be osteoarthritic. For minimally displaced fractures, if the orientation of the radiographic beam approximates the orientation of the fracture plane, a fracture line may be visible on radiographs. CT greatly enhances the sensitivity and precision of the diagnosis of these fractures. Incomplete ossification of the radial carpal bone may also not be visible on radiographs, and therefore a CT may be needed to diagnose the condition.

13.4 Carpal Hyperextension and Other Carpal Ligamentous Injuries

Carpal hyperextension is the term used to describe an increase of carpal extension. Excessive carpal extension can be developmental or acquired. Acquired carpal hyperextension is a frequent carpal joint problem that most often results from trauma (Bristow et al. 2015). The antebrachiocarpal joint is mainly stabilized by the radiocarpal and ulnarcarpal ligaments, the palmar carpal fibrocartilage stabilizes the distal carpal joints (Slocum and Devine 1982; Milgram et al. 2012), and the accessory metacarpal ligament as well as the accessory carpoulnar ligaments stabilizes the accessory carpal bone (Figure 13.6). With traumatic impact, the main structures supporting the normal angulation of the carpus become damaged, leading to the typical presentation of a palmigrade stance. Traumatic carpal hyperextension is generally treated with arthrodesis, since external coaptation does not seem to allow for healing of the ligaments. Depending on the level of injury, a partial carpal (i.e. fusion of the distal carpal joints, leaving the antebrachiocarpal joint intact) or pancarpal (i.e. fusion of all carpal joints) arthrodesis may be performed (Bristow et al. 2015).

Other, less common causes of carpal hyperextension include immune-mediated joint disease and hyperadrenocorticism (Cushing's syndrome; Parker et al. 1981; Lotsikas and Radasch 2006; Shaughnessy et al. 2016). Immune-mediated mono- or polyarthritis may be associated with carpal hyperextension and thus should be kept in mind during the diagnostic workup. Increased corticosteroid levels negatively impact tenocyte proliferation, inhibit collagen synthesis, decrease tenocyte migration, and induce tendon cell apoptosis (Galdiero et al. 2014). In affected dogs, joint instability and tendon rupture may also occur elsewhere.

Immobilization in a splint can also result in ligament laxity of the immobilized limb; in one report, carpal hyperextension was observed in dogs after only 10 days of immobilization (Altunatmaz and Guzel 2006).

Developmental carpal hyperextension is unusual but has been reported in growing Doberman Pinchers and Shar-Peis and various other breeds including German Shepherd Dogs (GSD) (Shires et al. 1985; Altunatmaz and Guzel 2006; Cetinkaya et al. 2007). The problem is often bilateral, and in severe cases the tarsi can also be affected.

CARPAL REGION

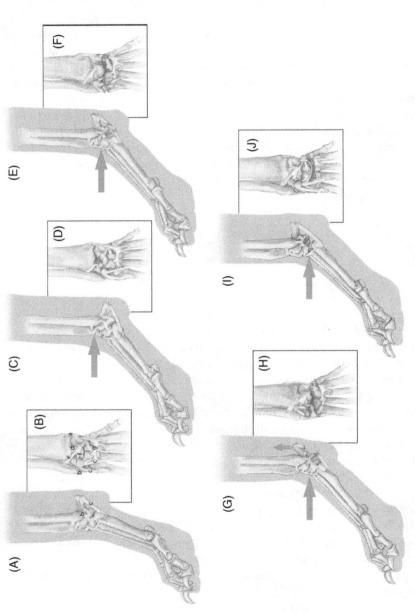

Figure 13.6 Illustration of carpal hyperextension: (A, B) normal appearance for the (a) medial collateral ligament, (b) lateral collateral ligament, (c) accessory metacarpal ligaments, (d) palmar radiocarpal ligament, (e) palmar ulnocarpal ligament, (f) intercarpal ligaments, (g) palmar fibrocartilage; (C, D) injury at the level of the antebrachiocarpal joint (red arrow), the accessory carpal and ulnar carpal bones are in a normal position indicating disruption of the radiocarpal and ulnocarpal ligaments only; (E, F) injury at the level of the middle carpal joint (red arrow) with proximal displacement of the accessory carpal bone and ulnar carpal bone suggested by an increased joint space between the ulnar carpal bone and fourth carpal bone indicating disruption of several intercarpal ligaments. In this dog, no disruption of the ligament between the accessory carpal and ulnar carpal bone is seen, indicating that the ligament connecting the two is intact; (G, H) injury at the level of the middle carpal joint (red arrow) with proximal displacement of the accessory carpal bone and ulnar carpal bone suggested by an increased joint space between the accessory carpal and ulnar carpal bone as well as between the ulnar carpal bone and fourth carpal bone indicating disruption of several intercarpal ligaments, the ligament connecting the accessory carpal and ulnar carpal bone, and the accessory metacarpal ligaments; and (I,J) injury at the level of the distal carpal (carpometacarpal) joint (white arrows) indicating disruption of the palmar fibrocartilage.

Other causes, including collateral ligament damage, fractures, and luxations of the carpal bones, as well as injuries to muscles and tendons traveling over the carpus, may also lead to chronic pain, decreased carpal function, and carpal hyperextension. Subluxation or luxation of carpal bones other than hyperextension injuries is rare. Luxations of the carpal joint are also rare but generally associated with severe trauma.

13.4.1 Signalment and History

Traumatic carpal hyperextension most often occurs in large-breed active dogs. However, small-breed dogs can also be affected. Carpal hyperextension is most commonly associated with a fall, jump, or motor vehicle accident (Denny and Barr 1991). Carpal injuries related to trauma can also be seen in competitive agility dogs (Levy et al. 2009; Cullen et al. 2013). The angle of the A-frame (a tall "contact" obstacle that agility dogs must overcome) has been hypothesized to be related to carpal hyperextension injury in these dogs. However, a prospective study evaluating the landing carpal extension angles refuted this hypothesis (Appelgrein et al. 2018). In that study, the antebrachiocarpal landing angle was approximately 240° for any given A-frame angle and it was concluded that this angle likely represents the maximum physiological carpal extension angle when contacting the A-frame.

Another cause for carpal injury could be from repetitive trauma as seen in Herding dogs (Jerram et al. 2009). A similar etiology could be considered for long-distance sled dogs. Indeed, carpal injury and an increased risk to be dropped from a team during marathon sled dog racing was found to be associated with increased training miles (von Pfeil et al. 2015).

Carpal hyperextension and collateral ligament injuries have no specific predisposition for age, weight, or breed. However, older working Collies have been suggested to potentially be predisposed to progressive degenerative hyperextension as a result of chronic, repetitive carpal injury (Jerram et al. 2009).

Regardless of the specific underlying traumatic cause, acutely affected dogs are in pain and exhibit varying degrees of lameness of the affected leg. Carpal swelling can be present, particularly if the injury is acute. Once the condition is more chronic, there is typically less discomfort. The main abnormality noted by owners is hyperextension and lameness of the affected thoracic limb. Depending on the severity of the injury, the degree of hyperextension can be mild or severe. In severe situations, patients may develop a palmigrade stance with the accessory carpal bone in contact with the ground (Video 13.1).

Video 13.1:

Video of patients with carpal hyperextension (traumatic and due to immune-mediated polyarthritis).

13.4.2 Physical Examination

Lameness can vary in severity, depending on the amount and location of damage and chronicity. The contralateral side is used to compare the carpal angle and the presence of swelling. Upon palpation of the carpus, soft tissue swelling and discomfort can be noted in addition to carpal hyperextension (Figure 13.7). The examiner should also evaluate the presence of crepitus and resistance and assess for collateral ligament instability (Figure 13.8), requiring knowledge of normal motion. Palpation of the dorsal surface of the carpus will help to detect minor swelling or

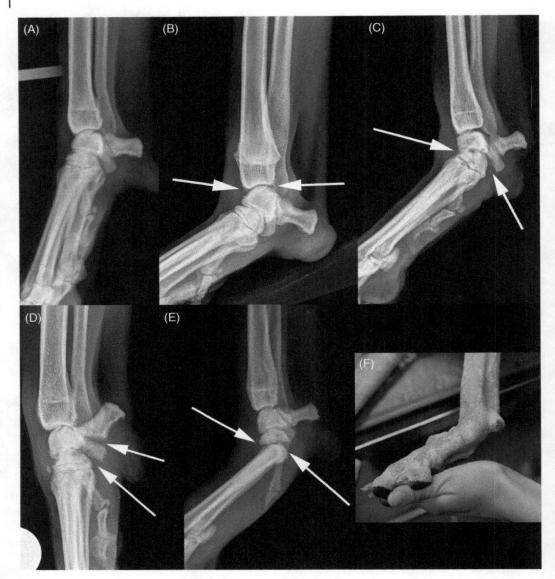

Figure 13.7 Radiograph images depicting ligaments affected by carpal hyperextension corresponding to illustrations in Figure 13.6: (A) normal appearance; (B) injury at the level of the proximal carpal joint (white arrows): the accessory carpal and ulnar carpal bones are in a normal position indicating disruption of the radiocarpal and ulnocarpal ligaments only; (C) injury at the level of the middle carpal joint with proximal displacement of the accessory carpal bone and ulnar carpal bone suggested by an increased joint space between the ulnar carpal bone and fourth carpal bone (white arrows) indicating disruption of several intercarpal ligaments. In this dog, no disruption of the ligament between the accessory carpal and ulnar carpal bone is seen, indicating that the ligament connecting the two is intact; (D) injury at the level of the middle carpal joint with proximal displacement of the accessory carpal bone and ulnar carpal bone suggested by an increased joint space between the accessory carpal and ulnar carpal bone as well as between the ulnar carpal bone and fourth carpal bone (white arrows) indicating disruption of several intercarpal ligaments and the accessory metacarpal ligaments; (E) injury at the level of the distal carpal (carpometacarpal) joint (white arrows) indicating disruption of the palmar fibrocartilage; and (F) typical appearance of carpal hyperextension when applying dorsal stress to the distal limb.

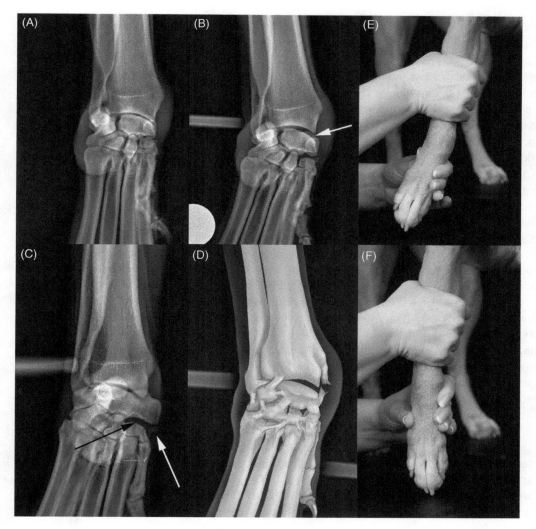

Figure 13.8 Traumatic medial collateral ligament injury in a 4-year-old GSD: (A–C) radiographs, (D) illustration of the injury, and (E, F) physical examination to detect collateral ligament injury by applying medial/later stress to these ligaments. (A) Radiographs of the affected limb showing soft tissue swelling on the medial aspect but no evidence of instability. (B) Stress radiograph of the affected limb showing an increased antebrachiocarpal joint space (white arrow) indicating disruption of the medial collateral ligament. (C) Stress radiograph of the unaffected, normal limb highlighting a normal antebrachiocarpal joint width. Note: while this is a similar stress view of the opposite limb, due to slightly different positioning, the sesamoid bone (arrow) within the abductor pollicis longus is more obvious due to lack of superimposition with other carpal bones. Similarly, the different positioning gives the appearance of a wider middle carpal joint (black arrow). (D) Illustration of image (B) depicting the torn collateral ligament and widened joint space. (E) Application of valgus stress and (F) varus stress to the carpus, testing the integrity of the medial ligament and lateral collateral ligament, respectively.

discomfort of tendons or joint areas. Goniometry and flexibility measurements of the carpal flexors should be measured to quantify the degree of hyperextension and establish a baseline (Chapter 5). For healthy Labrador Retrievers, the mean ($\pm$SD) normal range of motion in dogs is reported to be 32° ($\pm$2°) in flexion and 196° ($\pm$2°) in extension (Jaegger et al. 2002).

13.4.3 Diagnostics

Radiographs should be acquired in every patient as the first diagnostic step. When the problem is unilateral, orthogonal views of the unaffected, contralateral side are obtained for comparison purposes. Standing or stress views mimicking weight-bearing are imperative to identify the location of injury within the carpal joint (Figure 13.7). Stress views can be safely acquired using adhesive tape or ties to extend the carpus. Otherwise a wooden spoon can be used to provide counterpressure. This ensures a safe distance of the examiner's hands from the radiation beam, while simultaneously being able to provide the necessary amount of pressure needed to achieve appropriate stress view imaging. In addition to regional soft tissue swelling, based on the level of subluxation and associated supportive structures, injuries occur at three levels (Slocum and Devine 1982). Subluxation of the antebrachiocarpal level results from damage to the short oblique radial carpal, palmar radiocarpal, and palmar ulnarcarpal ligaments. Injuries to the intercarpal level result from rupture of the metacarpal accessory ligaments and the short intercarpal ligament between the accessory and ulnar carpal bones. Carpometacarpal joint injuries include rupture of the ligaments of the middle carpal- the carpometacarpal joints and the palmar fibrocartilage. In addition to flexed and hyperextended views, views with mediolateral stress (Figure 13.8) are also acquired to evaluate the medial and lateral collateral ligaments. Finally, oblique views acquired at 45° angles can help identify carpal bone fractures.

CT can be considered if there is concern for additional fractures of the carpal bones that may not be visible on radiographs or if stress views do not reveal a subluxation of any joint. MRI may reveal very subtle lesions and allow for evaluation of all periarticular soft tissue structures of clinical interest. Advanced imaging can aid in treatment decision and increase the success for each specific treatment, which depending on the damaged structures involved, may include partial or pancarpal arthrodesis. Ultrasound has also been used, albeit its value for the diagnosis of these injuries has not yet been established.

Arthrocentesis should be performed if infectious or inflammatory etiologies are possible. While infrequently reported in the literature, IMPA should be considered as a possible cause for carpal lameness (Lotsikas and Radasch 2006). With chronicity, affected dogs can progress to palmigrade stance, mimicking a traumatic hyperextension injury. Based on the authors' experience, Shelties and Welsh Corgies may be at increased risk of IMPA affecting the carpus, although other breeds are also affected. Arthroscopy of the carpus has also been suggested as a potential additional imaging technique, to aid in the diagnosis of hyperextension, infection, and IMPA (Warnock and Beale 2004).

13.4.4 Other Carpal Ligamentous Injuries

No ligament crosses the entire carpus. Rather, ligaments cross one or two carpal rows. The main carpal ligaments are the medial collateral ligament, the short radial lateral collateral ligament and the short oblique lateral collateral ligament. Medial collateral ligaments sprains can result from severe trauma or, more seldomly, from athletic activities. Lateral collateral injuries have been reported in racing Greyhounds and other dogs (Roe and Dee 1986; Guilliard and Mayo 2000). Dorsal carpal ligament sprains have also been reported in a series comprising two racing Greyhounds, one working Pointer, one working Border Collie, and one working Labrador Retriever (Guilliard 1997). Injuries to collateral and dorsal ligaments result in focal swelling in the short term and in focal fibrosis over time. Collateral injuries are detected by placing varus or valgus stress on the carpus with the joint extended and are confirmed by use of stress radiography (Figure 13.8) or diagnostic ultrasonography.

13.5   Deformities of the Carpal Region

Deformities of the distal aspect of the antebrachium are the most common limb deformities, with a reported prevalence of 0.74% of all orthopedic problems (Marcellin-Little et al. 1998). These deformities result from genetic problems, most commonly chondrodystrophy and chondrodysplasia (Parker et al. 2009; Brown et al. 2017). They can also result from developmental skeletal disorders or inflammatory bone diseases including hypertrophic osteodystrophy (HOD) or multiple epiphyseal dysplasia or premature growth plate closure.

Carpus valgus, a term used to describe lateral angulation originating in the distal portion of the antebrachium, is the most common antebrachial deformity. The lateral deviation of the manus is generally associated with excessive external rotation of the radius, and a loss of carpal flexion. Carpus valgus can also be associated with subluxation of the elbow joint, particularly distal humero-ulnar subluxation, and with a varus angulation of the proximal portion of the radius, resulting in biapical antebrachial deformity (Kwan et al. 2014).

Carpus varus, the medial deviation of the carpus, is much less common than carpus valgus and is most often the result of an injury to the distal radial physis.

13.5.1   Signalment and History

Deformities of the carpal region are common in chondrodystrophic and chondrodysplastic dog breeds (Parker et al. 2009; Brown et al. 2017). Genetically driven deformities are bilateral. However, one thoracic limb can be more severely affected than the contralateral thoracic limb (Kwan et al. 2014). Trauma to a radial or ulnar physis can lead to premature closure and result in antebrachial deformity. In one study, 7% of physeal injuries led to a limb deformity (Marretta and Schrader 1983). Antebrachial deformities secondary to trauma are generally unilateral.

13.5.2   Physical Examination

Antebrachial deformities are diagnosed by observation and palpation and are confirmed by use of radiographs. The deviation of the manus will vary when measured while standing, while sedated, and on radiographs (Kwan et al. 2014). The examination of a patient with antebrachial deformity includes the evaluation of varus or valgus; the presence of effusion, crepitus, and pain response to joint motion in the carpus and elbow; and the range of motion of the carpus and elbow measured using a goniometer (Chapter 5).

13.5.3   Diagnostics

Palpation and goniometry under sedation may be the most accurate way to evaluate valgus or varus deformities; standing measurements appear to overestimate it and radiographs appear to underestimate it. Radiographs should include the entire limb distal to the elbow. It is easiest to evaluate deformities if an attempt is made to provide a true lateral and craniocaudal view of the elbow, without attempting to correct the position of the distal limb (Figure 13.9). Complex deformities can be assessed using CT (Kwan et al. 2014), which allows the objective assessment of radial rotation, length deficit, and subluxation of the elbow and carpus.

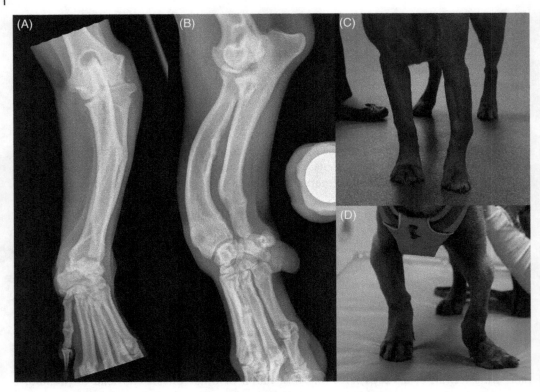

Figure 13.9 Typical radiographic appearance of an (A, B) angular limb deformity secondary to premature closure of the distal ulnar physis showing radius procurvatum, valgus deformity, and external rotation of the distal limb, elbow incongruity, and a shortened ulna. (C) Clinical appearance of (C) carpus *varus* secondary to premature radial physis closure, and (D) carpus *valgus* secondary to premature distal ulnar physis closure.

13.6 Tendinous and Muscular Lesions of the Carpal Region

Tendon and muscular injuries in the carpal region are sparsely described in the veterinary literature but, in the authors' experience, are a more common cause of lameness than previously thought. These injuries are unlikely to lead to severe disability, and lameness is generally moderate to mild. Most severe carpal tendon and muscular injuries result from trauma such as shearing injuries or penetrating wounds (e.g. bite wounds and gunshot wounds). The flexor tendons may be injured at any level, including caudal to the carpal joint and should therefore be palpated for swelling and pain (Chapter 12).

Flexor carpi ulnaris (FCU) *tendinopathy* or partial avulsions of the insertion site of the FCU on the accessory carpal bone occur in dogs, most often in large, athletic dogs. It has been reported in Greyhounds and a Weimaraner dog (Kuan et al. 2007). The FCU consists of two muscle bellies: the ulnar head originates from the proximal medial ulna, and the humeral head originates from the medial epicondyle of the humerus. Both insert as a combined tendon on the accessory carpal bone. FCU injuries result in a weight-bearing lameness. Upon palpation, a firm swelling is palpable proximal to the accessory carpal bone. Pain may be exacerbated if the muscle is stretched (e.g. carpal hyperextension). The diagnosis is confirmed using musculoskeletal ultrasound by seeing a disruption of collagen fibers and the presence of intratendinous fluid. Radiographs may show swelling or calcification if a chronic injury is present (Figure 13.10). Neoplasia has to be considered as a differential diagnosis and appropriate diagnostics (e.g. ultrasound, fine-needle aspirate (FNA), and biopsy) should be utilized on an individual basis.

Inflammation of the *abductor pollicis (digiti I) longus*, described as stenosing tenosynovitis, has also been reported as a cause of lameness (Hittmair et al. 2012). This muscle originates from the lateral surface of the radius and ulna as well as the interosseous membrane and curves medially to insert on the base of the first metacarpus. The muscle abducts and extends the first digit and as such adduction and flexion of the digit will stretch the muscle. This may result in a pain response in affected animals. Animals may present with a visual swelling (Figure 13.11) of the medial aspect of the carpus, and radiographs may show enthesopathy and bony proliferation in the area of the radial sulcus (that the muscle passes through). These changes result in stenosis of the tendon and may be associated with clinical symptoms, although they may also be nonclinical. Surgical (resection or release of the tendon) and nonsurgical treatments have been described.

13.7 Other Diseases Affecting the Carpal Region

13.7.1 Lack or Loss of Carpal Extension

Carpal laxity syndrome is a term used to describe loss of carpal extension or flexion. Lack of carpal extension, also termed "carpal flexural deformity" has been reported in growing large-breed dogs (Vaughan 1992; Altunatmaz and Guzel 2006; Cetinkaya et al. 2007). Although the cause of this lack of carpal extension is not known, malnutrition, lack of exercise, or a discrepancy between rapid bone growth and slower muscle growth leading to tightness of the antebrachial flexor muscles may possibly play a role. Affected dogs stand with the carpus flexed, potentially relieving the tension on their digital flexor tendons. Treatment with appropriate nutrition and exercise generally resolves the condition.

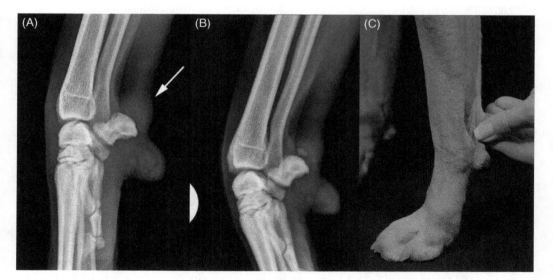

Figure 13.10 Radiographs of a dog affected with flexor carpi ulnaris (FCU) tendinopathy: (A) early stages showing soft tissue swelling only (white arrow); (B) chronic stages showing calcification of the tendon of insertion; and (C) location for palpation of FCU tendon insertion at the accessory carpal bone.

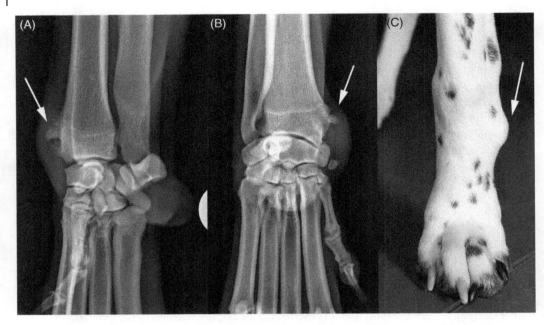

Figure 13.11 Images depict (A, B) radiographic and (C) clinical presentation of a dog with abductor pollicis longus tendinopathy; (A) osseous proliferation in the area of the radial sulcus visible on the lateral and (B) craniocaudal radiograph. Also note (C) typical soft tissue swelling associated with this tendinopathy.

Lack of carpal extension has also been described in dogs with neurologic injury (Holland 2005). It can occur in dogs with palsy of the distal (antebrachial) branch of the radial nerve. The loss of radial innervation leads to a lack of ability to extend the carpus and, with continued active flexion from antebrachial flexor muscles, a progressive loss of carpal extension can occur. This type of loss of carpal extension is seen in dogs with brachial plexus avulsion (Chapter 16) and in dogs with iatrogenic transection of the radial nerve.

Lack of carpal flexion while standing and walking is also seen in dogs with severe antebrachial deformities, a situation described as carpal buckling. A transient loss of carpal extension is routinely present after limb lengthening (Kwan et al. 2014).

Since full carpal extension is required while standing and walking, loss of carpal extension has a major clinical impact in dogs. A loss of approximately 30° of extension can make limb use impossible. Lack or loss of carpal extension is diagnosed by observing or videotaping dogs while standing and walking and using palpation and goniometry. Imaging is performed to identify or rule out underlying structural disease (in juvenile animals).

13.7.2   Lack or Loss of Carpal Flexion

Since complete carpal flexion is not required for locomotion and to perform activities of daily living, a loss of carpal flexion has minimal function impact in dogs. Lack of carpal flexion is frequently present in dogs with carpal osteoarthritis and as a consequence of fractures affecting the carpal region. Lack of carpal flexion is also present in the majority dogs with antebrachial deformities secondary to impaired physeal growth. In a case series, 6 of 7 dogs with antebrachial deformities were lacking carpal flexion with an average loss of flexion of 50° (Marcellin-Little et al. 1998). The authors have also observed lack of carpal flexion in geriatric, large-breed dogs without identifiable underlying disease.

13.7.3 Hypertrophic Osteodystrophy

HOD is an inflammatory disease affecting the metaphyseal region of long bones in growing dogs, particularly dogs of large and giant breeds. The disease is often limited to or is most severe in the distal portion of the antebrachium (if it extends beyond the distal region). Usually developing at 3–4 months of age, HOD is often associated with hyperthermia, anorexia, diarrhea, severe pain in the metaphyseal regions of long bones, and a loss of willingness to ambulate. The clinical signs often subside after a week or so. However, severely affected dogs may require hospitalization and supportive care. Episodes can recur every few weeks until the end of growth. The cause of HOD is not known. Factors implicated have included vitamin C deficiency and the presence of viral RNA in metaphyseal osteoblasts. In severe instances, HOD can lead to the formation of periosteal new bone and to antebrachial and crural deformities. Soft tissue mineralization has been reported in severely affected dogs. HOD is diagnosed by use of radiography (Figure 13.12). The distal radial

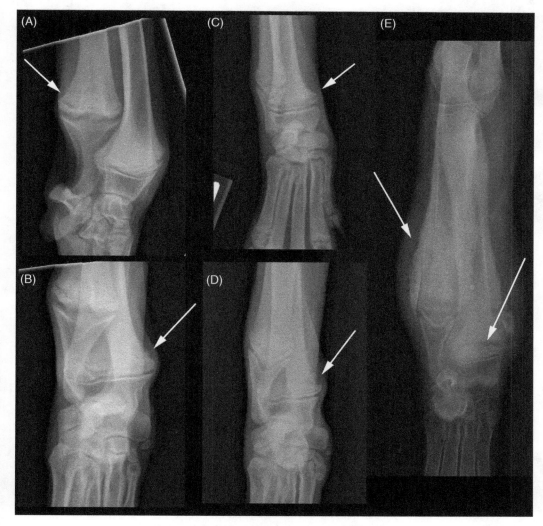

Figure 13.12 Hypertrophic osteodystrophy (HOD): (A, B) classic appearance of a lucent "double physis" line (white arrow) paralleling the distal radial and ulnar physes; (C, D) variations of a double physis; (C) a broader lucent line is visible particularly in the distal radius; (D) early changes with HOD, showing a faintly visible lucency adjacent to the physis; and (E) chronic appearance of HOD, note that the double physeal lines are still visible.

and ulna growth plate may be irregular or appear to be doubled (i.e. "double physis" sign as a result of impaired ossification of the metaphyseal region) and periosteal bone formation may be visible depending on the disease stages (Demko and Mclaughlin 2005).

13.7.4 Shearing Injuries

Shearing injuries routinely affect the carpal region (Benson and Boudrieau 2002) and often include a loss of tendon and collateral ligaments. The orthopedic examination of carpal region with

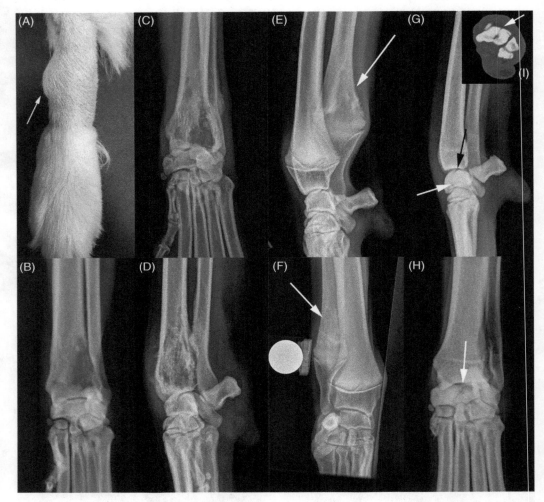

Figure 13.13 Other miscellaneous conditions of the carpal region. Images (A–D) depict distal radius osteosarcoma: (A) swelling associated with distal radius osteosarcoma; (B) craniocaudal radiograph of a dog showing predominantly osteolytic changes consistent with osteosarcoma; (C, D) radiographs of a dog showing typical osteolytic-osteoproliferative changes consistent with osteosarcoma. Images (E, F) depict radiographs of a dog with retained cartilaginous core of the ulna. Images (G–I) depict incomplete ossification of the radial carpal bone: (G) the lateral radiograph shows a very faint line (white arrow), note that the (black arrow) frequently identified line at the joint surface is normal and results from superimposition of the ulnar carpal bone over the radial carpal bone; (H) the craniocaudal view shows a lucent line that is suggestive of incomplete ossification; and (I) the craniocaudal view confirms the diagnosis (white arrow indicates the fissure line across the radial carpal bone).

shearing injuries includes the assessment of mediolateral and craniocaudal carpal instability. In most instances, the loss of carpal stability is medial and dorsal, and the joint will be stable once tissues heal as a result of periarticular fibrosis. Diagnosis is easily accomplished based on visualization but imaging may be required to detect the degree of soft tissue involvement (e.g. stress views to detect collateral ligament instability, etc.).

13.7.5 Carpal Region Neoplasia

By far, the most common neoplasia of the carpal region is osteosarcoma of the distal radius (Figure 13.13). Further information is provided in Chapters 11 and 17.

13.7.6 Miscellaneous Other Conditions

Idiopathic ischemic necrosis of the accessory carpal bone has been reported in one dog (Harris and Langley-Hobbs 2013).

Incomplete ossification of the radial carpal bone has been reported in several dog breeds, including Pointers, Setters, and Boxers (Gnudi et al. 2003; Perry et al. 2010). The intermedioradial carpal bone represents a fusion of the primitive radial, central, and intermediate carpal bones, and failure of this fusion can result in incomplete ossification. Radiographs may not show the lesion, but CT will clearly identify the separation (Figure 13.13).

Subluxation or *luxation of carpal bones* other than hyperextension injuries is rare. Two reports described luxations of numbered carpal bones (Guilliard and Mayo 2001; Comerford et al. 2006). One report described a dorsomedially luxated radial carpal bone (Palierne et al. 2008). Radiographs or CT are utilized to establish these diagnoses.

Retained cartilaginous cores of the ulna are cones of non-ossified cartilage that project into the distal metaphysis (Figure 13.13). Unless they are associated with premature closure of the distal ulnar growth plate, no treatment is needed for this condition.

References

Altunatmaz, K. and Guzel, O. (2006). Carpal flexural deformity in puppies. *Medycyna Wet* 62 (6): 649–651.

Appelgrein, C., Glyde, M.R., Hosgood, G. et al. (2018). Reduction of the A-frame angle of incline does not change the maximum carpal joint extension angle in agility dogs entering the A-frame. *Vet Comp Orthop Traumatol* 31 (2): 77–82.

Benson, J.A. and Boudrieau, R.J. (2002). Severe carpal and tarsal shearing injuries treated with an immediate arthrodesis in seven dogs. *J Am Anim Hosp Assoc* 38 (4): 370–380.

Brianza, S.Z., Delise, M., Maddalena Ferraris, M. et al. (2006). Cross-sectional geometrical properties of distal radius and ulna in large, medium and toy breed dogs. *J Biomech* 39 (2): 302–311.

Bristow, P.C., Meeson, R.L., Thorne, R.M. et al. (2015). Clinical comparison of the hybrid dynamic compression plate and the castless plate for pancarpal arthrodesis in 219 dogs. *Vet Surg* 44 (1): 70–77.

Brown, E.A., Dickinson, P.J., Mansour, T. et al. (2017). FGF4 retrogene on CFA12 is responsible for chondrodystrophy and intervertebral disc disease in dogs. *Proc Natl Acad Sci USA* 114 (43): 11476–11481.

Cetinkaya, M.A., Yardimci, C., and Saglam, M. (2007). Carpal laxity syndrome in forty-three puppies. *Vet Comp Orthop Traumatol* 20 (2): 126–130.

Comerford, E.J., Doran, I.C., and Owen, M.R. (2006). Carpal derangement and associated carpal valgus in a dog. *Vet Comp Orthop Traumatol* 19 (2): 113–116.

Cullen, K.L., Dickey, J.P., Bent, L.R. et al. (2013). Survey-based analysis of risk factors for injury among dogs participating in agility training and competition events. *J Am Vet Med Assoc* 243 (7): 1019–1024.

Demko, J. and Mclaughlin, R. (2005). Developmental orthopedic disease. *Vet Clin North Am Small Anim Pract* 35 (5): 1111–1135.

Denny, H.R. and Barr, A.R.S. (1991). Partial carpal and pancarpal arthrodesis in the dog: a review of 50 cases. *J Small Anim Pract* 32 (7): 329–334.

Dougherty, S.A., Center, S.A., Shaw, E.E., and Erb, H.A. (1991). Juvenile-onset polyarthritis syndrome in Akitas. *J Am Vet Med Assoc* 198 (5): 849–856.

Galdiero, M., Auriemma, R.S., Pivonello, R., and Colao, A. (2014). Cushing, acromegaly, GH deficiency and tendons. *Muscles Ligaments Tendons J* 4 (3): 329–332.

Gnudi, G., Mortellaro, C.M., Bertoni, G. et al. (2003). Radial carpal bone fracture in 13 dogs. *Vet Comp Orthop Traumatol* 16 (3): 178.

Goodrich, Z.J., Norby, B., Eichelberger, B.M. et al. (2014). Thoracic limb alignment in healthy Labrador Retrievers: evaluation of standing versus recumbent frontal plane radiography. *Vet Surg* 43 (7): 791–803.

Guilliard, M.J. (1997). Dorsal radiocarpal ligament sprain causing intermittent carpal lameness in high activity dogs. *J Small Anim Pract* 38 (10): 463–465.

Guilliard, M.J. and Mayo, A.K. (2000). Sprain of the short radial collateral ligament in a racing Greyhound. *J Small Anim Pract* 41 (4): 169–171.

Guilliard, M.J. and Mayo, A.K. (2001). Subluxation/luxation of the second carpal bone in two racing Greyhounds and a Staffordshire Bull Terrier. *J Small Anim Pract* 42 (7): 356–359.

Harris, K.P. and Langley-Hobbs, S.J. (2013). Idiopathic ischemic necrosis of an accessory carpal bone in a dog. *J Am Vet Med Assoc* 243 (12): 1746–1750.

Hittmair, K.M., Groessl, V., and Mayrhofer, E. (2012). Radiographic and ultrasonographic diagnosis of stenosing tenosynovitis of the abductor pollicis longus muscle in dogs. *Vet Radiol Ultrasound* 53 (2): 135–141.

Holland, C.T. (2005). Carpal hyperflexion in a growing dog following neural injury to the distal brachium. *J Small Anim Pract* 46 (1): 22–26.

Jacques, D., Cauzinille, L., Bouvy, B., and Dupré, G. (2002). A retrospective study of 40 dogs with polyarthritis. *Vet Surg* 31 (5): 428–434.

Jaegger, G., Marcellin-Little, D.J., and Levine, D. (2002). Reliability of goniometry in Labrador Retrievers. *Am J Vet Res* 63 (7): 979–986.

Jerram, R.M., Walker, A.M., Worth, A.J., and Kuipers Von Lande, R.G. (2009). Prospective evaluation of pancarpal arthrodesis for carpal injuries in working dogs in New Zealand, using dorsal hybrid plating. *N Z Vet J* 57 (6): 331–337.

Johnson, K.A. (1987). Accessory carpal bone fractures in the racing Greyhound. Classification and pathology. *Vet Surg* 16 (1): 60–64.

Johnson, K.A., Dee, J.F., and Piermattei, D.L. (1989). Screw fixation of accessory carpal bone fractures in racing Greyhounds: 12 cases (1981–1986). *J Am Vet Med Assoc* 194 (11): 1618–1625.

Johnson, K.C. and Mackin, A. (2012). Canine immune-mediated polyarthritis. *J Am Anim Hosp Assoc* 48 (2): 71–82.

Kuan, S.Y., Smith, B.A., Fearnside, S.M. et al. (2007). Flexor carpi ulnaris tendonopathy in a Weimaraner. *Aust Vet J* 85 (10): 401–404.

Kwan, T.W., Marcellin-Little, D.J., and Harrysson, O.L.A. (2014). Correction of biapical radial deformities by use of bi-level hinged circular external fixation and distraction osteogenesis in 13 dogs. *Vet Surg* 43 (3): 316–329.

Levy, M., Hall, C., Trentacosta, N., and Percival, M. (2009). A preliminary retrospective survey of injuries occurring in dogs participating in canine agility. *Vet Comp Orthop Traumatol* 22 (4): 321–324.

Li, A., Bennett, D., Gibbs, C. et al. (2000). Radial carpal bone fractures in 15 dogs. *J Small Anim Pract* 41 (2): 74–79.

Lotsikas, P.J. and Radasch, R.M. (2006). A clinical evaluation of pancarpal arthrodesis in nine dogs using circular external skeletal fixation. *Vet Surg* 35 (5): 480–485.

Lunn, K.F. (2001). Fever of unknown origin: a systematic approach to diagnosis. *Compendium* 23 (11): 976–992.

Marcellin-Little, D.J., Ferretti, A., Roe, S.C., and Deyoung, D.J. (1998). Hinged Ilizarov external fixation for correction of antebrachial deformities. *Vet Surg* 27 (3): 231–245.

Marretta, S.M. and Schrader, S.C. (1983). Physeal injuries in the dog: a review of 135 cases. *J Am Vet Med Assoc* 182 (7): 708–710.

Milgram, J., Milshtein, T., and Meiner, Y. (2012). The role of the antebrachiocarpal ligaments in the prevention of hyperextension of the antebrachiocarpal joint. *Vet Surg* 41 (2): 191–199.

Palierne, S., Delbeke, C., Asimus, E. et al. (2008). A case of dorso-medial luxation of the radial carpal bone in a dog. *Vet Comp Orthop Traumatol* 21 (2): 171–176.

Parker, H.G., Vonholdt, B.M., Quignon, P. et al. (2009). An expressed fgf4 retrogene is associated with breed-defining chondrodysplasia in domestic dogs. *Science* 325 (5943): 995–998.

Parker, R.B., Brown, S.G., and Wind, A.P. (1981). Pancarpal arthrodesis in the dog: a review of forty-five cases. *Vet Surg* 10 (1): 35–43.

Perry, K., Fitzpatrick, N., Johnson, J., and Yeadon, R. (2010). Headless self-compressing cannulated screw fixation for treatment of radial carpal bone fracture or fissure in dogs. *Vet Comp Orthop Traumatol* 23 (2): 94–101.

Roe, S.C. and Dee, J.F. (1986). Lateral ligamentous injury to the carpus of a racing Greyhound. *J Am Vet Med Assoc* 189 (4): 453–454.

Rutherford, S. and Ness, M.G. (2012). Dorsal slab fracture of the fourth carpal bone in a racing Greyhound. *Vet Surg* 41 (8): 944–947.

Shaughnessy, M.L., Sample, S.J., Abicht, C. et al. (2016). Clinical features and pathological joint changes in dogs with erosive immune-mediated polyarthritis: 13 cases (2004-2012). *J Am Vet Med Assoc* 249 (10): 1156–1164.

Shires, P.K., Hulse, D.A., and Kearney, M.T. (1985). Carpal hyperextension in two-month-old pups. *J Am Vet Med Assoc* 186 (1): 49–52.

Slocum, B. and Devine, T. (1982). Partial carpal fusion in the dog. *J Am Vet Med Assoc* 180 (10): 1204–1208.

Theyse, L.F., Voorhout, G., and Hazewinkel, H.A. (2005). Prognostic factors in treating antebrachial growth deformities with a lengthening procedure using a circular external skeletal fixation system in dogs. *Vet Surg* 34 (5): 424–435.

Tomlin, J.L., Pead, M.J., Langley-Hobbs, S.J., and Muir, P. (2001). Radial carpal bone fracture in dogs. *J Am Anim Hosp Assoc* 37 (2): 173–178.

Vaughan, L.C. (1992). Flexural deformity of the carpus in puppies. *J Sm Anim Pract* 33: 381–384.

Vedrine, B. (2013). Comminuted fracture of the ulnar carpal bone in a Labrador Retriever dog. *Can Vet J* 54 (11): 1067–1070.

von Pfeil, D.J., Liska, W.D., Nelson, S. et al. (2015). A survey on orthopedic injuries during a marathon sled dog race. *Vet Med (Auckl)* 6: 329–339.

Warnock, J.J. and Beale, B.S. (2004). Arthroscopy of the antebrachiocarpal joint in dogs. *J Am Vet Med Assoc* 224 (6): 867–874.

Yalden, D.W. (1970). The functional morphology of the carpal bones in carnivores. *Acta Anat (Basel)* 77 (4): 481–500.

CARPAL REGION

14

Elbow Region

Felix Michael Duerr

Department of Clinical Sciences, College of Veterinary Medicine and Biomedical Sciences, Colorado State University, Fort Collins, CO, USA

14.1 Introduction and Common Differential Diagnoses

Pathology in the elbow region is probably the most frequent source of chronic thoracic limb lameness in dogs. The elbow joint is a complex joint that is affected by many diseases. In general, elbow arthritis is more common and manifests in more severe clinical symptoms when compared to shoulder and carpal arthritis. In addition to the joint itself, soft tissue injuries of the region also cause lameness. Therefore, definitively identifying the source of lameness within the elbow region based on palpation can be very difficult and additional diagnostic tests are often necessary for establishing a diagnosis. The most commonly employed tests include CT and arthroscopy for the diagnosis of joint pathology. Figure 14.1 and Table 14.1 outline common differential diagnoses and diagnostic steps for the elbow region.

14.2 Normal Anatomy and Arthritis

The elbow (or cubital) joint is a hinge joint (with the main motion being limited to the sagittal plane, i.e. flexion and extension). The joint is formed by the radius, ulna, and humerus and divided into the following joints (Figures 14.2):

- Humeroradial joint, which is responsible for ~52% (Mason et al. 2005) of the weight-bearing forces of the elbow joint.
- Proximal radioulnar joint, which is responsible for ~48% (Mason et al. 2005) of the weight-bearing forces of the elbow joint and allows for supination and pronation.
- Humeroulnar joint, which is the responsible joint for restricting motion of the elbow to sagittal plane motion.

The medial (i.e. *trochlea*) and lateral (i.e. *capitulum*) humeral condyles articulate with the ulna and radial head, respectively (Figure 14.2). The *trochlea* is of greater size than the capitulum and sloped more distally, which becomes relevant for the pathophysiology of condylar fractures and elbow luxations (i.e. lateral condylar fractures and luxations are more common). In some dogs, the *sesamoid of*

Table 14.1 Key features for selected diseases affecting the elbow region.

Disease	Common signalment	Diagnostic test of choice	Exam findings	Treatment	Clinical pearls	Terminology
Fractures	Any (condylar fractures most common in small-breeds, approximately 4 months old)	Radiographs (orthogonal views needed – particularly to detect minimally displaced condylar fractures; Figure 14.4)	Pain, crepitus, non-weight-bearing lameness	Depends on location but frequently surgical fixation recommended	Articular fractures generally require surgical fixation, hence condylar fractures are generally treated surgically	Y-T fracture = inter- or bicondylar fracture
Incomplete ossification of the humeral condyle (IOHC)	Spaniel breeds	CT (Radiographs may show radiolucent line across condyles or smooth proliferation along lateral supracondylar crest)	Pain on elbow hyperextension or may be asymptomatic	Surgical fixation recommended (to avoid fracture)	Frequently bilateral – evaluate (and treat) both sides ASAP	DD: Progressive humeral intracondylar fissure (HIF) – same treatment
Incongruity	Same as MCD/UAP	CT or arthroscopy	Same as MCD/UAP	Same as MCD/UAP	Incongruity is contributing feature to Elbow dysplasia	Premature physeal closure may result in severe incongruity and angular limb deformity
Medial Compartment Disease (MCD)	Large-/giant-breeds, with Labrador Retrievers and Bernese Mountain Dogs are predisposed	Radiographs if secondary changes are present – CT during early stages or for "traumatic fractures of the coronoid process"	Pain upon ROM and Campbell's test, joint effusion, periarticular swelling or *no clear abnormalities*	Surgical treatment in combination with lifelong medical management or medical management	Adult dogs may present with *traumatic fractures of the coronoid process* – establishing a diagnosis in these patients requires CT/arthroscopy since radiographs are normal	Previously known as FCP – Fragmented Coronoid Process; other terminology includes (medial) coronoid disease
Osteochondrosis Dissecans (OCD)	Same as MCD	CT or arthroscopy	Same as MCD	Same as MCD	Generally not an isolated disease in the elbow but rather with MCD	"Kissing lesions" occur in the same location – these are due to coronoid pathology and not a true OCD lesion

Condition	Signalment	Diagnostics	Clinical signs	Treatment	Clinical notes	Other terms/comments
Ununited anconeal process (UAP)	German Shepherd Dogs, Bernese Mountain Dogs, and Mastiffs	Radiographs (after 4–5 months of age) sufficient – ideally CT to evaluate for MCD and incongruity	Pain on elbow manipulation (particularly hyperextension)	Surgical removal, reattachment ± ulna osteotomy or medical management	Ideally diagnose and treat prior to six months (greater chance of fusion of the UAP)	The Campbell's test is used to detect collateral ligament integrity (but also to detect pain in dogs with MCD)
Traumatic elbow luxation	Any	Radiographs	Non-weight-bearing lameness and severe pain	Closed or open reduction (if closed reduction fails or is contraindicated)	Dogs will hold limb in an abducted and externally rotated position	
Congenital elbow luxation	Juvenile small-breed (Type I) and large-breed (Type II) dogs	Radiographs (CT if surgery is performed)	Lameness and pain variable	Surgical or nonsurgical management	Generally have obvious abnormal bony conformation of elbow joint	
Panosteitis	Frequently seen in German Shepherd Dogs between 5 and 18 months of age	Radiographs (but may require CT during early stages) show intramedullary radiodensities	Pain on long bone palpation and shifting leg lameness	Rest and pain management	Disease should be self-limiting; if clinical symptoms continue in the same leg, further imaging should be considered	Other terms include eosinophilic panosteitis, juvenile osteomyelitis, and enostosis or medullary fibrosis
Septic arthritis	Postsurgical dogs and dogs with preexisting arthritis	Joint fluid analysis, culture, and physical exam findings	Moderate-to-severe pain on ROM, periarticular swelling, and pitting limb edema	Antibiotics and consider joint lavage	Dogs with preexisting joint disease (such as arthritis) are predisposed. A lack of fever or negative culture results do not rule out septic arthritis	
Flexor enthesopathy (FE)	Same as MCD	Radiographs may show calcification; however, ultrasound is required to diagnose noncalcified FE	Variable degree of lameness and pain upon palpation and stretching of flexor muscles	Address concomitant pathologies if present, nonsurgical management most common for primary form	Important to differentiate primary FE (i.e. no concomitant elbow pathology) and concomitant FE (i.e. together with, most commonly, MCD)	Other terms include ununited medial epicondyle and medial humeral condylar osteochondritis dissecans

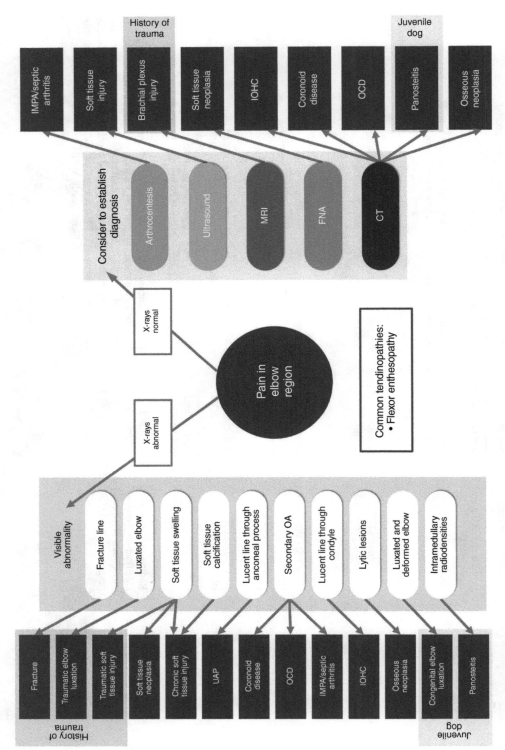

Figure 14.1   Schematic of common diseases affecting the elbow region and the steps necessary to establish a diagnosis.

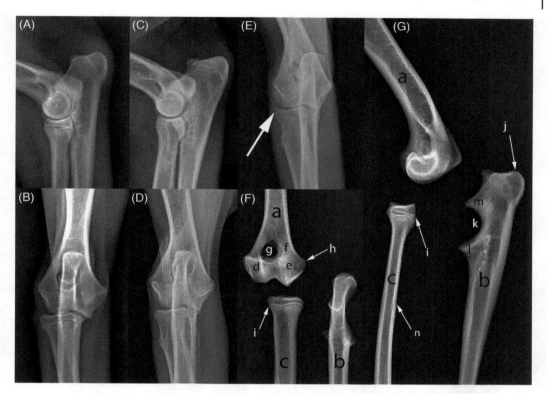

Figure 14.2   Normal anatomy of the elbow joint (Note: for all craniocaudal images, lateral is on the left): (A–E) radiographs of canine patients without elbow pathology; (A, B) note that the proximal radial physis is clearly visible in a 9-month-old dog; (C, D) note the appearance of the proximal radial physis in an adult dog; (E) note the sesamoid of the supinator muscle (white arrow), a normal structure that is visible in some dogs and should not be confused with a pathologic condition; and (F, G) normal anatomy of the bones contributing to the elbow joint: (a) humerus; (b) ulna; (c) radius; (d) lateral humeral condyle (=capitulum); (e) medial humeral condyle (=trochlea); (f) medial supracondylar crest; (g) olecranon fossa; (h) medial epicondyle; (i) proximal radial physis; (j) tuber olecranon; (k) trochlear notch; (l) coronoid process of the ulna; and (m) anconeal process.

the *supinator muscle* is present and can be identified radiographically (and should not be confused with a pathologic condition). The *coronoid process* of the ulna consists of a lateral and medial portion; pathology of the latter frequently results in lameness. It is in contact with the radius via the *radial incisure* (i.e. the notch of the ulna within which the radius can supinate and pronate). The *olecranon fossa*, located above the humeral condyles, accommodates the anconeal process during elbow extension. During development, a large apophysis (i.e. separate ossification center at site of tendon attachment) is visible at the tuber olecranon which should not be confused with a pathologic condition (e.g. fracture or ununited anconeal process [UAP]). The *triceps* muscle attaches at the tuber olecranon and is the major extender of the elbow joint. The *biceps* brachii muscle inserts on the radius and ulna and together with the brachialis muscle is one of the major flexors of the elbow joint. Normal range of motion (ROM) of the elbow joint is approximately 30–160° (Chapter 5). The digital *flexor and extensor muscles* originate from the area of the medial and lateral epicondyle, respectively. The *median and ulnar nerves* are located on the medial aspect of the elbow, with the ulnar nerve being superficial so that it can be palpated caudally. The *radial nerve* is located on the lateral aspect of the elbow.

Osteoarthritis (OA) of the elbow joint is generally thought to be the consequence of a primary problem such as elbow dysplasia (i.e. "secondary" osteoarthritis). One of the most common reasons for secondary osteoarthritis of the elbow joint is medial compartment disease (MCD). Reports of immune-mediated and infectious arthritis of the elbow joint exist (Chapter 13; Stull et al. 2008). Therefore, arthrocentesis and synovial fluid evaluation should be considered in cases where establishing a diagnosis is difficult.

14.3 Fractures of the Elbow Region

The most commonly observed fracture of the elbow region is a Salter-Harris Type IV of the lateral humeral condyle (Figure 14.3). These fractures are articular (Chapter 13 for review of Salter-Harris classification), and as such immediate surgical treatment is recommended. Typically, treatment for these fractures involves reducing them anatomically (i.e. perfect alignment of the joint surface is

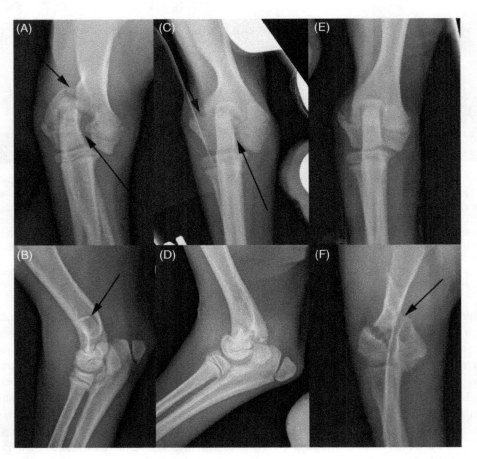

Figure 14.3 Examples of condylar fractures in three patients: *Patient I* (A, B) moderately displaced lateral condylar fracture. Note that the fracture lines are easily identified (black arrows) on the craniocaudal view, but difficult to identify on the lateral view; *Patient II* (C, D) minimally displaced lateral condylar fracture. While the fracture lines (black arrows) are visible on the craniocaudal view, the fracture is very difficult to identify on the lateral view. In such cases, comparing to the (E) normal, unaffected limb can be helpful; *Patient III* (F) Y-T fracture in an adult patient affecting both condyles (black arrow identifies the medial condylar fracture that is not present in the other two patients).

the goal) and stabilizing them with internal fixation utilizing a transcondylar lag screw in combination with pins or a plate (Perry et al. 2015). Medial humeral condylar fractures are observed less commonly but the diagnostic and treatment approaches are similar. If condylar fractures are observed in older animals, consideration should be given to incomplete ossification of the humeral condyle (IOHC) as an underlying disease. Less commonly observed fractures of the elbow region include Salter-Harris Type I fractures of the distal humerus and proximal radius, intercondylar (also described as T-Y fracture) and supracondylar fractures, as well as proximal ulna fractures with luxation of the radial head (i.e. Monteggia fracture).

14.3.1   Signalment and History

As for any fracture, trauma is the main cause which can happen to dogs of any age/signalment. However, fractures of the elbow region are frequently seen in immature dogs. In these patients, lateral humeral condylar fractures are most common because of the smaller-sized lateral (vs. medial) supracondylar crest (Figure 14.2). These fractures occur frequently in smaller breeds (with the French Bulldog being predisposed) and often occur with minor trauma. The peak age has been reported to be four months (Perry et al. 2015).

14.3.2   Physical Exam

Because of the acute nature of the injury, physical exam findings usually show severe pain upon elbow ROM. However, pain may present as less severe in stoic animals or when fractures are minimally displaced.

14.3.3   Diagnostics

Diagnosis of these fractures is readily accomplished with orthogonal radiographs, although the diagnosis can be missed if only a lateral view is taken (Figure 14.3).

14.4   Incomplete Ossification of the Humeral Condyle

IOHC is defined as failure of ossification of the lateral and medial aspects of the humeral condyle. This ossification should be completed during the first three months of growth, while the distal humeral physis (which is located proximally to the ossification centers) continues to grow until five to eight months. A lack of fusion of the medial and lateral condyles results in a fibrous band connecting the two parts of the condyle which creates a weak area predisposing for development of condylar fractures.

Recently, Farrell and others (2011) have reported that dogs may also suffer from a condition termed "progressive humeral intracondylar fissure (HIF)." The condition is very similar to IOHC; however, animals develop the separation of the condyles after normal ossification has occurred, thus indicating a fatigue fracture due to cyclic loading rather than a failure of fusion during development (Farrell et al. 2011). Because of the uncertainty about the difference in etiology, some authors use the term HIF to encompass both conditions, IOHC and stress fractures of the humeral condyle (Moores and Moores 2017).

Treatment of condylar fractures due to IOCH/HIF requires open reduction and surgical fixation like that used for traumatic condylar fractures. Ideally IOHC/HIF is identified prior to the patient

ELBOW REGION

developing a condylar fracture, in which case treatment is much simpler and associated with less cost and a better prognosis (Moores and Moores 2017). Treatment consists of surgical fixation across the condyles to prevent fracture development (Hattersley et al. 2011).

14.4.1 Signalment and History

Spaniel breeds are predisposed to IOHC (Moores et al. 2012), however, many other breeds (including Yorkshire Terriers, Labrador Retrievers, German Shepherd Dogs, Rottweilers, and Mastiff) may also be affected by this condition. Dogs typically present for lameness due to IOHC later in life with a peak age at presentation of three to four years. However, recent awareness of the condition (particularly in the United Kingdom) has allowed for earlier diagnosis prior to the patient showing clinical signs. Early clinical signs of lameness may result from micromovement of the condyles (without fracture), but if the condition remains undiagnosed, animals may present later with more acute lameness once condylar fractures occur (Figure 14.4; Witte et al. 2010). Therefore, the degree of lameness and acuity can be highly variable amongst the different patients presenting with this condition. Certain features of the patient history, taken together with the patient signalment, should alert the clinician to consider IOHC as an underlying cause when patients are presented with acute condylar fractures:

- Owners may have observed a lameness prior to the non-weight-bearing lameness associated with the fracture (prodromal lameness).
- Condylar fractures because of IOHC may occur after minimal trauma (similarly to condylar fractures in immature animals).

In such cases, diagnostics of the non-affected limb should be considered to evaluate whether prophylactic treatment should be considered (in addition to treating the affected limb).

14.4.2 Physical Exam

In patients with IOHC, pain is most pronounced with hyperextension of the elbow and in some cases upon palpation of the lateral epicondylar region. However, it is important to note that physical exam findings may be deceiving as in some cases, dogs with IOHC may possess normal ROM with no effusion, crepitus, or periarticular thickening (Butterworth and Innes 2001). Therefore, diagnostics should be recommended in any middle-aged Spaniel breed (or other predisposed breeds) with undiagnosed lameness even in face of a normal elbow examination.

14.4.3 Diagnostics

Diagnosing IOHC can be challenging and may require advanced imaging. Radiographs may show a radiolucent line extending through the condyles or a smooth proliferation along the lateral supracondylar crest indicating stress remodeling (Figure 14.4) of this area due to instability of the condyles (Marcellin-Little et al. 1994). If such findings are not observed, IOHC or HIF may not be ruled out and advanced imaging should be considered as the next step. It is most common to use CT, although MRI has also been reported (Piola et al. 2012). Since IOHC is bilateral in ~25% of the dogs, both limbs should be evaluated. This is easily accomplished using CT, thus making it the ideal imaging modality. Bilateral radiographs may be considered instead if CT is unavailable, recognizing that some lesions may be missed since the radiographic beam must be parallel to the fissure line to accomplish a diagnosis. Therefore, oblique radiographs (including a 15° craniomedial caudolateral view) should be performed if radiographs are used as the sole diagnostic tool (Hattersley et al. 2011).

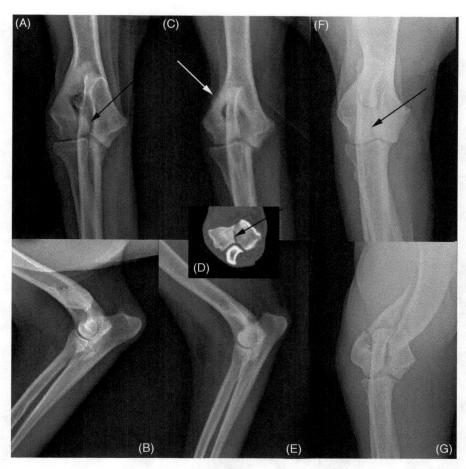

Figure 14.4   IOHC examples: *Patient I* (A, B) was diagnosed on radiographs with IOHC based on observation of a radiolucent line across the condylar area (black arrow); *Patient II* (C–E) was definitively diagnosed via CT as illustrated in (D) (black arrow) which was recommended after noting (C) smooth periosteal proliferation of the lateral supracondylar crest that is indicative of IOHC (white arrow); patients I and II underwent prophylactic transcondylar lag screw fixation without complications; *Patient III* (F, G): upon initial presentation, (F) the diagnosis of IOHC/HIF (black arrow) was missed and the condition progressed (G) to a Y-T fracture, illustrating the importance of careful evaluation of radiographs/the importance of pursuing advanced imaging.

14.5   Elbow Dysplasia/Incongruity

Elbow dysplasia (ED), also termed "developmental elbow disease," was defined as UAP, fragmented coronoid process (FCP), osteochondrosis dissecans (OCD), and incongruity by the International Elbow Working Group over 25 years ago (Michelsen 2013). However, the terminology has since changed particularly for FCP, and incongruity is now considered a contributing feature to the other three components of ED rather than an independent disease (Michelsen 2013). The following two types of incongruities (Figure 14.5) have been most commonly proposed to play a role in the pathophysiology of ED:

- Radioulnar incongruity – this incongruity describes a mismatch between the radius and ulna resulting in a step at the radioulnar joint. If the radius is shorter than the ulna, excessive pressure is placed on the coronoid process resulting in excessive loading and subsequent pathologic

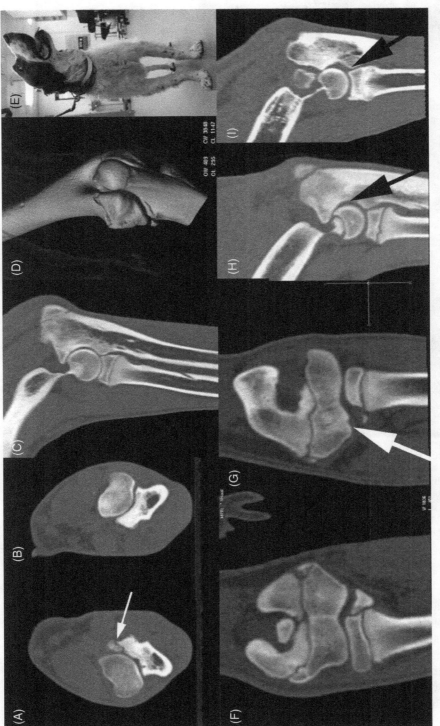

Figure 14.5 Elbow dysplasia CT: (A) transverse plane reconstruction; large fragment of the medial coronoid process and mild radioulnar incisure incongruity in a dog with medial compartment disease (MCD); (B) transverse plane reconstruction; normal appearance of the coronoid process; (C) sagittal plane reconstruction; congruent elbow; (D) 3D reconstruction; appearance of a fragment of the medial coronoid process; (E) typical bow-legged stance with external rotation of the limb in a clinical patient with chronic MCD; (F) dorsal plane reconstruction; normal appearance of the medial aspect of the humeral condyle; (G) dorsal plane reconstruction; the defect (white arrow) and subchondral sclerosis are consistent with OCD; (H) sagittal plane reconstruction; humeroulnar (notch) incongruity (black arrow); and (I) sagittal plane reconstruction; radioulnar incongruity (black arrow) resulting in UAP.

changes. In contrast, if the radius is longer than the ulna, excessive pressure is placed on the anconeal process which may result in lack of fusion of the process. These incongruities are generally subtle and consequently CT or arthroscopy is necessary to make the diagnosis of incongruity. Specific knowledge of the type of incongruity aids the treatment decision and therefore is highly valuable. These two types of incongruity may also be secondary to premature growth plate closures (i.e. short ulna = premature closure of the distal ulna physis; short radius = premature closure of either the proximal or distal radius physis). In cases where the degree of incongruity is severe, radiography is useful to detect which incongruity scenario applies.

- Humeroulnar incongruity – this incongruity describes either a mismatch between the ulna notch and the humeral trochlea or displacement of the humerus from the ulnar notch because of a long radius. CT or arthroscopy is preferred to make the diagnosis of humeroulnar incongruity, although in severe cases radiographs can be diagnostic.

Many other mechanisms for the pathophysiology of ED have been described, such as radioulnar incisure incongruity (i.e. a misshapen radial incisure that results in increased pressure on the coronoid; Figure 14.5), as well as excessive pressure on the coronoid because of traction forces caused by the biceps muscle (that attaches medially at the proximal ulna; Michelsen 2013). However, the influence that the different types of incongruities have on the development of ED is still being investigated. Further, it is important to understand that not every dog with ED will have detectable evidence of incongruity, even when advanced imaging is used. This can be explained by the inability of commonly used diagnostic modalities to identify dynamic (i.e. movement during motion) incongruity. Alternatively, transient incongruity (i.e. incongruity during development) may have resolved by the time imaging is performed.

ED results in debilitating elbow arthritis and since many animals are affected bilaterally, it poses one of the greatest treatment challenges in small animal orthopedics – amputation may not be a feasible option and function after successful elbow arthrodesis is questionable due to substantial mechanical lameness (Coppieters et al. 2015). Therefore, treatment decisions should carefully weigh the potential risks against short- and long-term benefit of any intervention. Because most animals with ED will develop a considerable amount of arthritis during their life span, lifelong medical management should be part of the treatment plan for any dog with ED.

14.6 Medial Compartment Disease

The terminology "fragmented medial coronoid process (FCP)" is used to describe fragmentation of the medial aspect of the coronoid process of the ulna (Figure 14.5A). This terminology is less commonly used nowadays since the pathologic changes encompass far more than pathology of the coronoid process. Such changes include disseminated cartilage and subchondral bone pathology of the entire joint, particularly the medial compartment resulting in variable degrees of lameness (Video 14.1). Therefore, some authors have used the term "(medial) coronoid disease." However, because some dogs may experience erosion of the medial compartment without fissuring or fragmentation of the coronoid process (Coppieters et al. 2015), "medial compartment disease" (MCD) is the currently preferred term to describe this condition (Michelsen 2013).

Video 14.1

Clinical lameness and conformation with elbow arthritis/dysplasia.

Treatment of MCD frequently includes arthroscopic debridement, although surgical treatment has been questioned by some since arthritis progression is expected even with surgical intervention (Burton et al. 2011; Barthélémy et al. 2014; Dempsey et al. 2019). Others have concluded that arthroscopy is superior to medical management and treatment via arthrotomy (Evans et al. 2008). The lack of definitive information regarding the ideal treatment is likely related to a lack of objective outcome measures and the wide variability seen with the disease complex of MCD (Fitzpatrick and Yeadon 2009). If traditional medical management is exhausted, novel treatment options such as joint injections, elbow resurfacing, load-shifting procedures, or total elbow replacement may therefore be considered despite a lack of sufficient long-term data to support their use (Coppieters et al. 2015).

14.6.1 Signalment and History

MCD is considered a developmental disease and diagnosed most commonly in juvenile patients. Nonetheless, some patients may not present until later in life when symptoms arise due to secondary elbow osteoarthritis. Large-/giant-breeds are predisposed, with Labrador Retrievers and Bernese Mountain Dogs most frequently affected. However, the disease has also been reported in smaller dogs (such as Dachshund and French Bulldog).

14.6.2 Physical Exam

Diagnosis of MCD is usually based on the following features: reduced ROM, discomfort on hyperflexion and -extension, joint effusion, and periarticular swelling (in chronic cases with secondary degenerative changes). Patients with MCD attempt to redirect the forces to the lateral compartment (to off-load the medial compartment), resulting in a typical bow-legged stance with external rotation of the limb (Figure 14.5E). Although it is not always palpable, joint effusion can be identified caudal to the humeral epicondyles (Figure 14.6). Diagnosis of MCD based on a pain response is difficult since some patients appear to show little to no response to palpation. To increase the odds of eliciting a pain response, the elbow should be evaluated during flexion, during hyperextension, and while performing a manipulation known as the "Campbell's test." This test was originally developed for detection of collateral ligament disruption (Farrell et al. 2007), but it can be particularly useful when screening for ED in young animals since other features of chronic elbow OA (e.g. periarticular swelling, reduced ROM, etc.) may not be present. For this test, the limb is pronated and supinated while keeping the carpus and elbow flexed at approximately 90° while applying gentle pressure at the area of the medial aspect of the coronoid process. This area is located approximately 1 cm distal to the medial epicondyle (which is easily palpated when the elbow is extended) in large-breed dogs. Hyperextension of the joint is performed by pushing cranially at the level of the elbow joint while keeping the shoulder in a consistent position (i.e. the ROM of the shoulder should not change when the elbow is extended). Pain on flexion can be tested while the animal is standing by simply flexing the elbow joint and evaluating for symptoms of pain and whether the dog "moves" away and hops towards the contralateral side (Videos 14.2 and 3.1).

Video 14.2

Clinical exams of elbow examination for detection of elbow pathology and how to differentiate elbow from shoulder pain.

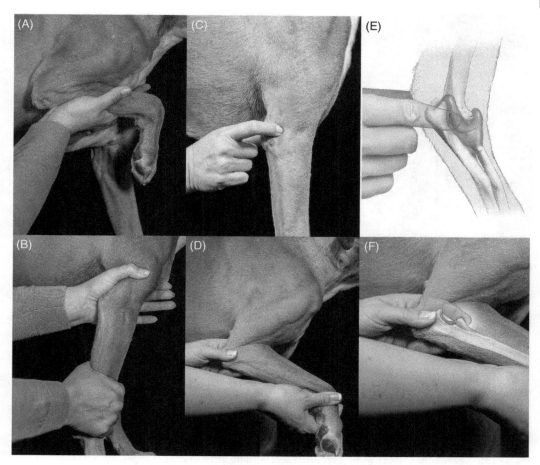

Figure 14.6   Examination to detect elbow dysplasia: (A) flexion of the elbow; (B) isolated hyperextension of the elbow without hyperextension of the shoulder; (C, E) palpation of joint effusion caudal to the humeral epicondyles; (D, F) the "Campbell's test" is performed by pronating and supinating the limb while keeping the carpus and elbow flexed at approximately 90° and applying gentle pressure to the area of the medial aspect of the coronoid process.

14.6.3   Diagnostics

Unfortunately, establishing a diagnosis in the juvenile patient frequently requires advanced imaging since radiographs may only show subtle changes. Such changes may include sclerosis of the ulnar trochlear notch, an indistinct coronoid process, incongruity, and mild degenerative changes (Figure 14.7). Once osteoarthritis is established, the diagnosis is easily accomplished with radiography. Although a CT is generally recommended in juvenile patients to accomplish a diagnosis, it is important to consider that even this modality is not 100% accurate with a reported specificity of 85–93% (Groth et al. 2009; Villamonte-Chevalier et al. 2015). Hence, the diagnosis of MCD may require arthroscopy in addition to CT, particularly for cases that are suffering from cartilage changes only (Coppieters et al. 2015). Additional diagnostic steps may include intra-articular injection of mepivacaine (Chapter 8). This diagnostic tool is helpful if a positive effect is observed (i.e. to confirm the diagnosis of ED) but has been shown to have an approximately 10% chance of false-negative results (Van Vynckt et al. 2012).

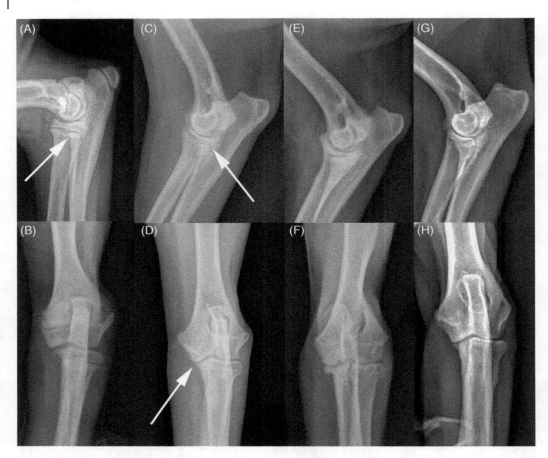

Figure 14.7   Examples of MCD: (A, B) juvenile patient with no degenerative changes, the only subtle abnormality is the lack of a clear distinction of the coronoid process on the lateral view (white arrow); (C, D) 11-month-old dog with mild sclerosis (C; lateral view, white arrow) and irregularity in the area of the medial coronoid process (D; craniocaudal view and white arrow); (E, F) adult dog with degenerative changes secondary to MCD; (G, H) 7-year-old dog with normal-appearing radiographs that was diagnosed with traumatic fracture of the medial coronoid process based on CT.

14.7   Traumatic Fracture of the Medial Coronoid Process

Fragmentation of the coronoid process has also been described in adult patients without degenerative changes (Meyer-Lindenberg et al. 2002; Tan et al. 2016). Termed "traumatic fracture of the medial coronoid process," this presentation is also referred to as "adult-onset FCP" or "jump-down syndrome" (Tan et al. 2016). This disease has been proposed to be associated with traumatic descents or concussive activities such as agility or fly ball. It is unknown to date whether these patients suffer from nonclinical, developmental ED prior to the traumatic event or whether the disease is exclusively traumatic in origin. Regardless of the etiology, it is important to note that adult dogs can suffer from coronoid disease even if radiographs are normal (Figure 14.7). Establishing a diagnosis follows the same diagnostic pathway as for juvenile dogs with MCD (i.e. CT and/or arthroscopy). Treatment with arthroscopic fragment removal carries a good prognosis based on the limited information available (Tan et al. 2016).

14.8   Osteochondrosis Dissecans

Osteochondrosis/osteochondritis dissecans (OCD) of the elbow joint affects the medial humeral condyle (trochlea). In contrast to OCD lesions of other joints, elbow OCD is frequently diagnosed together with MCD. Similar to OCD lesions in other joints, OCD of the elbow is the consequence of an endochondral ossification failure resulting in excessive thickness of the cartilage that may detach (and develop a flap). Cartilage pathology affecting the trochlea may also develop secondary to a mismatch between the humerus and ulna, as well as from erosion from the opposing coronoid pathology. Such lesions are termed "kissing lesions" and can be difficult to distinguish from true OCD lesions in some cases (Cook and Cook 2009). Although OCD of the elbow can sometimes be identified with radiography, most often CT (Figure 14.5) or arthroscopy is used to establish a final diagnosis. The use of these technologies also allows to identify concurrent incongruity and coronoid pathology. Because the prognosis for elbow OCD is questionable, treatment is somewhat controversial, with most authors recommending surgical debridement of the lesion (and addressing concurrent elbow pathology if indicated).

14.9   Ununited Anconeal Process

Failure of fusion of the ossification center of the anconeal process is defined as UAP. The pathophysiology of UAP is unclear, but premature distal ulnar physis closure frequently results in UAP indicating that radioulnar incongruity may play a substantial role. Ossification of the anconeal process should be completed by 20 weeks during normal development, although fusion frequently occurs earlier. UAP has been reported to occur together with MCD in 16% of the cases (Meyer-Lindenberg et al. 2006). A wide variety of treatment options are available including ulnar osteotomy procedures, lag screw fixation, or removal of the anconeal process.

14.9.1   Signalment and History

Any large-/giant-breed dog is susceptible to UAP, especially German Shepherd Dogs, Bernese Mountain Dogs, and Mastiffs. Nevertheless, even small dog breeds, including French Bulldogs and Dachshunds, have been diagnosed with UAP. Animals with unilateral disease usually present before they reach maturity. Bilateral disease, which is present in 20–25% of the cases, may make the lameness harder to identify for owners and hence these animals may present later in life due to advanced degenerative disease (Cross and Chambers 1997).

14.9.2   Physical Exam

Dogs with UAP generally have more obvious physical exam findings compared to dogs presenting with MCD. Significant joint effusion is generally palpable, and pain is most evident with hyperextension of the joint.

14.9.3   Diagnostics

In contrast to the other forms of ED, UAP is easily diagnosed with radiographs. If a lack of anconeal fusion is observed after 20 weeks of age, the diagnosis is confirmed (Figure 14.8). The flexed lateral radiographic view (Figure 14.8A) eliminates superimposition of the anconeal process and

ELBOW REGION

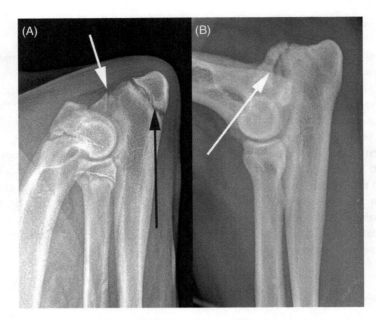

Figure 14.8 UAP: (A) 7-month-old dog with UAP (white arrow); the black arrow indicates the normal appearance of the apophysis of the tuber olecranon; (B) 12-month-old dog with UAP (white arrow) – note the different appearance compared to the patient shown in image (A).

the humerus, thereby simplifying observation of the radiolucent line separating the anconeal process. However, since the treatment recommendations differ if concurrent incongruity and MCD are diagnosed, a CT is generally recommended if available.

14.10 Elbow Luxation

Elbow luxation is categorized into traumatic and congenital etiologies. It is important to differentiate the two etiologies since treatment and prognosis differ greatly. Treatment for traumatic elbow luxations (TELs) generally consists of immediate closed reduction (if no articular fractures or chronic degenerative changes are present). Open (surgical) reduction is performed if closed reduction fails. On the other hand, congenital elbow luxations (CELs) cannot be treated with closed reduction since the osseous and soft tissue anatomy is altered. Treatment options for CEL include surgical and non-surgical management depending on clinical factors and type of luxation (Figure 14.9). CEL can be categorized into three forms: *Type I* is defined as caudolateral luxation of the radial head without disruption of the humeroulnar joint (i.e. the ulna is in a normal position); *Type II* is defined as a lateral rotation and subluxation of the ulna; *Type III* is associated with severe skeletal deformities and defined as luxation of radius and ulna. Outlined below are the diagnostic criteria and features of both TEL and CEL etiologies to assist the reader in differentiating between them.

14.10.1 Signalment and History

TEL is most commonly a result from vehicular accidents or falls and, therefore, can happen in dogs of any signalment. Congenital luxations are generally seen in juvenile animals, although mild forms may not present clinically until later in life. Type I luxation more typically manifests

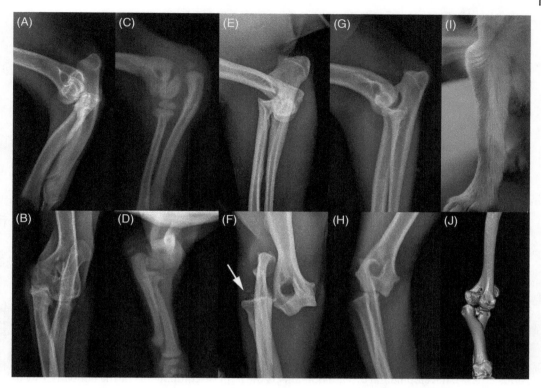

Figure 14.9   Elbow luxation: (A, B) Type I congenital elbow luxation (caudolateral luxation of the radial head); (C, D) Type II congenital elbow luxation (lateral rotation and subluxation of the ulna); (E, F) traumatic, lateral elbow luxation (note the collateral ligament avulsion fragments, white arrow); (G, H) traumatic, lateral subluxation of the elbow; and (I, J) clinical picture and 3D-CT reconstruction of the patient shown in images (A, B).

in large-breed dogs but is also described in Yorkshire Terriers. Type II luxations occur more often in small-breed dogs (Rahal et al. 2000). Of the three variants of CEL, Type III luxation occurs less frequently and is poorly described, but it is known to occur in small-breed dogs with a case study in Cavalier King Charles Spaniel reported (McDonell 2004).

14.10.2   Physical Exam

TELs are generally associated with severe pain and non-weight-bearing lameness. Most TELs are lateral (i.e. the radius and ulna are lateral to the humerus) because of the larger-sized and distally sloped trochlea (medial humeral condyle; Figure 14.2) making the radial head easily palpable and the lateral epicondyle less distinct. Patients with lateral TEL present with their limb in an abducted and externally rotated position. Congenital luxations may cause various degrees of lameness and degrees of pain. Depending on the severity and chronicity, limited ROM and crepitus may be present. Palpation of the elbow (for both types) allows palpation of the abnormal/displaced anatomic structures. In extension, the anconeal process is located within the olecranon fossa, making the elbow inherently stable. When the elbow is flexed, Campbell's test can be used to evaluate the integrity of the medial and lateral collateral ligament. This is done by flexing the elbow and carpus to 90° and evaluating the maximum angles of pronation (testing medial collateral ligament integrity) and supination (testing lateral collateral ligament). Normal values for Campbell's test have been described to change pronation from approximately 30–60° after transection of the medial collateral ligament and supination from approximately 45–70° after transection of the lateral collateral ligament. However, a large inter-animal variation was also reported (Farrell et al. 2007). Therefore, comparison to the contralateral limb is recommended. NOTE: this test is also used to evaluate for a pain response in dogs with ED as discussed in Section 14.6.2.

14.10.3   Diagnostics

Elbow luxations (congenital and traumatic) are generally suspected based on history (for traumatic luxations) and palpation; the diagnosis is easily confirmed via radiography. For TEL, craniocaudal projections clearly show displacement of the radius/ulna while lateral projections may be less obvious. The observer should also evaluate the radiographs for evidence of chronic changes (such as osteoarthritis) or avulsion fragments of the collateral ligament (Figure 14.9F) or other fractures since these findings may pose a contraindication for closed reduction and require surgical intervention. For CEL, radiographic changes vary based on the type of luxation and severity. If surgical treatment is planned, further imaging (CT) may be indicated to assess the integrity of the coronoid process and degree of elbow incongruity, and to aid in surgical planning.

14.11   Panosteitis

Panosteitis is a developmental disease that affects the adipose components of the bone marrow of long bones. The disease has also been reported in the literature as eosinophilic panosteitis, juvenile osteomyelitis, as well as enostosis (i.e. medullary fibrosis). Histologically, the disease cycles through a phase where adipose bone marrow is replaced with osseous tissue followed by regeneration of the bone marrow to its original constitution. The disease was once thought to be of bacterial or viral origin; however, currently the etiology is controversial, and newer theories have included an association with high-protein diets and osseous compartment syndrome (Schawalder et al. 2002). Moreover, the high incidence in German Shepherd Dogs suggests a genetic component. The disease is self-limiting and generally not associated with systemic signs. Treatment consists of rest and pain management.

14.11.1   Signalment and History

Dogs affected with panosteitis most commonly present symptomatically between 5 and 18 months of age, although the disease has been reported in patients up to 5 years of age. Lameness can be of varying degrees of severity and may affect one or multiple limbs simultaneously or sequentially since the disease frequently affects multiple bones (Bohning et al. 1970). The latter explains one of the hallmark signs of panosteitis, a lameness that shifts from one leg to another. Since the disease is self-limiting, owners may also report that the symptoms resolved without treatment. Recurrence may occur, yet in most cases subsequent episodes are less severe. Panosteitis is seen most frequently in German Shepherds (with a male predisposition), although many other large/giant breeds and even small-breed dogs are reported to be affected. As such, the disease should be considered a differential for any juvenile dog presented with shifting leg lameness (Towle-Millard and Breur 2018).

14.11.2   Physical Exam

Panosteitis can affect all long bones, most commonly the bones of the elbow region (radius, ulna, and humerus) followed by bones of the stifle region (Towle-Millard and Breur 2018). These long bones should be carefully evaluated for pain upon deep palpation. When performing long bone palpation, it is important to be aware of the local anatomy, since compression of the nerves may result in a false-positive pain response. The disease starts in the location of the nutrient foramina; however, the entire diaphysis and areas of the metaphysis can be affected. Physical exam should also evaluate for any concomitant disease (such as ED).

14.11.3   Diagnostics

Radiographs are used most frequently to confirm the clinical suspicion of panosteitis. Radiographic changes vary depending on the stages of the disease and are most visible in the location of the nutrient foramina. During the early stages, a decreased radiodensity of the medullary cavity has been reported (Towle-Millard and Breur 2018). However, the hallmark feature of panosteitis is an intramedullary increase in radiodensity (Figure 14.10) since the early stages are frequently missed. Specific lesions include opacities of the medullary canal (these can be well demarcated or diffuse, i.e. "medullary blurring"), loss of normal trabecular pattern (i.e. "trabecular coarsening"), and changes to the endosteum (the layer that lines the medullary cavity, i.e. "endosteal roughening;" Stead et al. 1983).

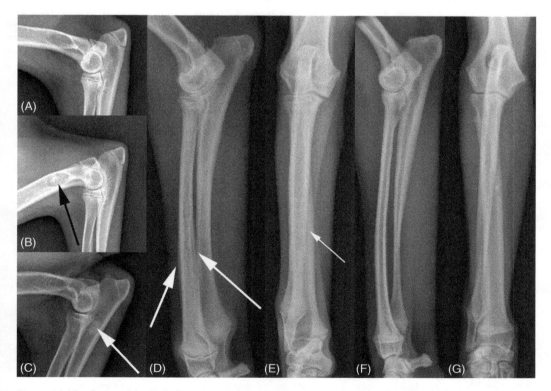

Figure 14.10   Panosteitis: (A, F, G) normal radiographs for comparison; (B–E) radiographs consistent with panosteitis illustrating the variable radiographic appearance of this disease: (B) increased intramedullary opacity and loss of trabecular pattern (black arrow); (C) well-demarcated intramedullary opacity (white arrow); and (D, E) endosteal roughening and diffuse intramedullary opacities (white arrows).

ELBOW REGION

Early stages of the disease may not be detectable with radiography. If panosteitis is suspected, yet no radiographic changes are evident, advanced imaging such as CT or nuclear scintigraphy may be utilized. Alternatively, repeat radiographs in two to four weeks in combination with an improvement in clinical symptoms may verify the diagnosis.

14.12   Septic Arthritis

Septic (or infectious) arthritis results from one of three general mechanisms: direct introduction (i.e. via surgery or trauma), hematogenous seeding, or local spread of infectious organisms into the synovium/joint space. Regardless of the mechanism, the most common cause of infection is bacterial. However, fungal, protozoal, mycoplasmal, mycobacterial, and rickettsial infections have all been reported and should therefore be considered as differential diagnoses particularly if treatment with antibiotics is unsuccessful. Since lameness associated with septic arthritis requires a change of the treatment plan, it is an important differential diagnosis to consider.

Septic arthritis resulting from direct introduction via surgery is probably the most common form of septic arthritis in dogs, yet the incidence is fairly low (approximately 1–5%). The stifle, elbow, and carpus have been reported to be most commonly affected.

Hematogenous septic arthritis is likely the second most common form of septic arthritis in dogs. Two different types have been described: a juvenile form in dogs <1 year of age (Fitch et al. 2003) and an adult form, recently also termed "spontaneous septic arthritis," that is described in middle-aged dogs with preexisting joint disease (e.g. osteoarthritis; Benzioni et al. 2008; Mielke et al. 2018). Regardless of the type, in small animals with hematogenous septic arthritis, most often a single joint is affected. The juvenile form appears to be rare, but large-/giant-breed dogs appear predisposed and the elbow is most frequently affected (Fitch et al. 2003). Spontaneous septic arthritis of both the elbow and hip joint has been described (Benzioni et al. 2008; Mielke et al. 2018). It is unknown why preexisting joint disease predisposes to hematogenous spread to the joint, although, increased synovial vascularity/blood flow due to chronic osteoarthritis may ease hematogenous introduction of bacteria into the joint (Clements et al. 2005).

Joint infection causes local inflammation followed by release of catabolic enzymes and loss of glycosaminoglycan resulting in further deterioration of the joint. As such, early intervention including at least joint aspiration, culture, and antibiotic therapy should be instituted as soon as possible. Other treatment options such as joint irrigation, arthroscopic debridement/lavage, and local antibiotics may also be considered.

14.12.1   Signalment and History

Most dogs with septic arthritis have a history of surgical intervention, trauma, or previous osteoarthritis in the affected joint. Particularly in the latter case, it can be difficult for owners to differentiate infection from the variable severity of clinical signs associated with osteoarthritis. Dogs presenting for septic arthritis after surgery can be of any age and breed. Infection after surgery is observed frequently during the early postoperative phase but may also be seen months–years after surgery with low-grade infections. Dogs with septic arthritis secondary to chronic osteoarthritis are frequently middle-aged to older medium large-breed dogs (Clements et al. 2005; Milgram et al. 2018). If acute worsening of a dog with previously diagnosed osteoarthritis is observed, spontaneous septic arthritis should be considered an important differential diagnosis.

14.12.2 Physical Exam

Lameness associated with septic arthritis is generally severe and associated with substantial pain upon joint manipulation. Periarticular joint swelling (in severe cases pitting edema) and local heat is common and can be severe at times (Video 14.3). Other symptoms associated with postsurgical septic arthritis may include discharge (varying from serous purulent) from the incision site, licking of the surgical site, or exposure of the implant. Some animals present with pyrexia and/or local lymphadenopathy; however, a lack of either or both does not rule out septic arthritis as a diagnosis.

> **Video 14.3**
>
>
>
> Clinical presentation of septic elbow arthritis mimicking a neurologic problem.

14.12.3 Diagnostics

A diagnosis of septic arthritis is made based on a combination of clinical symptoms, physical exam findings, cytology, and joint fluid culture. However, cytologic findings in septic arthritis vary (Chapter 9) and rarely show the pathognomonic finding of intracellular bacteria. Similarly, a negative culture has been reported in up to 50% of dogs with septic arthritis (Clements et al. 2005). Therefore, because some cases with suspected septic arthritis may not be diagnosed definitively, response to antibiotic therapy may be used to solidify a tentative diagnosis.

Radiographs may be used to diagnose chronic changes associated with ongoing septic arthritis. Such changes may include secondary degenerative or erosive changes and signs of osteomyelitis (Figure 14.12C). For some joints (such as stifle), substantial joint effusion can be seen radiographically and be a helpful indicator of intra-articular disease.

14.13 Flexor Enthesopathy

Flexor enthesopathy (FE) is defined as pathologic changes of the flexor muscles originating at the medial epicondyle of the humerus (De Bakker et al. 2012). The disease has previously been reported under the names ununited medial epicondyle and medial humeral condylar osteochondritis dissecans. This disease can be a single disease entity (primary FE) or may occur together with other elbow pathologies such as MCD (concomitant or secondary FE). Treatment of the primary form focuses on treating the affected muscles while the concomitant form is frequently treated by addressing the concomitant pathologies (De Bakker et al. 2013).

14.13.1 Signalment and History

FE has been described in several large medium-sized breeds. The incidence has been reported to be 15% in nonclinical Labrador Retrievers (Paster et al. 2009) and 40% in dogs presented for lameness thought to be due to elbow pathology (De Bakker et al. 2012).

14.13.2 Physical Exam

Palpation of the origin of the flexor muscles may reveal thickening and occasionally the calcified bodies can be palpable. Pain upon stretching of the flexor muscles (carpal extension while flexing the elbow; Chapter 5) may be elicited, while hyperextension of the elbow joint is non-painful with the primary form. Medial compartment palpation may indicate MCD (i.e. indicating the secondary form of FE; Section 14.6).

14.13.3 Diagnostics

A diagnosis of FE can be made if radiographs show calcification in the area of the medial epicondyle (Figure 14.11). However, radiographs do not always allow to differentiate primary from concomitant FE. For this purpose, CT is generally recommended in dogs with radiographic evidence of FE to evaluate for MCD. Arthroscopy can be used to evaluate the origin of the flexor muscles, nonetheless in one study it was unable to allow differentiation of the two forms (De Bakker et al. 2013). If no radiographic calcification is present, ultrasound is a useful tool to identify

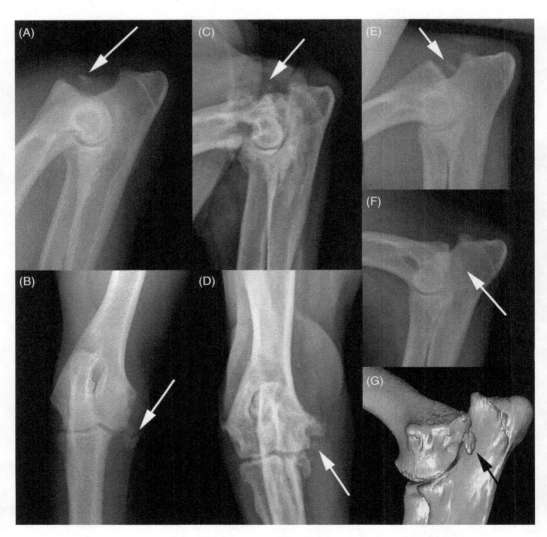

Figure 14.11 Flexor enthesopathy (FE): (A, B) primary FE (white arrow); (C, D) concomitant FE with MCD resulting in severe osteoarthritis; (E, F) primary FE, note the difficulty in identifying the calcification if it is superimposed over other osseous structures (F, white arrow); (G) primary FE calcification (black arrow) in 3D reconstruction of a CT.

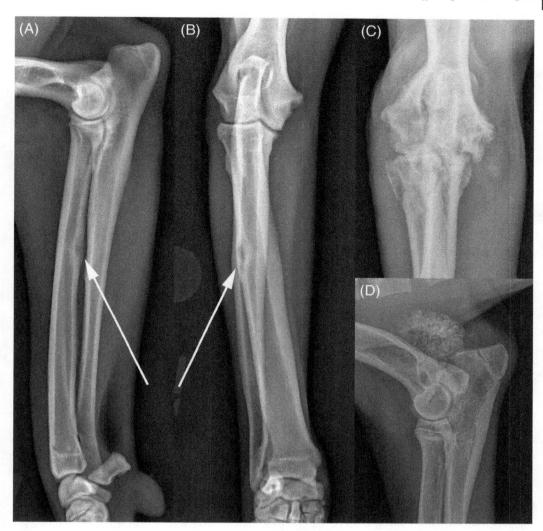

Figure 14.12   Other diseases affecting the elbow region: (A, B) radioulnar ischemic necrosis (RUIN), note the focal, ill-defined cortical lucency and adjacent endosteal bone formation (white arrows); (C) severe osseous remodeling and soft tissue swelling in a dog with chronic, septic arthritis. The visible changes could also be consistent with a synovial neoplasm; (D) calcinosis circumscripta.

smaller areas of calcification or structural abnormalities of the flexor muscles. Other reported imaging modalities for the differentiation of FE include MRI, HisPECT, and scintigraphy.

14.14   Other Diseases Affecting the Elbow Region

14.14.1   Calcinosis Circumscripta

Calcinosis circumscripta (also termed tumoral calcinosis; Figure 14.12D) is defined as ectopic deposition of calcium salts resulting in formation of mineralization in the soft tissues (Tafti et al. 2005). The condition has been described in young large-breed dogs with the German Shepherd

Dog apparently predisposed. Lesions may occur anywhere in the body, with the pelvic limb and tongue most commonly affected (Tafti et al. 2005). Recently a case report described calcification of the triceps muscle in a Rottweiler (Tambella et al. 2013).

Mineralization occurs because of deposition of serum calcium areas of tissue damage due to trauma (including surgical intervention), necrosis, inflammation, or neoplasia. The patient should be evaluated for elevated calcium levels and screened for neoplasia. Surgical excision has been reported.

In people, a similar well-recognized condition, heterotopic ossification (defined as the formation of ectopic lamellar bone in soft tissues), is categorized as traumatic, neurogenic, and genetic (Balboni et al. 2006).

14.14.2 Radioulnar Ischemic Necrosis

Radioulnar ischemic necrosis (RUIN) (Figures 14.12A, B) describes an osteolytic lesion at the level of the interosseous ligament (Lisbeth et al. 2018). The disease has been described in a Jack Russell Terrier and Golden Retriever (Deffontaines et al. 2016), although the authors have seen this finding in several other breeds. Although the etiology is unknown, tearing of the ligament with secondary desmitis/enthesiopathy and potential ischemia is suspected. This condition is an important differential diagnosis since presence of the osteolytic lesion may rise suspicion of fungal or neoplastic disease. The location at the radioulnar ligament is key for differentiation of these from RUIN. In both reported cases, the patients presented with a thoracic limb lameness that resolved after treatment (nonsurgical or ulna ostectomy).

14.14.3 Triceps Tendon Disruption

Rupture or avulsion of the triceps tendon has been described in approximately 20 cases in the veterinary literature (Earley et al. 2018), with most of these dogs presenting with a history of trauma. In addition, prior surgery or steroid administration has also been reported. The most frequently reported treatment consists of surgical repair followed by immobilization of the elbow with a trans-articular fixator or splint. Important differential diagnoses include a fracture of the olecranon or soft tissue neoplasia weakening the muscle predisposing it to rupture. Therefore, diagnostics should include at least radiographs and ideally ultrasound to evaluate the muscle for structural abnormalities inconsistent with a traumatic rupture. Advanced imaging such as MRI has also been reported.

14.14.4 Elbow Region Neoplasia

Neoplasia of the elbow region is observed infrequently. Nonetheless, tumors of the synovium and triceps muscle should be considered as differential diagnoses. Both are difficult to diagnose with radiography and therefore additional imaging and/or diagnostics should be considered if neoplasia is suspected. Further details about neoplastic conditions affecting the region are provided in Chapters 11 and 17.

14.14.5 Miscellaneous Other Conditions

Other rare causes of lameness associated with pathology in the elbow region include a subchondral bone cyst of the ulnar trochlear notch (Makielski et al. 2015); bilateral bone cysts affecting the humeral condyles (Choate and Arnold 2011); and ossifying myositis of the extensor carpi radialis origin (Morton et al. 2015). Brachial plexus avulsion (Chapter 16) may be confused with disease of the elbow region. The author has diagnosed insertional biceps tendinopathy, although this has not been reported in peer-reviewed literature.

References

Balboni, T.A., Gobezie, R., and Mamon, H.J. (2006). Heterotopic ossification: pathophysiology, clinical features, and the role of radiotherapy for prophylaxis. *Int J Radiat Oncol Biol Phys* 65 (5): 1289–1299.

Barthélémy, N.P., Griffon, D.J., Ragetly, G.R. et al. (2014). Short- and long-term outcomes after arthroscopic treatment of young large breed dogs with medial compartment disease of the elbow. *Vet Surg* 43 (8): 935–943.

Benzioni, H., Shahar, R., Yudelevitch, S., and Milgram, J. (2008). Bacterial infective arthritis of the coxofemoral joint in dogs with hip dysplasia. *Vet Comp Orthop Traumatol* 21 (3): 262–266.

Bohning, R.H. Jr., Suter, P.F., Hohn, R.B., and Marshall, J. (1970). Clinical and radiologic survey of canine panosteitis. *J Am Vet Med Assoc* 156 (7): 870–883.

Burton, N.J., Owen, M.R., Kirk, L.S. et al. (2011). Conservative versus arthroscopic management for medial coronoid process disease in dogs: a prospective gait evaluation. *Vet Surg* 40 (8): 972–980.

Butterworth, S.J. and Innes, J.F. (2001). Incomplete humeral condylar fractures in the dog. *J Small Anim Pract* 42 (8): 394–398.

Choate, C.J. and Arnold, G.A. (2011). Elbow arthrodesis following a pathological fracture in a dog with bilateral humeral bone cysts. *Vet Comp Orthop Traumatol* 24 (5): 398–401.

Clements, D.N., Owen, M.R., Mosley, J.R. et al. (2005). Retrospective study of bacterial infective arthritis in 31 dogs. *J Small Anim Pract* 46 (4): 171–176.

Cook, C.R. and Cook, J.L. (2009). Diagnostic imaging of canine elbow dysplasia: a review. *Vet Surg* 38 (2): 144–153.

Coppieters, E., Gielen, I., Verhoeven, G. et al. (2015). Erosion of the medial compartment of the canine elbow: occurrence, diagnosis and currently available treatment options. *Vet Comp Orthop Traumatol* 28 (1): 9–18.

Cross, A.R. and Chambers, J.N. (1997). Ununited anconeal process of the canine elbow. *Compend Contin Educ Pract Vet* 19 (3): 349–361.

De Bakker, E., Samoy, Y., Coppieters, E. et al. (2013). Arthroscopic features of primary and concomitant flexor enthesopathy in the canine elbow. *Vet Comp Orthop Traumatol* 26 (5): 340–347.

De Bakker, E., Saunders, J., Gielen, I. et al. (2012). Radiographic findings of the medial humeral epicondyle in 200 canine elbow joints. *Vet Comp Orthop Traumatol* 25 (5): 359–365.

Deffontaines, J.-B., Lussier, B., Bolliger, C. et al. (2016). Chronic desmitis and enthesiophytosis of the radio-ulnar interosseous ligament in a dog. *Can Vet J* 57 (5): 487.

Dempsey, L.M., Maddox, T.W., Comerford, E.J. et al. (2019). A comparison of owner-assessed long-term outcome of arthroscopic intervention versus conservative management of dogs with medial coronoid process disease. *Vet Comp Orthop Traumatol* 32 (1): 1–9.

Earley, N.F., Ellse, G., Wallace, A.M. et al. (2018). Complications and outcomes associated with 13 cases of triceps tendon disruption in dogs and cats (2003–2014). *Vet Rec* 182 (4): 108.

Evans, R.B., Gordon-Evans, W.J., and Conzemius, M.G. (2008). Comparison of three methods for the management of fragmented medial coronoid process in the dog. A systematic review and meta-analysis. *Vet Comp Orthop Traumatol* 21 (2): 106–109.

Farrell, M., Draffan, D., Gemmill, T. et al. (2007). In vitro validation of a technique for assessment of canine and feline elbow joint collateral ligament integrity and description of a new method for collateral ligament prosthetic replacement. *Vet Surg* 36 (6): 548–556.

Farrell, M., Trevail, T., Marshall, W. et al. (2011). Computed tomographic documentation of the natural progression of humeral intracondylar fissure in a cocker Spaniel. *Vet Surg* 40 (8): 966–971.

Fitch, R.B., Hogan, T.C., and Kudnig, S.T. (2003). Hematogenous septic arthritis in the dog: results of five patients treated nonsurgically with antibiotics. *J Am Anim Hosp Assoc* 39 (6): 563–566.

Fitzpatrick, N. and Yeadon, R. (2009). Working algorithm for treatment decision making for developmental disease of the medial compartment of the elbow in dogs. *Vet Surg* 38 (2): 285–300.

Groth, A.M., Benigni, L., Moores, A.P., and Lamb, C.R. (2009). Spectrum of computed tomographic findings in 58 canine elbows with fragmentation of the medial coronoid process. *J Small Anim Pract* 50 (1): 15–22.

Hattersley, R., Mckee, M., O'Neill, T. et al. (2011). Postoperative complications after surgical management of incomplete ossification of the humeral condyle in dogs. *Vet Surg* 40 (6): 728–733.

Lisbeth, S., Andrea, K., Nikola, K. et al. (2018). Imaging diagnosis: radiography and computed tomography of radioulnar ischemic necrosis in Jack Russell. *Vet. Radiol. Ultrasound* 59 (1): E7–E11.

Makielski, K., Muir, P., and Bleedorn, J. (2015). Focal defect resembling a subchondral bone cyst of the ulnar trochlear notch in a dog. *J Am Anim Hosp Assoc* 51 (1): 20–24.

Marcellin-Little, D.J., DeYoung, D.J., Ferris, K.K., and Berry, C.M. (1994). Incomplete ossification of the humeral condyle in Spaniels. *Vet Surg* 23 (6): 475–487.

Mason, D.R., Schulz, K.S., Fujita, Y. et al. (2005). In vitro force mapping of normal canine humeroradial and humeroulnar joints. *Am J Vet Res* 66 (1): 132–135.

McDonell, H.L. (2004). Unilateral congenital elbow luxation in a Cavalier King Charles Spaniel. *Can Vet J* 45 (11): 941–943.

Meyer-Lindenberg, A., Fehr, M., and Nolte, I. (2006). Co-existence of ununited anconeal process and fragmented medial coronoid process of the ulna in the dog. *J Small Anim Pract* 47 (2): 61–65.

Meyer-Lindenberg, A., Langhann, A., Fehr, M., and Nolte, I. (2002). Prevalence of fragmented medial coronoid process of the ulna in lame adult dogs. *Vet Rec* 151 (8): 230–234.

Michelsen, J. (2013). Canine elbow dysplasia: aetiopathogenesis and current treatment recommendations. *Vet J* 196 (1): 12–19.

Mielke, B., Comerford, E., English, K., and Meeson, R. (2018). Spontaneous septic arthritis of canine elbows: twenty-one cases. *Vet Comp Orthop Traumatol* 31 (6): 488–493.

Milgram, J., Yudelevitch, S., Shahar, R., and Benzioni, H. (2018). Bacterial infective arthritis of the coxofemoral joint in dogs with hip dysplasia. *Vet Comp Orthop Traumatol* 21 (3): 262–266.

Moores, A.P., Agthe, P., and Schaafsma, I.A. (2012). Prevalence of incomplete ossification of the humeral condyle and other abnormalities of the elbow in English Springer Spaniels. *Vet Comp Orthop Traumatol* 25 (3): 211–216.

Moores, A.P. and Moores, A.L. (2017). The natural history of humeral intracondylar fissure: an observational study of 30 dogs. *J Small Anim Pract* 58 (6): 337–341.

Morton, B.A., Hettlich, B.F., and Pool, R.R. (2015). Surgical treatment of traumatic myositis ossificans of the extensor carpi radialis muscle in a dog. *Vet Surg* 44 (5): 576–580.

Paster, E.R., Biery, D.N., Lawler, D.F. et al. (2009). Un-united medial epicondyle of the humerus: radiographic prevalence and association with elbow osteoarthritis in a cohort of Labrador Retrievers. *Vet Surg* 38 (2): 169–172.

Perry, K.L., Bruce, M., Woods, S. et al. (2015). Effect of fixation method on postoperative complication rates after surgical stabilization of lateral humeral condylar fractures in dogs. *Vet Surg* 44 (2): 246–255.

Piola, V., Posch, B., Radke, H. et al. (2012). Magnetic resonance imaging features of canine incomplete humeral condyle ossification. *Vet Radiol Ultrasound* 53 (5): 560–565.

Rahal, S.C., De Biasi, F., Vulcano, L.C., and Neto, F.J. (2000). Reduction of humeroulnar congenital elbow luxation in 8 dogs by using the transarticular pin. *Can Vet J* 41 (11): 849–853.

Schawalder, P., Andres, H., Jutzi, K. et al. (2002). Canine panosteitis: an idiopathic bone disease investigated in the light of a new hypothesis concerning pathogenesis. Part 1: Clinical and diagnostic aspects. *Schweiz Arch Tierheilkd* 144 (3): 115–130.

Stead, A., Stead, M.C., and Galloway, F.H. (1983). Panosteitis in dogs. *J Small Anim Pract* 24 (10): 623–635.

Stull, J.W., Evason, M., Carr, A.P., and Waldner, C. (2008). Canine immune-mediated polyarthritis: clinical and laboratory findings in 83 cases in western Canada (1991–2001). *Can Vet J* 49: 1195–1203.

Tafti, A.K., Hanna, P., and Bourque, A.C. (2005). Calcinosis circumscripta in the dog: a retrospective pathological study. *J Vet Med A Physiol Pathol Clin Med* 52 (1): 13–17.

Tambella, A.M., Palumbo Piccionello, A., Dini, F. et al. (2013). Myositis ossificans circumscripta of the triceps muscle in a Rottweiler dog. *Vet Comp Orthop Traumatol* 26 (2): 154–159.

Tan, D.K., Canapp, S.O. Jr., Leasure, C.S. et al. (2016). Traumatic fracture of the medial coronoid process in 24 dogs. *Vet Comp Orthop Traumatol* 29 (4): 325–329.

Towle-Millard, H.A. and Breur, G.J. (2018). Miscellaneous orthopedic conditions. In: Veterinary Surgery: Small Animal, 2e (eds. S.A. Johnston and K.M. Tobias), 1299–1315. St. Louis: Elsevier.

Van Vynckt, D., Verhoeven, G., Saunders, J. et al. (2012). Diagnostic intra-articular anaesthesia of the elbow in dogs with medial coronoid disease. *Vet Comp Orthop Traumatol* 25 (4): 307–313.

Villamonte-Chevalier, A., Van Bree, H., Broeckx, B. et al. (2015). Assessment of medial coronoid disease in 180 canine lame elbow joints: a sensitivity and specificity comparison of radiographic, computed tomographic and arthroscopic findings. *BMC Vet Res* 11: 243.

Witte, P.G., Bush, M.A., and Scott, H.W. (2010). Propagation of a partial incomplete ossification of the humeral condyle in an American Cocker Spaniel. *J Small Anim Pract* 51 (11): 591–593.

ELBOW REGION

15

Shoulder Region
Kristina M. Kiefer[1] and Dirsko J.F. von Pfeil[2,3]

[1] *Veterinary Surgery and Sports Medicine Assistance, Research and Tutelage, St. Paul, MN, USA*
[2] *Small Animal Surgery Locum, PLLC, Dallas, TX, USA*
[3] *Sirius Veterinary Orthopedic Center, Omaha, NE, USA*

15.1 Introduction and Common Differential Diagnoses

Shoulder disease is becoming a more frequently recognized cause of thoracic limb lameness. Shoulder pathology can be difficult to localize and distinguishing between elbow and shoulder pain is a challenge that can frustrate even the most seasoned orthopedists. Osteochondrosis is one example of a common shoulder disease that is easily identified diagnostically, as radiographs are frequently sufficient to establish a diagnosis. However, many sources of shoulder pain arise from soft tissue injuries and show no radiographic pathology. As such, other types of diagnostic imaging are frequently a component in evaluation of shoulder lameness. If the clinician is struggling to identify a painful reaction in a dog with a thoracic limb lameness, a neurologic examination evaluating cervical pain, brachial plexus palpation, and neuromuscular reflexes should also be evaluated, as root signatures of the thoracic limb are not an uncommon finding.

Figure 15.1 and Table 15.1 outline common differential diagnoses and diagnostic steps for this region.

15.2 Normal Anatomy and Osteoarthritis

The joint surfaces of the canine shoulder comprise the concave glenoid cavity of the scapula and the convex surface of the humeral head (Figure 15.2). Shoulder stability depends on a complex interaction between numerous structures, which can be divided into passive (i.e. static components that are unable to contract) and active (i.e. dynamic components that can actively contract) stabilizers. *Passive* shoulder stability is provided through appropriate synovial fluid volume, the concave and convex joint surfaces of the glenoid and humeral head, and the medial and lateral glenohumeral ligaments (MGL and LGL, respectively; Figures 15.3 and 15.4). These ligaments are intra-articular structures and act as collateral ligaments of the shoulder joint. Another passive stabilizer is the joint capsule, which travels from the scapular glenoid to the humeral head. *Active* shoulder-stabilizing structures include some of the so-called "(rotator) cuff muscles," such as the

SHOULDER REGION

Table 15.1 Key features for selected diseases affecting the shoulder region.

Disease	Common signalment	Diagnostic test of choice	Exam findings	Treatment	Clinical pearls	Terminology
Fractures	Any breed or age	Radiographs (orthogonal views)/CT	Pain, crepitus, and non- or minimally weight-bearing lameness	Depends on location	Articular fractures require surgical fixation; scapular fractures depend on location	
Medial shoulder instability	Adult hunting and agility dogs	Arthroscopy/MRI	Abduction pain, ±muscle atrophy, and ±increased abduction angles	Nonsurgical and surgical for severe cases	Frequently not identified without advanced imaging or arthroscopy	Medial shoulder syndrome/disease
Shoulder luxation	History of traumatic incident	Radiographs (orthogonal views)	ROM pain, soft tissue swelling, and increased distance between acromion and humeral head	Closed reduction or surgical reconstruction	Luxation of shoulder without a traumatic incident should be evaluated for glenoid dysplasia	
Biceps brachii tendinopathy	Large-breed, active dogs	Ultrasound/MRI	Pain with shoulder flexion and elbow extension, and ±pain on direct palpation of tendon	Depends on severity: medical management versus surgical release	Pain with this disease is highly variable – biceps is intra-articular (e.g. joint blocks/injection can be pursued)	Classified as calcifying and non-calcifying
Supraspinatus tendinopathy	Large-breed, active dogs	Ultrasound/MRI	Pain with shoulder flexion (without elbow extension)	Medical management versus surgical release	Calcification can be incidental – need to correlate with clinical symptoms	Classified as calcifying and non-calcifying
Infraspinatus disease	Hunting breeds	Classical gait and palpation – ultrasound to confirm diagnosis	Swelling and pain at infraspinatus, incapable of internal rotation with contracture	Medical management or surgical release at acute phase and tendon release with contracture	Can be a biphasic disease process, acute (often missed), followed by contracture	Infraspinatus contracture; fibrotic myopathy of infraspinatus
Osteochondrosis/ osteochondrosis dissecans	Young large- or giant-breed dogs	Radiographs (orthogonal views) and arthroscopy	Pain on shoulder ROM and ±weight-bearing lameness	Arthroscopic debridement	Radiographs are typically diagnostic, while arthroscopy confirms and allows therapy	

Condition	Signalment	Diagnostics	Clinical signs	Treatment	Notes	Other
Caudal glenoid fragments	Any dog but Rottweilers may be overrepresented for accessory caudal glenoid ossification center	Radiographs (orthogonal views)	Weight-bearing lameness, pain on ROM of joint	Nonsurgical management or surgical removal	This can be an incidental finding and may be a sign of osteoarthritis rather than developmental	Accessory caudal glenoid ossification center; incomplete ossification of caudal glenoid
Glenoid dysplasia	Young dogs, mini and toy Poodles overrepresented	Radiographs (orthogonal views)	Non- or weight-bearing lameness, humeral head medial to scapula	Nonsurgical or excision arthroplasty or shoulder arthrodesis		
Adhesive capsulitis	Unknown	Ultrasound or MRI	Chronic lameness, ROM pain, and limited shoulder mobility	Unknown	Rare	Frozen shoulder
Neoplasia	Older dogs	Radiographs (orthogonal views), ±MRI or CT scan	Pain and non- or weight-bearing lameness	Depends on location and neoplasia	Proximal humerus is predilection site	

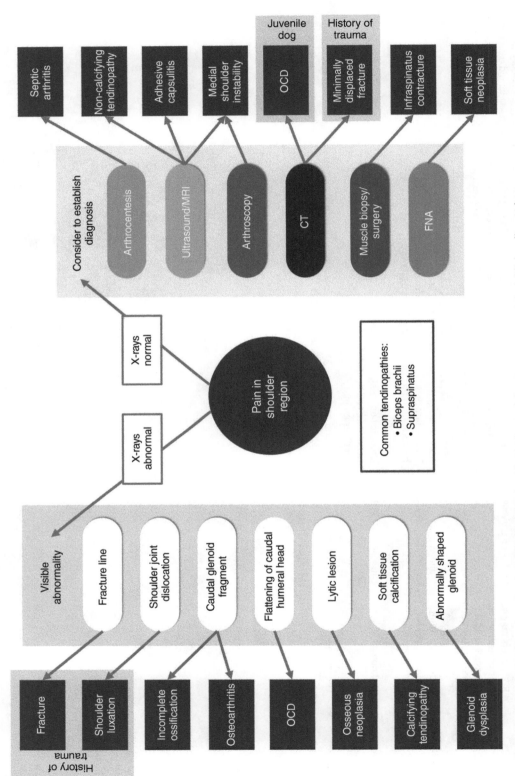

Figure 15.1 Schematic of common diseases affecting the shoulder region and the steps necessary to establish a diagnosis.

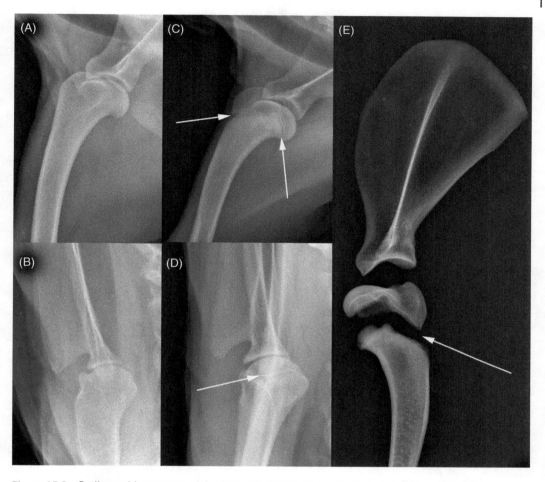

Figure 15.2 Radiographic anatomy of the (normal) shoulder joint: (A) lateral and (B) craniocaudal radiographic view of a normal adult shoulder; (C) lateral and (D) craniocaudal radiographic view of an immature dog, wherein the white arrows indicate normal appearance of the proximal humerus physis; (E) separation of the humerus in a cadaver, to illustrate normal shape of the proximal physis of the humerus (white arrow).

infraspinatus, supraspinatus, subscapularis, and teres minor muscles. The teres major, biceps brachii, caput longum of the triceps, the coracobrachialis, and the deltoideus muscles have also been suggested to provide minor active support.

The tendon of the biceps brachii, subscapularis muscle, and the MGL are located intra-articularly and therefore can be evaluated arthroscopically. The supraspinatus is located extra-articularly. The main stabilizers of the medial shoulder are the MGL and subscapularis, while the tendons of the supraspinatus, infraspinatus, and teres minor muscles and the LGL provide the majority of the lateral stability.

Osteoarthritis of the shoulder joint is generally thought to be associated with common shoulder pathologies (e.g. osteochondrosis, medial shoulder instability [MSI], and tendinopathies) indicating a secondary (i.e. due to underlying disease) etiology. Interestingly, a study found that over 50% of dogs necropsied for unrelated reasons showed cartilage erosion of the caudal humeral head, of

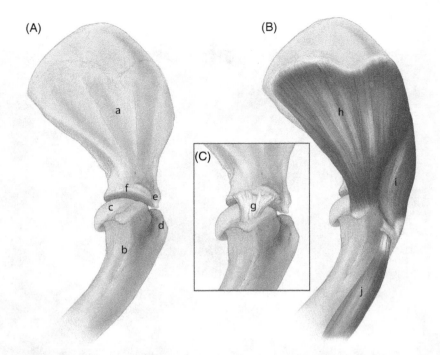

Figure 15.3 Normal anatomy of the medial shoulder for (A) osseous structures; (B) muscles; and (C) the collateral ligament of the medial shoulder: (a) scapula; (b) humerus; (c) humeral head; (d) greater tubercle; (e) supraglenoid tubercle; (f) glenoid; (g) medial glenohumeral ligament; (h) subscapularis; (i) supraspinatus; and (j) biceps brachii.

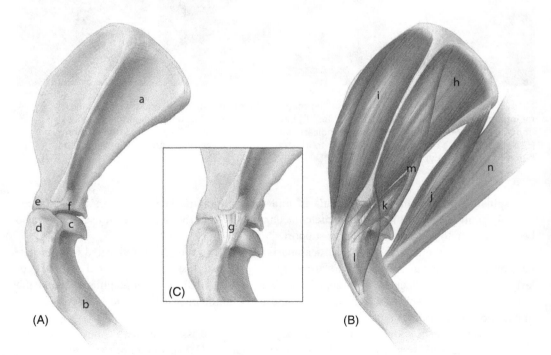

Figure 15.4 Normal anatomy of the lateral shoulder for (A) osseous structures; (B) muscles; and (C) the collateral ligament of the lateral shoulder: (a) scapula; (b) humerus; (c) humeral head; (d) greater tubercle; (e) supraglenoid tubercle; (f) glenoid; (g) lateral glenohumeral ligament; (h) infraspinatus; (i) supraspinatus; (j) teres major; (k) teres minor; (l) acromial part and (m) scapular part of the deltoideus; and (n) latissimus dorsi.

which only 0.1% were due to osteochondrosis (Craig and Reed 2013). These findings suggest that primary osteoarthritis (i.e. without a known cause) may be common in canine shoulder joints. Probably because of its less confined anatomy, osteoarthritis of the shoulder joint appears to be tolerated better than arthritis of other joints (e.g. elbow).

15.3   Fractures of the Shoulder Region

Fractures of the shoulder joint are generally associated with a history of trauma, unless they are pathologic (Chapter 17). Most humeral fractures involve the diaphysis or distal aspect of the humerus; fractures of the proximal, mature humerus are a rarity if no underlying pathology such as bone neoplasia is present (Rochat 2018). Proximal Salter-Harris (SH) fractures should be considered as a differential in juvenile patients and can be mistaken for shoulder luxation (Figures 15.5

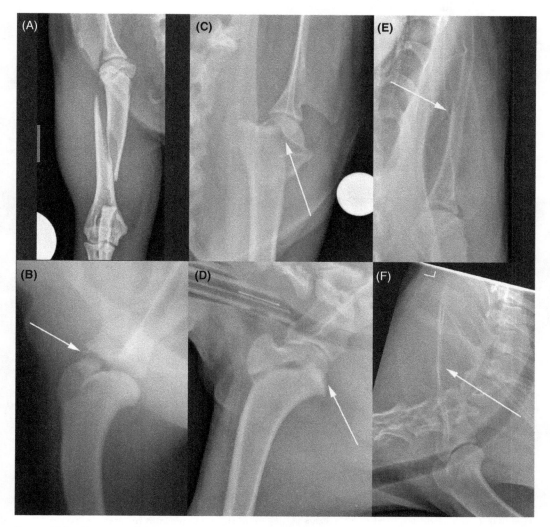

Figure 15.5   Fractures of the shoulder region: (A) mid-diaphyseal, long-oblique humeral fracture; (B) supraglenoid tubercle avulsion fracture (white arrow); (C, D) proximal humeral Salter-Harris Type I fracture (white arrow); and (E, F) minimally displaced mid-body scapular fracture.

SHOULDER REGION

and 15.9). Fractures close to the shoulder joint more commonly consist of scapular fractures. Avulsion fractures of the supraglenoid tubercle (the origin of the biceps brachii) become more obvious when performing a fully flexed view of the shoulder with the elbow extended, causing greater displacement of the fracture due to the pull of the biceps tendon. Physical exam findings usually reveal moderate to non-weight-bearing lameness, soft tissue swelling that may range from minimal to severe, and significant pain on shoulder range of motion (ROM) and/or direct palpation of bony structures.

As a general note, it is important to realize that the shoulder can be a challenging joint to isolate during manipulation and ROM, making it difficult to distinguish it from the elbow as the source of pain. This caveat particularly applies for less painful conditions (e.g. osteochondrosis and mild arthritis), though it may also pertain when minimally displaced fractures are present. When the shoulder is passively extended, the elbow also extends passively (Figure 15.6) and while it is most convenient to flex the shoulder joint by grasping the antebrachium, this approach simultaneously flexes the elbow. However, with conscious recognition of anatomy, it is possible to eliminate flexion of the elbow by intentionally grasping the humerus when flexing the shoulder joint.

Most fractures can be diagnosed with radiographs but scapular fractures can sometimes be difficult to identify (Figure 15.5). Given the frequent traumatic nature of presentation, they may first be identified on thoracic radiographs obtained during initial assessment and stabilization of a traumatic patient. If the fracture is complex, a CT scan is valuable to clearly assess the extent of the fracture as well as formulate therapeutic planning. Articular fractures and proximal humeral fractures (including SH fractures) generally should be surgically stabilized. Minimally displaced scapular body fractures are frequently amenable to external coaptation for management. Severely comminuted fractures involving the articular surfaces may require arthrodesis.

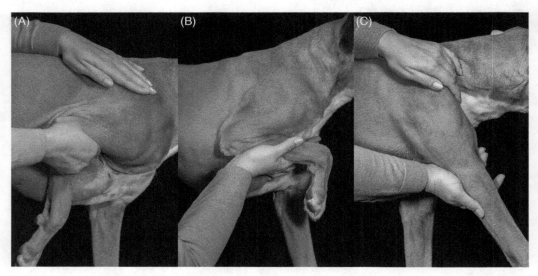

Figure 15.6 Physical examination of the shoulder: flexion of the joint to assess for a pain response attributable specifically to the shoulder requires intentional isolation of the joints. This is best achieved by (A) grasping the humerus and drawing it caudodorsally toward the body of the scapula, rather than (B) grasping the antebrachium. Note that it is impossible to isolate the elbow from the shoulder during extension, so that (C) passive extension of the shoulder joint results in passive extension of the elbow.

15.4   Medial Shoulder Instability

MSI describes a condition of reduced stability of the shoulder, caused by pathology of the medial structures of this joint. MSI is the most common type of canine shoulder instability and a frequent cause of shoulder-related lameness (Cogar et al. 2008). Lateral and multidirectional shoulder instability has been reported to occur in about 25% of shoulder instability cases (Franklin et al. 2013).

MSI is believed to result from repetitive trauma. Depending on the amount and magnitude of involved forces, the structures supporting the shoulder can become strained, frayed, disrupted, or broken down completely. This results in various degrees of instability, including subluxation or complete luxation (covered in 15.5) of the scapulohumeral joint. As MSI does not always result in detectable instability, the term "medial shoulder syndrome or disease" has been suggested in the non-peer-reviewed literature. While the official nomenclature may change in the future, for the scope of this chapter, MSI will be used throughout.

The anatomy of the shoulder and its stabilizers needs to be understood to diagnose MSI. The two most important structures affected with MSI include the subscapularis tendon (SST) and MGL. Based on the degree of disruption of these structures, a grading system (Table 15.2) has been proposed (O'Donnell et al. 2017).

The suggested causes for MSI include slipping, falling, and other unusual high-impact stress, as well as chronic repetitive activity, overuse, or repetitive micro-trauma. Collectively, these all lead to abduction of the shoulder joint with the shoulder stabilizers tested to their limits. The main stress seems to be concentrated on the medial joint capsule, the MGL, and the SST. While it has been suggested that the MGL provides the majority of medial shoulder stability (Sidaway et al. 2004), an experimental study in purpose bred laboratory Beagles reported no instability after isolated transection of the cranial band of the MGL (Fujita et al. 2013). Six weeks after transection, villous hyperplasia and vascularization of the medial compartment were found. These findings suggest that an inflammatory response caused by partial disruption of the ligament may eventually result in MSI. This observation is consistent with descriptions of patients who were clinically normal, but surprisingly had severe damage to the MGL and SST during arthroscopic examination (Rochat 2018). The SST can also be damaged or inflamed, which can affect medial shoulder stability. In one study, significant MSI was detected in cadavers after transection of the SST (Pettitt et al. 2007). Muscle atrophy, damage to other shoulder cuff muscles and congenital abnormalities such as loss of concavity of the glenoid or a misshapen proximal humerus, can also contribute to instability. The latter is a common cause for shoulder instability in small-breed dogs (Vaughan and Jones 1969).

Treatment of MSI can be nonsurgical or surgical with the choice of treatment depending on the degree of injury and on which structures are damaged. Nonsurgical treatment generally includes

Table 15.2   Medial shoulder instability (MSI) grading scheme.

Grade	Description	Definition
1	Mild MSI	Laxity without gross tearing of the medial glenohumeral ligament (MGL) or subscapularis tendon (SST)
2	Moderate MSI	Partial tear of MGL, SST, or both
3	Severe MSI	Complete tear of MGL, SST, or both
4	Luxation	Complete tear of MGL, SST, and complete displacement of humeral head

Source: Adapted from O'Donnell et al. (2017).

SHOULDER REGION

rehabilitation, Velpeau slings, or the use of a shoulder stabilization system ("shoulder hobbles") that prevent abduction (Henderson et al. 2015). Severe instability such as subluxation and complete luxation typically require surgery. Surgical options reported comprise thermal capsulorrhaphy, intra-articular reconstruction, and arthroscopically assisted or open placement of prosthetic ligaments.

15.4.1 Signalment and History

MSI is most commonly seen in middle-aged working dogs with hunting, field trial, or competitive agility dogs seemingly predisposed. Agility dogs must overcome jumps and A-frames, pass weave poles, and perform quick turns, which is believed to result in damage to the medial shoulder stabilizers. The reported mean age of affected dogs is four to five years (Cook et al. 2005b; O'Donnell et al. 2017).

History and clinical signs with MSI consist of varying degrees of lameness and depend on the severity and time since injury. Clinical signs may be very mild and only noted during performance. Owners may observe a shortened stride and reduced level of performance, avoiding certain activities such as quick turns. However, particularly with high-grade MSI, dogs may also show more severe symptoms such as non-weight-bearing lameness. Typically, lameness is worse after exercise or heavy work. Further, despite rest and administration of nonsteroidal anti-inflammatories, these signs often do not improve and return quickly once activity levels are increased.

15.4.2 Physical Exam

Pain and muscle spasm upon regional palpation, atrophy of the shoulder muscles, and restricted ROM (particularly in extension) are frequently noted upon examination of patients with MSI. Discomfort upon abduction and increased abduction angles (as identified during the abduction test; Figure 15.7) are also common but may not always be present.

The *abduction test* quantifies the degree of abduction of the shoulder. This assessment should be performed with the patient awake as well as sedated. Although sedation provides the most accurate measurement, evaluating the patient while awake allows the clinician to assess the degree of discomfort. The latter can be performed with the dog standing or in lateral recumbency. To properly perform the abduction test, the elbow and shoulder are extended so that the humerus and spine of the scapula are axially aligned. The center of the goniometer is located over the shoulder joint. One limb of the goniometer is aligned with the spine of the scapula and the other extends over the lateral aspect of the antebrachium, placed parallel to the humerus. One hand holds the antebrachium at the level of the elbow and abducts the shoulder while the other hand holds the shoulder joint/spine of the scapula. This allows the clinician to ascertain that the shoulder and elbow joints are both extended; allowing for flexion of either joint will result in an abnormally high value (Figure 15.7). Abduction is performed until resistance by the soft tissues is detected. The measured goniometer value (considering straight would be 0) at that point is reported. To avoid variations based on improper technique, it is important to always perform the abduction test following the same protocol. The frequently referenced normal values are based on a previous study that evaluated 33 medium to large-breed dogs with clinical MSI and 26 control dogs. The authors reported mean abduction angles of ~54° in the MSI group and ~33° in the control group (Cook et al. 2005a). While these values are still used as a general reference, recent work suggests that there are likely breed variations as well as significant variability between observers (Devitt et al. 2007; George et al. 2017). For example, a recent study in sled dogs ($n = 130$ shoulders) reported a median shoulder abduction angle of ~45° in clinically normal dogs (George et al. 2017). This dis-

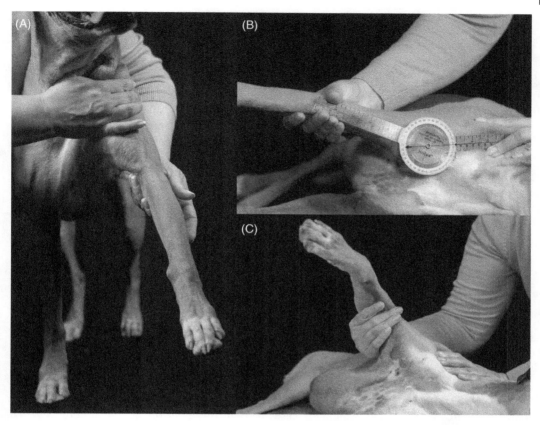

Figure 15.7   Shoulder abduction test: (A) subjective evaluation of the degree of shoulder abduction during stance which also allows to evaluate for a pain response; (B) goniometric evaluation in lateral recumbency – for the measurements to be accurate, the elbow and shoulder must be fully extended; the center of the goniometer is placed over the shoulder joint, the two limbs of the goniometer are aligned with the spine of the scapula and the humerus; (C) note, if the elbow is not fully extended as illustrated in the image, an (false) increased goniometric measurement may result.

crepancy may be due to breed variability and function, or inclusion of dogs that were affected by nonclinical MSI, or discrepancy of measurement techniques. An increased abduction angle makes a diagnosis of MSI more likely (Devitt et al. 2007); however, a "normal" shoulder abduction angle does not rule out MSI. Like cranial cruciate ligament disease, partial tearing of the MGL and SST may not result in detectable instability. Although in the authors' experience, these patients frequently show a more pronounced pain response during abduction.

Because of the subjective nature and variability associated with the shoulder abduction test, it should only be used as a guide in making a diagnosis of MSI and considered in combination with other diagnostics. In unilaterally affected dogs, abduction angles should be evaluated by comparing the affected and non-affected side. A diagnosis of MSI is more likely if a patient has significantly higher abduction on the side the patient is lame compared to the non-lame side.

Despite these possible limitations of goniometric assessment of abduction angles to help diagnose MSI, it remains the mainstay of diagnosis since definitive tests are more costly and involved. The authors therefore recommend applying this test to any dog presenting with thoracic limb lameness, keeping its limitations in mind.

15.4.3 Diagnostics

As mentioned above, the shoulder abduction test may result in a tentative diagnosis of MSI, but advanced imaging is necessary to confirm this diagnosis. The diagnostic modalities of choice include ultrasound, magnetic resonance imaging (MRI), and arthroscopy, or a combination of these. Radiographs and CT can be used to rule out other diseases.

Currently, orthogonal survey *radiographs* of the shoulder are mainly recommended to rule out diseases that are easily detected radiographically (such as primary bone tumors). Dogs with MSI frequently show no radiographic abnormalities and therefore radiographs are not very sensitive to help diagnose MSI (or other soft tissue pathology of the shoulder). Notably, one study in particular found up to 45% of shoulder radiographs to be normal despite severe intra-articular or periarticular disease, such as synovitis, MGL disease, SST inflammation, or tears (Bardet 1998). The most commonly seen radiographic abnormality in dogs with MSI is mild osteoarthritis (Figure 15.8). On the other hand, radiographs have recently been suggested as a more objective means of measuring shoulder abduction angles. One cadaveric study described a technique aiming to provide a standardized radiographic measurement for shoulder abduction angles, using a specific positioning and a restraint device (Livet et al. 2018). Clinical evaluation of this technique has not been described yet but it may become a clinically valuable tool to help diagnose MSI in the future. Because of the low sensitivity of radiographs to detect MSI, advanced imaging such as musculoskeletal ultrasound and/or MRI should be considered to establish a diagnosis.

Magnetic resonance imaging is a sensitive imaging modality for canine shoulder conditions that allows for evaluation of the entire joint and surrounding structures. Unfortunately, MRI typically requires full anesthesia, is time-consuming, and is costly. Recent developments in MRI technology will likely facilitate the development of shorter protocols that can be performed under sedation but currently, MRI is not a routine diagnostic for detection of MSI at the authors' institutions. However, particularly in diagnostically challenging cases or if involvement of the spinal cord, regional nerves, and the brachial plexus is suspected, MRI is strongly recommended.

Ultrasound is frequently used to assess the soft tissue structures of the shoulder, particularly the lateral muscles and tendons which are easily accessible. The medial compartment of the shoulder

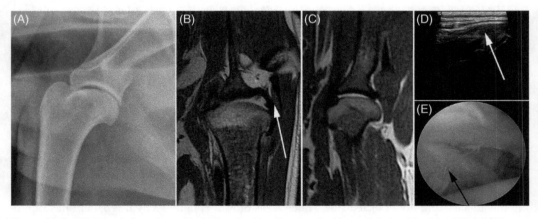

Figure 15.8   Diagnostic imaging techniques of a dog diagnosed with medial shoulder instability (MSI): (A) lateral radiograph showing minimal osteoarthritic changes; (B) MRI (sequence: Dorsal Proton Density) illustrating typical thickening along the medial aspect of the shoulder joint (white arrow), at the attachment of the medial glenohumeral ligament (MGHL) and subscapularis; (C) a normal shoulder MRI of a different patient for comparison; (D) ultrasound images showing thickening and ill-defined MGHL and subscapularis (white arrow); and (E) arthroscopic image showing tearing of the MGHL (black arrow).

is more difficult to assess, particularly in overweight dogs. In one study, poor correlation between ultrasonographic and arthroscopic evaluation of the SST was described (Cogar et al. 2008). To facilitate evaluation of the MGL and SST, sedation and a hockey-stick probe are recommended (Cook 2016). Benefits of ultrasound include the relatively low cost, ability to perform the examination without general anesthesia, and possibility of performing a dynamic assessment. However, interpretation of the images can be challenging and requires advanced training. If both, MRI and ultrasound are performed, MRI should ideally be done prior to ultrasound to avoid creation of artifacts.

Shoulder *arthroscopy* has been recommended as the gold standard for diagnosing MSI (Devitt et al. 2007). Arthroscopy allows excellent assessment of the intra-articular shoulder structures, including the intra-articular components of the MGL and the SST. These structures can also be placed under stress by abduction of the shoulder during arthroscopy or palpated with a probe. Arthroscopy can also help identify concurrent shoulder pathologies, for example changes to the biceps tendon that may occur secondary to the inflammation associated with MSI. Such changes (secondary biceps tendinopathy) must be differentiated from primary biceps tendon disease as this may influence the treatment. Standard arthroscopy allows to establish a diagnosis and proceed with potential treatment at the same time, if indicated. The disadvantage of arthroscopy is that the evaluation is limited to the intra-articular structures.

Since treatment for MSI is frequently nonsurgical, *needle arthroscopy* may also be used if the focus is on the diagnostic aspect. This technique was initially reported as a diagnostic tool in horses and uses a smaller arthroscope that can be used under sedation (Frisbie et al. 2014). Needle arthroscopy has recently been assessed for diagnostic exploration in dogs (Fournet et al. 2018) and is becoming more commonly used in small animal practice. The author uses needle arthroscopy if advanced imaging has not revealed a diagnosis and if it is not clear that standard arthroscopy is indicated. The current technical difficulty associated with needle arthroscopy is obtaining high-resolution images similar to those acquired when using standard arthroscopy.

While *CT* (and CT arthrography) is a convenient and more readily available imaging modality, it is of limited use for the diagnosis of MSI (Eivers et al. 2018). However, CT is useful in ruling out other diseases (such as shoulder osteochondrosis dissecans [OCD] and elbow dysplasia). A recent report suggested that adding epinephrine to the contrast medium may improve image sharpness by delaying diffusion of the contrast (De Simone et al. 2013). Similarly, while *joint fluid analysis* can be helpful for other joints, dogs with significant pathology may show no cytological abnormalities in their joint fluid (Akerblom and Sjostrom 2007).

15.5 Traumatic Shoulder Luxation

Shoulder luxation (Figure 15.9) is an uncommon condition that is typically a consequence of traumatic injury in dogs. This condition is different than the above-described low-grade, chronic instability of the shoulder joint (MSI). Luxation direction (based on the location of the humerus) is most commonly medial, although lateral, cranial, and caudal have all been reported. Congenital deformities (Section 15.10.2) may also result in luxation, which tend to be medially displaced. These must be differentiated from traumatic luxations since the treatment is different (i.e. closed reduction is not indicated). Acute, traumatic luxations can often be managed with closed (manual) reduction followed by external coaptation (e.g. Velpeau sling for medial luxation; spica splint for all others). If the joint is grossly unstable even after reduction, or medical management fails, surgical stabilization is recommended.

SHOULDER REGION

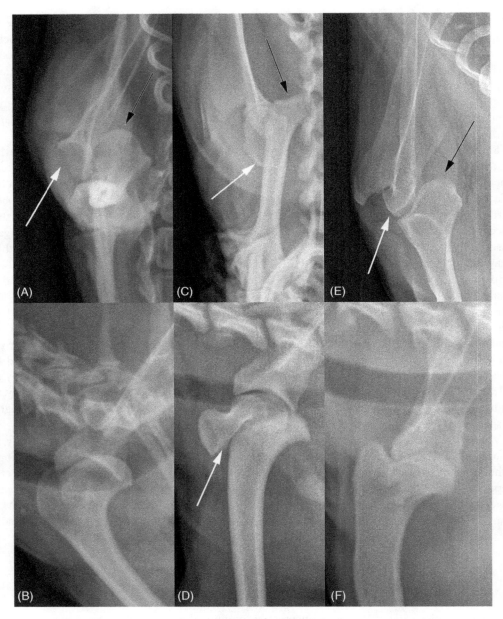

Figure 15.9 Shoulder luxation: (A, B) patient with traumatic medial shoulder luxation; (C, D) patient with Salter-Harris Type I fracture of the proximal humerus; and (E,F) patient with glenoid dysplasia. (A) The humeral head (black arrow) is obviously displaced medially to the glenoid cavity (white arrow) of the scapula on the craniocaudal radiographs, which is (B) less obvious on the lateral view. However, the caudal aspect of the glenoid has significant overlap with the caudal humeral head, indicating displacement. (C) A physeal fracture of the proximal humerus may be mistaken for traumatic luxation. The fracture line (white arrow) and the remaining proximal humerus (black arrow) may mimic the appearance of a luxation. However, the humeral head within the glenoid cavity can be visualized radiographically (compare (C) to (A)); (D) the lateral view clearly depicts the humeral head within the glenoid cavity, while the diaphysis of the humerus is displaced caudally. (E) Medial luxation secondary to glenoid dysplasia; the glenoid cavity (white arrow) is lacking a distinct concave surface (glenoid fossa) and the humeral head (black arrow) is abnormally shaped (compare (E) to (A)). (F) The lateral view shows significant overlap of the humeral head over the glenoid and abnormal osseous anatomy.

15.5.1 Signalment and History

Shoulder luxation is generally a consequence of trauma (e.g. vehicular accident), therefore any dog may be affected. In some cases, the history (including knowledge of any trauma event) may be unknown. A thorough investigation into preexisting lameness may be indicated, particularly if congenital conditions are considered as differential diagnoses.

15.5.2 Physical Exam

The physical exam on patients with traumatic luxation should prioritize systemic stability of the patient, given vehicular trauma is likely to create other comorbidities. The luxation itself may be challenging to appreciate if there is a large amount of soft tissue swelling. The limb is frequently non-weight-bearing, with flexion of the elbow. The distal limb may be in abduction (medial luxation) or adduction (lateral luxation). When palpable, the acromion and the greater tubercle of the head of the humerus will have increased distance between them, relative to normal. Palpation of these structures on the contralateral limb can give a reference of a "normal" spatial relationship between landmarks. Patients will be resistant to normal ROM of the shoulder joint. If luxation is achieved, severe crepitation throughout manipulation may be noted. Increased abduction may be appreciated for medial luxation, and for very unstable joints, the humeral head may palpably shift in multiple directions relative to the scapula (e.g. the examiner may elicit cranial drawer with cranial instability).

15.5.3 Diagnostics

Radiographs clearly demonstrate dislocation of the humeral head from the glenoid cavity (Figure 15.9). Radiographs should be assessed for any evidence of fractures or underlying/preexisting disease. In contrast to animals with congenital conditions (glenoid dysplasia), the radiographic appearance of the humeral head and glenoid cavity are normal. Further diagnostics are rarely needed to diagnose the problem, unless mild instability, rather than a true luxation is suspected. If the joint is extremely unstable, and the clinician is suspicious that the joint is continuously dislocating and reducing, fluoroscopy (if available) or serial digital radiographs may be utilized to evaluate the relationship between the humeral head the glenoid cavity. Although MRI or ultrasound are generally not necessary, they may benefit assessing the extent of soft tissue damage as well as aiding surgical planning.

15.6 Biceps Brachii Tendinopathy

Biceps tendinopathy is one of the more common etiologies of shoulder pain. As our diagnostic capacity has grown and workups of shoulder disease become more advanced, there is question as to whether this disease has been overdiagnosed (i.e. structural pathology may be an incidental finding). This condition is frequently referred to as biceps tenosynovitis, although this terminology may be inappropriate since an inflammatory component is not present in all cases (Gilley et al. 2002). Biceps tendinopathies can be primary or secondary in origin. Primary etiologies include strains, sprains, or tears (i.e. a primary problem of the biceps brachii). Secondary etiologies include impingement by extra-articular structures such as an enlarged supraspinatus muscle or intra-articular structures such as loose bony, fibrous, or cartilage fragments (i.e. pathology of the biceps is caused by a different underlying condition). In general, biceps tendinopathy indicates a chronic degenerative condition. However, rupture of the biceps tendon may be acute and can produce similar symptoms. Nonetheless, rupture of the biceps tendon is rare and presumed to be of traumatic etiology, which can occur within the substance of the tendon or as an avulsion from the supraglenoid tubercle (Figure 15.5). Complete rupture may be asymptomatic, as the strain on the injured tissue has been released (Wiemer et al. 2007).

Biceps tendinopathies may be classified as calcifying (i.e. if bony mineralization is present within the tendon) or non-calcifying, thereby indicating whether the pathologic changes include calcification of the muscle or tendon. This is particularly important from a diagnostic point of view since non-calcifying tendinopathies can be missed if radiographs are used as the only diagnostic tool. Calcifying tendinopathy implies chronicity. Although it is an anticipated progression of unaddressed disease (Bardet 1999), ambiguity remains in the literature as to whether this is a subset of biceps tendinopathies, or its own entity.

Nonsurgical management (e.g. restricted activity, anti-inflammatories and rehabilitation, and joint injections) or surgical treatment (e.g. biceps tendon release or tenodesis) has been reported (Bergenhuyzen et al. 2010). If secondary biceps tendinopathy is present, the primary condition should be addressed. For example, if impingement of the biceps tendon by the supraspinatus is present, treating the supraspinatus may alleviate the symptoms associated with the biceps.

15.6.1 Signalment and History

Biceps disease is largely associated with large-breed, active dogs, which are middle-to-older aged. Apart from biceps rupture, a specific traumatic event is rarely noted. The patient may present with an acute thoracic limb lameness, a chronic lameness that worsens with activity, or an intermittent lameness. Lameness is generally weight-bearing particularly with chronic cases, but a non-weight-bearing lameness may be observed with acute tears. Noting the chronicity may give some assistance in choosing an appropriate therapeutic option and predicting prognosis.

15.6.2 Physical Exam

External structures that can generally be distinguished on physical examination of the shoulder region include the tendon of the biceps brachii, the infraspinatus, supraspinatus, triceps and deltoid muscles, acromion, scapular spine and body, and the greater tubercle of the humerus. The biceps tendon may be palpated on physical exam by identifying its site of origin, the supraglenoid tubercle on the cranial margin of the articular space. A round, thick tendon should be palpable coursing distally from the supraglenoid tubercle, crossing the bicipital groove of the humeral head (Figure 15.10). The supraspinatus tendon is more lateral than the biceps but covers the medially located biceps origin substantially in some dogs (Figure 15.10). Additionally, the transverse ligament covers the origin complicating palpation of the biceps origin. Care should be taken to identify the correct tendon when possible. If the patient is well muscled, or over conditioned, palpation may be challenging, and flexion of the shoulder may aid in identifying this structure.

Muscle atrophy of the shoulder, producing a prominent scapular spine, may be present in chronic lameness cases as frequently seen with biceps tendinopathy. However, this is an unspecific finding, and a tentative diagnosis of biceps tendinopathy based on physical exam is most commonly based on a pain response during manipulation. The sensitivity of the patient's response to shoulder manipulation and biceps brachii palpation is highly variable and likely dependent upon severity, chronicity, and patient disposition. More severely affected individuals may react merely to palpation of the biceps tendon origin. Many will respond to palpation of the tendon, while the shoulder is flexed and the elbow simultaneously extended, placing the greatest strain on the tendon (Figure 15.11 and Video 3.1). This test is generally known as the "biceps test" and palpation of the

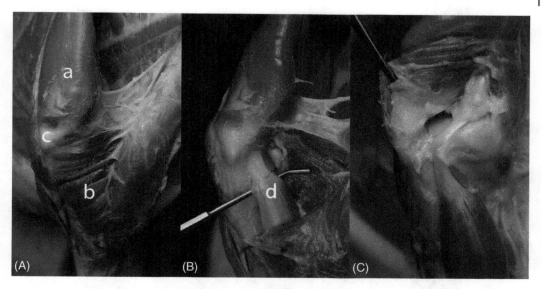

Figure 15.10   Cadaveric specimen demonstrating the biceps brachii anatomy of the medial aspect of the shoulder: (A) superficial dissection illustrating the structures overlaying the biceps tendon; (B) exposure of the biceps after removal of the pectoralis musculature; and (C) after transaction of the transverse humeral ligament and elevation of the supraspinatus muscle, the entire tendon of the biceps brachii can be seen deeply seated in the intertubercular groove: (a) supraspinatus muscle; (b) superficial pectoralis; (c) greater tubercle; and (d) biceps brachii.

entire muscle should be performed in this position. Some dogs may resist this test in a standing position because of other pathologies in the contralateral limb. As it is typically not known if there is bilateral disease or not, it is recommended to also perform the same exam with the dog in lateral recumbency. A painful response upon stretching of the muscle by itself or when performing direct palpation indicates potential biceps brachii pathology. If complete rupture of the biceps is present, the distal limb may be elevated caudodorsally beyond normal, without restriction (Video 15.1).

Video 15.1

Biceps stretch with complete biceps tear.

Other tests described include the shoulder drawer test and the biceps retraction test. The shoulder drawer test has been suggested to indicate biceps tendon rupture, although most commonly it is used to evaluate for craniocaudal shoulder instability. The biceps tendon retraction test is performed to evaluate for a pain response when pulling the tendon caudally with the dog in a weight-bearing position. A positive response indicates biceps tendinopathy (Rochat 2018).

15.6.3   Diagnostics

The pros, cons, and choice of diagnostics are similar to those described for diagnosing MSI. If the physical exam findings indicate biceps disease, radiographs are a logical first step to rule out other diseases and to potentially accomplish a diagnosis. However, if non-calcifying tendinopathy is present, *radiographs* may be completely normal. In chronic stages of the disease, sclerosis of the

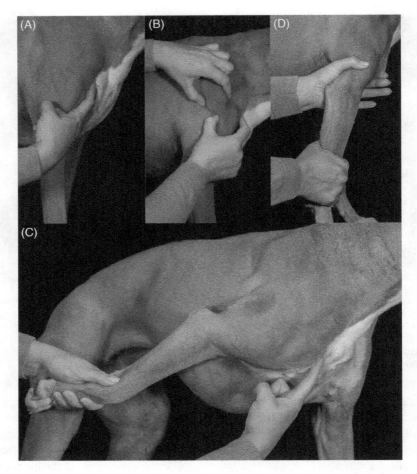

Figure 15.11 Biceps brachii palpation: (A) the biceps tendon can be digitally palpated, just medially to the greater tubercle; (B) shoulder drawer test is performed by stabilizing the scapula with one hand, while the other hand attempts to displace the humeral head cranially, relative to the supraglenoid tubercle; (C) biceps disease can frequently be detected by eliciting a painful response when placing the shoulder in flexion and hyperextending the elbow, while applying digital pressure to the biceps tendon, the so-called biceps test; (D) a painful response during the biceps test may be due to elbow disease since the elbow is hyperextended. This can easily be differentiated by performing isolated elbow hyperextension.

humeral intertubercular groove and/or mineralization of the biceps tendon and osteophytosis can be appreciated (Figure 15.12). *Skyline views* (Figure 15.13) may aid in identifying biceps pathology in addition to distinguishing biceps disease from supraspinatus disease.

Contrast arthrography has been reported, but because of its invasive nature and due to the increased use of ultrasound, this technique is less frequently performed. It may reveal incomplete or narrowed contrast flow within the biceps tendon sheath, irregular biceps tendon definition, or impingement of the biceps tendon (Davidson et al. 2000).

Ultrasound (Figure 10.2) is a useful tool to diagnose pathology of the biceps tendon, especially if the ultrasonographer is skilled at musculoskeletal evaluation (Kramer et al. 2001; Barella et al. 2018). Ultrasound is the only imaging modality that can be performed in a dynamic fashion and

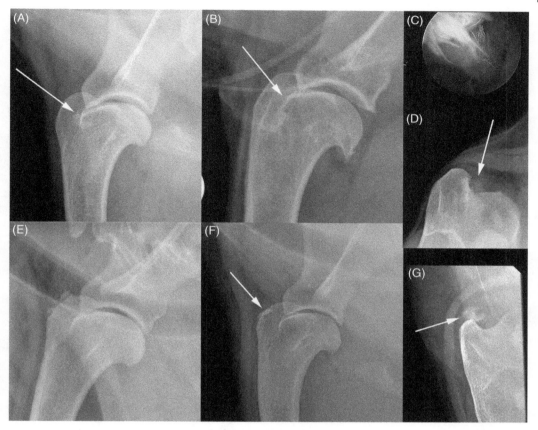

Figure 15.12 Imaging features of (A–D) biceps and (E–G) supraspinatus tendinopathy: (A) faint mineralization present in the bicipital groove, indicating likely biceps tendinopathy; (B) sclerosis along the bicipital groove, a common finding with chronic bicipital tendinopathy. This dog is also suffering from severe osteoarthritic changes; (C) arthroscopic view of the biceps tendon showing partial rupture; (D) skyline view of the shoulder, demonstrating calcification present within the intertubercular groove, this location is consistent with biceps tendinopathy rather than supraspinatus disease; (E, F) calcification of the supraspinatus tendon can be visualized at the cranial aspect of the scapulohumeral joint; (G) skyline view of the shoulder, demonstrating calcification present lateral to the intertubercular groove, this location is consistent with supraspinatus tendinopathy rather than biceps disease.

SHOULDER REGION

thereby allows for the diagnosis of adhesions of the biceps tendon to the tendon sheath or joint capsule (Cook 2016).

CT of the canine shoulder is frequently performed to rule out other diseases but it is not considered a primary imaging modality for biceps tendinopathy. CT arthrography is reported to be of more diagnostic value than CT alone in diagnosing biceps pathology, and CT arthrography with epinephrine appears to improve image sharpness, particularly if imaging is delayed (De Simone et al. 2013; Eivers et al. 2018).

MRI (Figure 10.5) is a sensitive diagnostic tool for identifying both primary biceps tendinopathy and biceps impingement (Murphy et al. 2008).

Arthroscopy has the distinct advantage to be able to combine diagnostic value with potential immediate therapy (e.g. biceps tendon release).

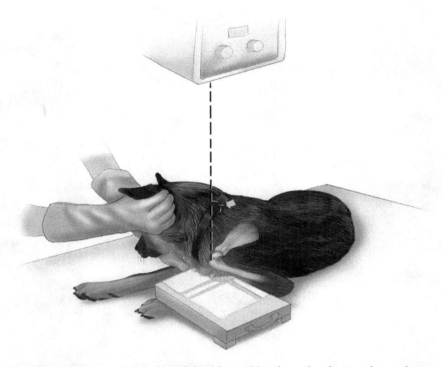

Figure 15.13   When obtaining a skyline view of shoulder, position the patient in sternal recumbency with the patient's head and neck placed on midline, or toward the contralateral shoulder, to prevent superimposition. With the shoulder and elbow joints of the limb of interest kept in alignment, flex the elbow, and position the radius and ulna laterally. The humerus should be parallel to the table top. Center the radiographic beam on the shoulder joint, collimated to either side and several centimeters cranial and caudal to the shoulder joint.

15.7   Supraspinatus Tendinopathy

Similar to biceps tendinopathy, supraspinatus tendinopathy has also been described as a calcifying and non-calcifying tendinopathy (Lafuente et al. 2009; Canapp et al. 2016). While there is some confusion whether these conditions are separate or a continuum of the disease, the term supraspinatus tendinopathy encompasses all conditions affecting the tendon. This may include partial, complete, or micro-tears of the tendon (tendinosis) as well as the chronic phases which may result in calcification of the tendon. The condition may go unidentified, or be misdiagnosed as a different shoulder injury, and therefore may be under-recognized. On the other hand, calcification may be an incidental finding (Maddox et al. 2013) and therefore radiographic abnormalities must be correlated with clinical signs. Although the pathogenesis of supraspinatus tendinopathy is not clearly understood, repetitive microtrauma has been suggested. Medical management of supraspinatus tendinopathy is most frequently performed but surgical resection for calcifying supraspinatus tendinopathy has also been reported (Lafuente et al. 2009).

15.7.1   Signalment and History

Supraspinatus tendinopathy most commonly occurs in medium- to large-breed, active dogs, functioning as pet, working, and agility dogs (Lafuente et al. 2009; Canapp et al. 2016). A unilateral lameness is more common than bilateral, and the disease can present acutely or after a chronic history. Dogs frequently are reported to have failed medical management therapy and have chronic intermittent or waxing and waning lameness.

15.7.2 Physical Exam

Patients generally present with a weight-bearing lameness. Pain on direct palpation of the supraspinatus may be found. Dogs commonly have pain on flexion of the shoulder, since this stretches the muscle. The entire muscle should be palpated starting with the origin in the supraspinatus fossa to the insertion on the greater tubercle. This palpation should be performed while the shoulder is flexed. Direct palpation of the muscle insertion (i.e. the most common location of pathology) can be difficult to differentiate from biceps pathology, given their close proximity. Differentiation between the two conditions may be possible by adding elbow extension to the manipulation. This maneuver stretches the biceps, which crosses both joints, whereas the supraspinatus crosses only the shoulder, and thus extension of the elbow should not change the pain response for supraspinatus pathology.

15.7.3 Diagnostics

Radiographic identification of supraspinatus tendinopathy is only apparent when calcification is present. In some cases, it can be challenging to determine if the calcification is supraspinatus or biceps tendon; however, supraspinatus calcification is generally identified more cranial and lateral than biceps calcification (Figure 15.12). In a recent case series, supraspinatus calcification was identified in 13% of the cases (Canapp et al. 2016). Radiographs are also useful to rule out other disease processes such as osseous neoplasia.

Similar to biceps brachii tendinopathy, other modalities used in identifying supraspinatus tendinopathy are ultrasound, MRI, and CT. *Ultrasound* is the most practical and cost-effective imaging modality. It allows distinction of supraspinatus disease from biceps disease and detects cases with minor calcification (Mistieri et al. 2012). Ultrasound findings may include increased diameter of the supraspinatus tendon, increased fluid content, and displacement of the biceps tendon medially (LaFuente et al. 2009; Mistieri et al. 2012). *MRI* is also an effective means of diagnosing supraspinatus tendinopathy, with similar abnormalities identified as ultrasound. Tendon volume can be measured and was consistently found to be larger in affected than normal supraspinatus tendons (Spall et al. 2016). *CT* has not been as thoroughly described for this particular disease but may be useful to rule out other disease processes. Since the supraspinatus is an extra-articular structure, arthroscopy is generally not considered a primary diagnostic methodology. However, intra-articular compression of the biceps tendon, termed a supraspinatus bulge, may be observed (Canapp et al. 2016).

15.8 Infraspinatus Disease

Infraspinatus disease is an uncommon cause of thoracic limb lameness, generally referred to as *infraspinatus contracture*, the result of permanent shortening (i.e. contracture not contraction) of the muscle. The condition manifests in two phases, the *acute* phase when the muscle is injured and the *chronic* phase once contracture has matured. The latter causes a mechanical lameness that results in a pathognomonic gait (Video 15.2). Animals are generally presented during the chronic phase. However, this may change with advances in diagnostic capabilities and knowledge about the disease progression.

Video 15.2

Infraspinatus contracture – gait and surgery.

Because of its location within the infraspinous fossa, osteofascial compartment syndrome has been hypothesized to be a component of the disease process. This condition occurs when muscles that are confined to a tight osteofascial space are injured. The hemorrhage and inflammation result in a substantial increase in pressure within the compartment. This pressure is hypothesized to cause decreased blood supply, necrosis, and ultimately contracture of the muscle (Devor and Sorby 2006).

Early diagnosis is key since treatment options differ greatly if animals are diagnosed during the acute phase. The contracted infraspinatus can be treated with tenectomy of the insertion of the infraspinatus tendon. A good-to-excellent outcome is anticipated for infraspinatus contracture release, making this condition the only fibrotic myopathy with a favorable prognosis. However, surgical treatment may potentially be avoided if therapy is initiated during the acute phase. Therapy for this phase is not well studied but may include a fascial release to decrease the pressure and avoid progression of the disease (Devor and Sorby 2006).

15.8.1 Signalment and History

Hunting dogs are most commonly afflicted with infraspinatus contracture. Frequently, they are reported to have an acute lameness that resolves with rest and medical therapy, followed by a recurrent, persistent, static, and non-painful lameness occurring several weeks later. The first stage is thought to be related to the original pain when the muscle is acutely injured. The inflammation and associated pain then subside, and the abnormal gait is appreciated when fibrotic changes have occurred. Patients typically have a unilateral lameness; bilateral infraspinatus disease is reported but extremely rare (Franch et al. 2009).

15.8.2 Physical Exam

Physical exam findings vary depending on the phase of infraspinatus injury. During the acute phase, mild swelling and varying degrees of pain may be identified on direct palpation and stretching of the infraspinatus muscle. The infraspinatus originates in the infraspinous fossa of the scapula (i.e. caudal to the scapular spine), crosses the shoulder joint, and inserts on the proximolateral surface of the humerus (i.e. on the cranial aspect of the proximal humerus). Given this location, the concentric action of the muscle varies depending on the shoulder joint position. For instance, when the shoulder joint is flexed, the muscle extends the joint. But when extended, the muscle flexes the joint. It is also an abductor and lateral rotator of the joint. Stretching of the muscle, therefore, can be performed by either extending or flexing the shoulder joint, while adducting and internally rotating the shoulder. This can be accomplished by examining the "down" leg in recumbent position (Figure 15.14). If performed during extension and examining the "up" leg, the entire muscle can be palpated. The emphasis of this palpation should be placed on the myotendinous portion, which is located approximately at the level of the acromion. However, this area may not be palpable because of the overlying deltoid muscle, particularly in well-muscled dogs.

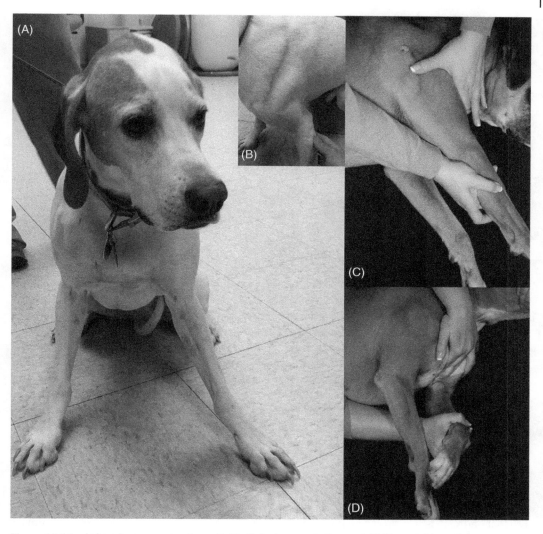

Figure 15.14 Infraspinatus contracture: (A, B) clinical presentation and (C, D) stretching of the infraspinatus muscle: (A) classic stance showing external rotation of the lower limb with elbow adduction; (B) severe infraspinatus muscle atrophy; (C) stretching and palpation of the muscle with extension of the shoulder joint while performing limb adduction and internal rotation; (D) stretching of the muscle with flexion of the shoulder joint while performing limb adduction and internal rotation, note that palpation of the muscle is not possible when manipulating the "down" limb to create excessive adduction and internal rotation.

When infraspinatus contracture occurs, the patient has a very distinctive appearance of their limb carriage. During ambulation, the elbow is adducted and the patient circumducts the limb, while flipping the paw to place it (Videos 15.2 and 15.3). When static, the distal antebrachium and paw can be observed to be externally rotated, while the elbow remains adducted, with varying degrees of shoulder abduction (Figure 15.14). This may also manifest in an elevated limb (i.e. abducted) if the patient is placed in lateral recumbency. Severe, visible muscle atrophy isolated to the infraspinatus muscle is also generally present.

Video 15.3

Infraspinatus contracture – gait comparison before and after surgery.

Palpation shows that the humerus is incapable of internal rotation (pronation) relative to the scapula, because the contracted infraspinatus prevents medial rotation. This can be evaluated by stabilizing the scapula and attempting internal rotation of the humerus/limb. Alternatively, one may internally rotate the limb without stabilizing the scapula: a patient that has a contracted infraspinatus will show elevation of the caudal scapula during this maneuver. The contralateral limb, when normal, provides a good reference point for what internal rotation capacity should be.

15.8.3 Diagnostics

Physical exam findings with mature contractures are unique enough that diagnosis of infraspinatus contracture is generally convincing on physical examination. Although further advanced diagnostics are typically not required specifically for the contracture, advanced imaging is beneficial to assess for other soft tissue injuries as well. For example, radiographs are a reasonable initial diagnostic tool to screen for other shoulder pathology, yet are expected to be normal with infraspinatus contracture.

In contrast, acute injury of the infraspinatus can be challenging to identify on physical exam. Ultrasound or MRI is a necessary diagnostic tool if the clinician is suspicious of early infraspinatus injury and seeks a diagnosis prior to contracture to attempt preemptive therapy to avoid progression of dysfunction. Ultrasound is the most affordable and clinically relevant imaging tool to confirm a diagnosis of infraspinatus contracture. MRI is reported to have 100% agreement and concordance with surgical findings of infraspinatus disease (Murphy et al. 2008).

15.9 Osteochondrosis Dissecans

Osteochondrosis is a disorder of the endochondral ossification process of developing animals. Normal endochondral ossification is the process whereby cartilage transforms into metaphyseal or epiphyseal bone. In *osteochondrosis*, the transformation into bone is disrupted, leaving a defect in the interface between cartilage and subchondral bone. Over time, this defect may allow the formation of a fissure or flap of cartilage over its surface, known as *osteochondrosis dissecans* (OCD). This flap can dissociate, which typically leads to joint effusion, synovitis, lameness, and arthritis (Ytrehus et al. 2007). The most likely site of OCD in the canine shoulder is the caudal surface of the humeral head, however, it has been reported infrequently to occur in the glenoid cavity (Lande et al. 2014; Bilmont et al. 2018). In general, surgical removal of the flap (osteochondroplasty) is recommended for treatment of shoulder OCD, which is associated with favorable outcomes.

15.9.1 Signalment and History

Given the developmental nature of the disease, most clinical symptoms occur early in the dog's life, with most animals presenting between 4 and 8 months of age. Large- and giant-breed dogs are most commonly affected, and high-protein, high-calorie diets have been implicated as an associated factor (Richardson and Zentek 1998). On occasion, evidence of osteochondrosis may become apparent incidentally, as the disease progresses with secondary osteoarthritis, or if OCD affects other structures (bicipital impingement secondary to joint mouse). Patients are typically lame in one limb, with the lameness worsening with exercise or intensive activity. In spite of the tendency for unilateral symptoms, approximately half of patients will have bilateral lesions (Rochat 2018).

15.9.2 Physical Exam

Most animals present with a mild-moderate weight-bearing lameness. Muscle atrophy may be present if symptoms have been noted for a prolonged period. Patients experience pain most commonly on flexion of the shoulder joint; however, some dogs react on extension as well. It is important to carefully examine the contralateral limb, given the frequency of bilaterality. An absence of pain reaction does not rule out the presence of osteochondrosis or OCD.

15.9.3 Diagnostics

Radiographs are the first-line diagnostic of choice. OCD lesions typically are readily appreciated on the caudal surface of the humeral head as a defect in the subchondral continuity. The flap is not actually visualized radiographically unless it has mineralized. Subchondral sclerosis can be appreciated with osteochondrosis or OCD. Positioning of the shoulder joint relative to other structures should be heeded, as summation may challenge interpretation. The lateral view is best obtained with the shoulder joint pulled distally away from the neck, and the contralateral thoracic limb pulled caudally away from the radiographic beam. If OCD is suspected, but not apparent radiographically, lateral views with pronation and supination of the limb can improve visualization of the caudal humeral head surface and delineate a lesion not otherwise apparent (Figure 15.15; Wall et al. 2015). In some cases, the OCD flap may be displaced or completely dislodged and relocated within the joint space. This is challenging to evaluate radiographically unless the dislodged flap is mineralized, which can occur with chronicity.

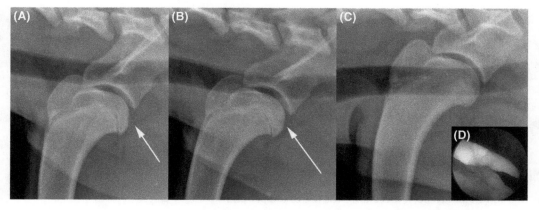

Figure 15.15 Shoulder images of a single dog with (A-D) OCD illustrating that radiographic positioning substantially changes the appearance of the lesion: (A) lateral, supinated radiograph demonstrating characteristic OCD lesion of the caudal humeral head. There is flattening of the subchondral surface, with minimal calcification of the flap; (B) lateral, neutral radiograph – note the mild lucency of the caudal humeral head and flattening of the surface; (C) lateral, pronated view – there is very mild lucency of the caudal humeral head but the lesion can easily be missed on this view; and (D) arthroscopic view of the OCD flap.

SHOULDER REGION

Arthrography, ultrasound, CT, and MRI have all been reported and evaluated for imaging osteochondrosis/OCD. One study reported reasonable success at identifying cartilage flaps of OCD lesions with arthrography and ultrasound, when the flap was not mineralized, and thus not identified radiographically (Vandevelde et al. 2006). Another study reported both ultrasound and MRI had better sensitivity (but not specificity) than radiographs at accurately diagnosing the presence or absence of shoulder OCD (Wall et al. 2015). CT is a frequently used imaging modality since it allows rapid investigation of the two most commonly observed pathologies in juvenile patients: shoulder OCD and elbow dysplasia. Furthermore, it aids to detect other, less commonly observed differential diagnoses, such as panosteitis.

Arthroscopy is also an extremely valuable tool in diagnosing OCD, since it allows for evaluation of the cartilage surface itself. It is also the only diagnostic method that allows therapeutic intervention. Since most OCD lesions are readily identified on radiographs, clinicians will frequently proceed to arthroscopy as the next diagnostic of choice, to also allow surgical correction of the disease.

15.10 Other Diseases Affecting the Shoulder Region

15.10.1 Caudal Glenoid Fragments

Lameness resulting from a fragment in the area of the caudal glenoid has been reported although different terminologies have been used. The condition was originally described as *accessory caudal glenoid ossification center* (Olivieri et al. 2004) whereas other authors have described it as "calcification of the caudal rim of the glenoid" (Van Vynckt et al. 2013). Regardless, these caudal glenoid fragments may be asymptomatic, if they are not freely movable. The fragment can be identified radiographically (Figure 15.16), although advanced imaging is prudent to ensure other causes of lameness are not present. Arthroscopic examination can identify the degree of mobility of the fragment, further validating diagnosis. It can also be utilized to remove the fragment and is reported to successfully alleviate lameness in some dogs (Olivieri et al. 2004).

15.10.2 Glenoid Dysplasia

Glenoid dysplasia (i.e. congenital shoulder luxation) describes a congenital deformity of the scapular glenoid cavity, which eliminates the normal articulation and stability of the shoulder joint. The resulting consequence is usually medial shoulder luxation in juvenile dogs (Vaughan and Jones 1969). Cases are usually detected in dogs less than a year of age. Miniature and toy Poodles appear to be a predisposed breed. Physical examination findings include a significant lameness to non-weight-bearing function of the limb. On palpation, the humeral head is detected medial to the scapula. Definitive diagnosis is accomplished with radiographs, which depict a distorted glenoid cavity, displacement of the humeral head, and in some cases, a distorted humeral head (Figure 15.9). Therapy may include surgical (excisional arthroplasty or shoulder arthrodesis) or nonsurgical treatment, depending on severity. Identification of this disease process in a mature dog, that has previously been asymptomatic, warrants a thorough investigation for other causes of lameness, as this condition has been present for the life of the patient.

15.10.3 Adhesive Capsulitis

Adhesive capsulitis, also termed "frozen shoulder," describes a condition of pain and loss of ROM caused by fibrosis of the joint capsule and adhesion formation within the joint. In people, it may arise spontaneously or secondary to other shoulder conditions or immobilization. Importantly, the condition has been described to undergo multiple phases, including a final "thaw" phase, with return of shoulder ROM and function regardless of intervention (Eljabu et al. 2016). This condition is well described in people and has recently been reported in eight canine patients (Carr et al. 2016). All patients were reported to have a chronic, severe thoracic limb lameness with pain on shoulder manipulation and severe decrease in ROM. None of the patients responded to treatment. Diagnostic imaging such as MRI, ultrasound, and arthroscopy may be utilized to identify underlying pathology. A tentative diagnosis is made if excessive joint capsule fibrosis, scar tissue, or adhesion formation is observed (Figure 15.16). If other shoulder conditions are observed, it is difficult to know whether the observed fibrotic changes are consequences of the other disease processes or a separate disease process. Successful treatment of adhesive capsulitis has not yet been identified in dogs. However, the thawing phase in people is reached one to three years after initial onset of symptoms (Eljabu et al. 2016) and it is unknown when or if this phase occurs in dogs.

15.10.4 Shoulder Region Neoplasia

The most common neoplasia of the shoulder is proximal humeral osteosarcoma. Brachial plexus neoplasia may also mimic a shoulder lameness. These conditions should be considered as differential diagnoses in any patient and are described in Chapters 11, 16, and 17.

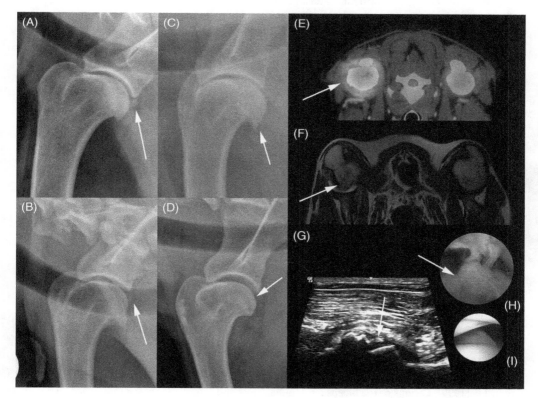

Figure 15.16 Other shoulder conditions: (A) caudal glenoid fragment (white arrow); (B) radiograph of a dog with severe osteoarthritis, biceps disease, and a caudal glenoid fragment; (C) radiograph of a dog with moderate osteoarthritis (white arrow); (D-H) diagnostic imaging of a dog with adhesive capsulitis, biceps tendinopathy, and a chronic OCD lesion: (D) lateral radiograph showing flattening of the humeral head (white arrow), mineralization in the bicipital tendon sheath, and degenerative changes; (E) positron emission tomography (PET)/CT showing increased uptake (white arrow) of the shoulder; (F) MRI showing a thickened joint capsule (white arrows); (G) ultrasound; (H) arthroscopy showing extensive synovial proliferation and adhesions (white arrow) and (I) a normal joint for comparison.

15.10.5 Miscellaneous Other Conditions

Avulsion of the supraspinatus and infraspinatus tendon has been reported in a case series of juvenile Labrador dogs. Radiographs may aid the diagnosis if an osseous avulsion fragment is present. Ultrasound, CT, or MRI is reasonable next diagnostics to verify the diagnosis (Mikola et al. 2018).

Ossification of the infraspinatus tendon-bursa has been reported in a case series of adult Labrador Retrievers (Mckee et al. 2007). Radiographs may demonstrate mineralized bodies lateral to the humeral head most easily visible on the craniocaudal view. Ultrasound, CT, or MRI can diagnose the condition if mineralization is not radiographically apparent.

Medial displacement of the tendon of origin of *biceps brachii* is recognized to occur following rupture of the transverse humeral ligament, which holds the biceps brachii securely within the intertubercular groove (Boemo and Eaton-Wells 1995). Medial displacement of the tendon can typically be detected while palpating the tendon and placing the shoulder through full ROM. Occasionally, a "popping" noise of the tendon displacing through this ROM may be heard. Ultrasound may be very useful, as it allows dynamic assessment.

Rupture of biceps tendon sheath has been reported in two cases with thoracic limb lameness. It was diagnosed by leakage of contrast material from the biceps tendon sheath on contrast arthrography (Innes and Brown 2004).

A single case of *abnormal ossification of the supraglenoid tubercle* and cranial glenoid cavity has been reported. The dogs showed irregular margination and supraglenoid tubercle separation from the scapula on CT (De Simone et al. 2013).

A single case report of *teres minor myopathy* exists (Bruce et al. 1997). Diagnosis was obtained with ultrasound imaging of the shoulder.

Scapular luxation results from traumatic rupture of the serratus ventralis muscle. This condition is generally diagnosed by observation of a dorsally displaced scapula (see Video 15.4), but CT or MRI can further elucidate the degree of damage (Jones et al. 2017; Frye et al. 2018).

Video 15.4

Scapular luxation.

References

Akerblom, S. and Sjostrom, L. (2007). Evaluation of clinical, radiographical and cytological findings compared to arthroscopic findings in shoulder joint lameness in the dog. *Vet Comp Orthop Traumatol* 20 (2): 136–141.

Bardet, J.F. (1998). Diagnosis of shoulder instability in dogs and cats: a retrospective study. *J Am Anim Hosp Assoc* 34 (1): 42–54.

Bardet, J.F. (1999). Lesions of the biceps tendon diagnosis and classification. *Vet Comp Orthop Traumatol* 12 (4): 188–195.

Barella, G., Lodi, M., and Faverzani, S. (2018). Ultrasonographic findings of shoulder teno-muscular structures in symptomatic and asymptomatic dogs. *J Ultrasound* 21 (2): 145–152.

Bergenhuyzen, A.L., Vermote, K.A., Van Bree, H., and Van Ryssen, B. (2010). Long-term follow-up after arthroscopic tenotomy for partial rupture of the biceps brachii tendon. *Vet Comp Orthop Traumatol* 23 (1): 51–55.

Bilmont, A., Mathon, D., and Autefage, A. (2018). Arthroscopic management of osteochondrosis of the glenoid cavity in a dog. *J Am Anim Hosp Assoc* 54 (5): e54503.

Boemo, C.M. and Eaton-Wells, R.D. (1995). Medial displacement of the tendon of origin of the biceps brachii muscle in 10 greyhounds. *J Small Anim Pract* 36 (2): 69–73.

Bruce, W.J., Spence, S., and Miller, A. (1997). Teres minor myopathy as a cause of lameness in a dog. *J Small Anim Pract* 38 (2): 74–77.

Canapp, S.O., Canapp, D.A., Carr, B.J. et al. (2016). Supraspinatus tendinopathy in 327 dogs: a Retrospective Study. *Vet Evid* 1 (3).

Carr, B.J., Canapp, S.O., Canapp, D.A. et al. (2016). Adhesive capsulitis in eight dogs: Diagnosis and management. *Front Vet Sci* 3: 55.

Cogar, S.M., Cook, C.R., Curry, S.L. et al. (2008). Prospective evaluation of techniques for differentiating shoulder pathology as a source of thoracic limb lameness in medium and large breed dogs. *Vet Surg* 37 (2): 132–141.

Cook, C.R. (2016). Ultrasound imaging of the musculoskeletal system. *Vet Clin Small Anim Pract* 46 (3): 355–371.

Cook, J.L., Renfro, D.C., Tomlinson, J.L., and Sorensen, J.E. (2005a). Measurement of angles of abduction for diagnosis of shoulder instability in dogs using goniometry and digital image analysis. *Vet Surg* 34 (5): 463–468.

Cook, J.L., Tomlinson, J.L., Fox, D.B. et al. (2005b). Treatment of dogs diagnosed with medial shoulder instability using radiofrequency-induced thermal capsulorrhaphy. *Vet Surg* 34 (5): 469–475.

Craig, L.E. and Reed, A. (2013). Age-associated cartilage degeneration of the canine humeral head. *Vet Pathol* 50 (2): 264–268.

Davidson, E.B., Griffey, S.M., Vasseur, P.B., and Shields, S.L. (2000). Histopathological, radiographic, and arthrographic comparison of the biceps tendon in normal dogs and dogs with biceps tenosynovitis. *J Am Anim Hosp Assoc* 36 (6): 522–530.

De Simone, A., Gernone, F., and Ricciardi, M. (2013). Imaging diagnosis-bilateral abnormal ossification of the supraglenoid tubercle and cranial glenoid cavity in an English Setter. *Vet Radiol Ultrasound* 54 (2): 159–163.

Devitt, C.M., Neely, M.R., and Vanvechten, B.J. (2007). Relationship of physical examination test of shoulder instability to arthroscopic findings in dogs. *Vet Surg* 36 (7): 661–668.

Devor, M. and Sorby, R. (2006). Fibrotic contracture of the canine infraspinatus muscle. *Vet Comp Orthop Traumatol* 2 (2): 117–121.

Eivers, C.R., Corzo-Menendez, N., Austwick, S.H. et al. (2018). Computed tomographic arthrography is a useful adjunct to survey computed tomography and arthroscopic evaluation of the canine shoulder joint. *Vet Radiol Ultrasound* 59 (5): 535–544.

Eljabu, W., Klinger, H.M., and Von Knoch, M. (2016). Prognostic factors and therapeutic options for treatment of frozen shoulder: a systematic review. *Arch Orthop Trauma Surg* 136 (1): 1–7.

Fournet, A., Manassero, M., Decambron, A., and Viateau, V. (2018). Needle arthroscopy for shoulder joint exploration. A cadaveric study in dogs. *Proceedings of the 27th Annual Scientific Meeting of the European College of Veterinary Surgeons*, Athens, Greece (4–6 July 2018). Vet Surg, E 37.

Franch, J., Bertran, J., Remolins, G. et al. (2009). Simultaneous bilateral contracture of the infraspinatus muscle. *Vet Comp Orthop Traumatol* 22 (3): 249–252.

Franklin, S.P., Devitt, C.M., Ogawa, J. et al. (2013). Outcomes associated with treatments for medial, lateral, and multidirectional shoulder instability in dogs. *Vet Surg* 42 (4): 361–364.

Frisbie, D.D., Barrett, M.F., Mcilwraith, C.W., and Ullmer, J. (2014). Diagnostic stifle joint arthroscopy using a needle arthroscope in standing horses. *Vet Surg* 43 (1): 12–18.

Frye, C.W., Hansen, C.M., Gendron, K., and von Pfeil, D.J.F. (2018). Successful medical management and rehabilitation of exercise-induced dorsal scapular luxation in an ultramarathon endurance sled dog with magnetic resonance imaging diagnosis of grade II serratus ventralis strain. *Can Vet J* 59 (12): 1329–1332.

Fujita, Y., Yamaguchi, S., Agnello, K.A., and Muto, M. (2013). Effects of transection of the cranial arm of the medial glenohumeral ligament on shoulder stability in adult Beagles. *Vet Comp Orthop Traumatol* 26 (2): 94–99.

George, C., Secrest, S., Davis, M. et al. (2017). Forelimb lameness localization and ultrasonographic assessment of the shoulder in Iditarod sled dogs. *Proceedings of the International Working Dog Conference*, Banff, Alberta Canada (2–6 April 2017). https://iwdc.iwdba.org/sites/default/files/11iditarod_2017_banff_iwdc.pdf (accessed 6 May 2019).

Gilley, R.S., Wallace, L.J., and Hayden, D.W. (2002). Clinical and pathologic analyses of bicipital tenosynovitis in dogs. *Am J Vet Res* 63 (3): 402–407.

Henderson, A.L., Latimer, C., and Millis, D.L. (2015). Rehabilitation and physical therapy for selected orthopedic conditions in veterinary patients. *Vet Clin North Am Small Anim Pract* 45 (1): 91–121.

Innes, J.F. and Brown, G. (2004). Rupture of the biceps brachii tendon sheath in two dogs. *J Small Anim Pract* 45 (1): 25–28.

Jones, S.C., Tinga, S., Porter, E.G., and Lewis, D. (2017). Surgical management of dorsal scapular luxation in three dogs. *Vet Comp Orthop Traumatol* 30 (1): 75–80.

Kramer, M., Gerwing, M., Sheppard, C., and Schimke, E. (2001). Ultrasonography for the diagnosis of diseases of the tendon and tendon sheath of the biceps brachii muscle. *Vet Surg* 30 (1): 64–71.

Lafuente, M.P., Fransson, B.A., Lincoln, J.D. et al. (2009). Surgical treatment of mineralized and nonmineralized supraspinatus tendinopathy in twenty-four dogs. *Vet Surg* 38 (3): 380–387.

Lande, R., Reese, S.L., Cuddy, L.C. et al. (2014). Prevalence of computed tomographic subchondral bone lesions in the scapulohumeral joint of 32 immature dogs with thoracic limb lameness. *Vet Radiol Ultrasound* 55 (1): 23–28.

Livet, V., Harel, M., Taroni, M. et al. (2018). Stress radiography for the diagnosis of medial glenohumeral ligament rupture in canine shoulders. *Proceedings of the 27th Annual Scientific Meeting of the European College of Veterinary Surgeons*, Athens, Greece (4–6 July 2018). Vet Surg, E 47.

Maddox, T.W., May, C., Keeley, B.J., and Mcconnell, J.F. (2013). Comparison between shoulder computed tomography and clinical findings in 89 dogs presented for thoracic limb lameness. *Vet Radiol Ultrasound* 54 (4): 358–364.

Mckee, W.M., Macias, C., May, C., and Scurrell, E.J. (2007). Ossification of the infraspinatus tendon-bursa in 13 dogs. *Vet Rec* 161 (25): 846–852.

Mikola, K., Piras, A., and Hakala, L. (2018). Isolated avulsion of the tendon of insertion of the infraspinatus and supraspinatus muscles in five juvenile Labrador Retrievers. *Vet Comp Orthop Traumatol* 31 (4): 285–290.

Mistieri, M.L., Wigger, A., Canola, J.C. et al. (2012). Ultrasonographic evaluation of canine supraspinatus calcifying tendinosis. *J Am Anim Hosp Assoc* 48 (6): 405–410.

Murphy, S.E., Ballegeer, E.A., Forrest, L.J., and Schaefer, S.L. (2008). Magnetic resonance imaging findings in dogs with confirmed shoulder pathology. *Vet Surg* 37 (7): 631–638.

O'Donnell, E.M., Canapp, S.O. Jr., Cook, J.L., and Pike, F. (2017). Treatment of medial shoulder joint instability in dogs by extracapsular stabilization with a prosthetic ligament: 39 cases (2008–2013). *J Am Vet Med Assoc* 251 (9): 1042–1052.

Olivieri, M., Piras, A., Marcellin-Little, D.J. et al. (2004). Accessory caudal glenoid ossification centre as possible cause of lameness in nine dogs. *Vet Comp Orthop Traumatol* 17 (3): 131–135.

Pettitt, R.A., Clements, D.N., and Guilliard, M.J. (2007). Stabilisation of medial shoulder instability by imbrication of the subscapularis muscle tendon of insertion. *J Small Anim Pract* 48 (11): 626–631.

Richardson, D.C. and Zentek, J. (1998). Nutrition and osteochondrosis. *Vet Clin North Am Small Anim Pract* 28 (1): 115–135.

Rochat, M. (2018). The shoulder. In: Veterinary Surgery: Small Animal, 2e (eds. S.A. Johnston and K.M. Tobias), 800–820. St. Louis: Elsevier.

Sidaway, B.K., Mclaughlin, R.M., Elder, S.H. et al. (2004). Role of the tendons of the biceps brachii and infraspinatus muscles and the medial glenohumeral ligament in the maintenance of passive shoulder joint stability in dogs. *Am J Vet Res* 65 (9): 1216–1222.

Spall, B.F., Fransson, B.A., Martinez, S.A., and Wilkinson, T.E. (2016). Tendon volume determination on magnetic resonance imaging of supraspinatus tendinopathy. *Vet Surg* 45 (3): 386–391.

Van Vynckt, D., Verhoeven, G., Samoy, Y. et al. (2013). Anaesthetic arthrography of the shoulder joint in dogs. *Vet Comp Orthop Traumatol* 26 (4): 291–297.

Vandevelde, B., Van Ryssen, B., Saunders, J.H. et al. (2006). Comparison of the ultrasonographic appearance of osteochondrosis lesions in the canine shoulder with radiography, arthrography, and arthroscopy. *Vet Radiol Ultrasound* 47 (2): 174–184.

Vaughan, L.C. and Jones, D.G. (1969). Congenital dislocation of the shoulder joint in the dog. *J Small Anim Pract* 10 (1): 1–3.

Wall, C.R., Cook, C.R., and Cook, J.L. (2015). Diagnostic sensitivity of radiography, ultrasonography, and magnetic resonance imaging for detecting shoulder osteochondrosis/oteochondritis dissecans in dogs. *Vet Radiol Ultrasound* 56 (1): 3–11.

Wiemer, P., Van Ryssen, B., Gielen, I. et al. (2007). Diagnostic findings in a lame-free dog with complete rupture of the biceps brachii tendon. A case report in a unilaterally affected working Labrador Retriever. *Vet Comp Orthop Traumatol* 20 (1): 73–77.

Ytrehus, B., Carlson, C., and Ekman, S. (2007). Etiology and pathogenesis of osteochondrosis. *Vet Pathol* 44 (4): 429–448.

SHOULDER REGION

16

Neurological Disease of the Thoracic Limb
Lisa Bartner

Department of Clinical Sciences, College of Veterinary Medicine and Biomedical Sciences, Colorado State University, Fort Collins, CO, USA

16.1   Introduction

When presented with a patient displaying a thoracic limb lameness, neurologic dysfunction should always be considered a differential diagnosis and a systematic approach is necessary to determine the cause of the gait abnormality. While there are many conditions affecting *both* thoracic limbs, these conditions are generally less confusing to differentiate from orthopedic disease than a dog presenting with *monoparesis* or unilateral *neurogenic lameness* (see Chapter 4 for definitions, Box 4.1). Furthermore, as described in Chapter 4, the same condition may result in monoparesis and/or unilateral neurogenic lameness if the dorsal and ventral nerve roots are affected, because of the close juxtaposition between sensory and motor components supplied by these two. For example, a nerve sheath tumor affecting the nerve root may cause inability to support weight (ventral root involvement) and pain during weight support (dorsal root involvement). The focus of this chapter is diseases that cause symptoms that can easily be confused with orthopedic causes of lameness (in its broader applied terminology). For nervous system conditions, an anatomic diagnosis must be reached before making a list of etiologic diagnoses; Chapter 4 described the neurologic examination and localization (i.e. anatomic diagnosis). Table 16.1 outlines common differential diagnoses and diagnostic steps for neurological diseases causing monoparesis or neurogenic lameness of the thoracic limb.

Video 16.1

Complete brachial plexus avulsion: clinical exam and presentation.

16.2   Relevant Anatomy

Branches of the sixth, seventh, eighth cervical, and the first and second thoracic spinal nerves fuse and form the brachial plexus. There is variability among individual animals where some can either have the fifth cervical and/or or lack the second thoracic spinal nerve(s), sometimes referred to as

Table 16.1 Key features of select neurologic diseases causing monoparesis or neurogenic lameness of the thoracic limb.

Disease	Common signalment	Diagnostic test of choice	Clinical presentation and course	Distinguishing exam findings	Treatment	Clinical pearls
Intervertebral Disc (IVD) extrusion (Hansen Type I)	Young- to middle-aged adults; chondrodystrophic	History and examination MRI	Acute, progressive, or wax/wane	Depends on severity and location; spinal hyperesthesia common	Depends on clinical signs; conservative or surgical	Common cause of lameness or monoparesis; frequently lateralized and acute
Acute non-compressive nucleus pulposus extrusion (ANNPE)	Older, large-breed	History and examination MRI	Peracute, nonprogressive after 24 h	May be painful on exam but non-painful after 24 h; symmetric or asymmetric signs	Conservative	Less commonly results in lameness or monoparesis; more often affects multiple limbs
Fibrocartilaginous embolism (FCE)	Young- to middle-aged, large- and giant-breed	History and examination MRI	Peracute, nonprogressive after 24 h	Usually non-painful and asymmetric signs	Conservative	Occasionally results in lameness or paresis (mono- or hemiparesis)
Neoplasia of the spinal nerve or spinal cord	Older but any age	History and examination Radiographs MRI CT Electrodiagnostics	Acute or chronic, progressive	Sensory exam (cutaneous testing) and muscle atrophy	Conservative; surgical; and radiation therapy	Common cause of monoparesis or lameness
Brachial plexus injury	Any	History and examination MRI Electrodiagnostics	Peracute to acute Nonprogressive after 24 h	Sensory exam (cutaneous testing) and muscle atrophy	Conservative; typically amputation in severe cases	Commonly causes lameness or monoparesis (if history supports)

Peracute = several hours; acute = several days; chronic = weeks or longer.
CT, computed tomography; CSF, cerebrospinal fluid; and MRI, magnetic resonance imaging.

a pre- or post-fixed plexus, respectively. Nevertheless, two or three spinal nerve branches combine to form the major named nerves of the brachial plexus, specifically the suprascapular, subscapular, axillary, musculocutaneous, radial, median, ulnar, and lateral thoracic nerves. Table 16.2 provides a summary of each nerve and the spinal cord segments from which they arise. Wide variations exist among individuals but as a general guideline, nerves exiting cranially in a plexus will innervate more cranial and proximal muscle groups of the limb, while more caudally exiting nerves will innervate caudal and distal muscle groups of the limb.

The *flexors* of the shoulder joint (infraspinatus, teres major, deltoideus, and teres minor) are innervated by the suprascapular and axillary nerves with small contributions from the radial nerve (Hermanson 2013). Elbow flexion is facilitated through activation of the biceps brachii and brachialis muscles innervated by the musculocutaneous nerve. Lastly, carpal and digit flexion are mediated by median and ulnar nerve innervation to the palmar antebrachial muscles (flexor carpi radialis and flexor carpi ulnaris muscles, and superficial digital flexor and interosseous muscles).

Muscles and their respective nerves responsible for *extension* of the thoracic limb include the shoulder extensors (supraspinatus, biceps brachii, and coracobrachialis) supplied by suprascapular, axillary, and musculocutaneous nerves; the elbow extensors in the caudal brachial muscle group (triceps brachii, anconeus, tensor fasciae antebrachia, and extensor carpi radialis) all innervated by the radial nerve; and the carpal and digital extensors belonging to the craniolateral antebrachial muscles (extensor carpi radialis, ulnaris lateralis, common digital extensor, lateral digital extensor, extensor digiti, and pollicis longus) supplied by the radial nerve (Hermanson 2013). Compromise to these muscles and/or nerves, particularly the radial nerve responsible for elbow extension, will affect the weight-bearing abilities of the limb. Injury to the other nerves may cause gait abnormalities but the animal will be able to support its own weight.

16.3 Neurological Diseases Affecting the Thoracic Limb

Signalment and clinical progression are key factors in considering likely causes of monoparesis or lameness affecting the thoracic limb. Commonly encountered conditions include Type I intervertebral disc (IVD) extrusion, neoplasia, fibrocartilaginous embolism (FCE), myelitis/meningomyelitis, and brachial plexus injury (Table 16.1).

16.3.1 Myelopathies and Radiculopathies

Unilateral injury or damage to the C6–T2 spinal cord segments forming the cervical intumescence (i.e. a myelopathy) or to the associated nerve roots (i.e. a radiculopathy) can cause gait abnormalities that are either restricted to only one thoracic limb, such as a lameness or monoparesis, or that are more pronounced in both thoracic limbs (e.g. short-strided gait).

Damage to the motor neuron cell bodies in the ventral gray matter of the cervical intumescence causes a lower motor neuron (LMN) paresis in the thoracic limbs characterized by a stiff, short-strided gait with symmetric lesions, or a monoparesis if the lesion is unilateral. Cervical myelopathies often also involve the white matter, containing the caudally directed general proprioceptive/upper motor neuron (GP/UMN) pathways to the ipsilateral pelvic limb causing a hemiparesis, or to both pelvic limbs causing a paraparesis (Figure 4.1); a GP ataxia may also be noted in either scenario. Deficits to GP/UMN tracts manifest as a long-strided gait in the pelvic limbs and, when present with a short choppy LMN thoracic limb stride, this combination is referred to as a

Table 16.2 Summary of the major motor and sensory distribution of the brachial plexus.

Nerve	Spinal cord segments	Muscle innervated	Motor function	Cutaneous areas	Segmental spinal reflex	Signs of dysfunction
Suprascapular	C6, C7	Supra- and infraspinatus	Extension and lateral support of the shoulder	None	None	Little gait abnormality Pronounced atrophy of supraspinatus and infraspinatus muscles
Brachiocephalicus	C5, C6, C7	Cleidobrachialis	Advance limb	Lateral, cranial, and medial brachium	None	Little gait abnormality Anesthesia of cranial brachium
Musculocutaneous	C6, C7, C8	Biceps brachii, brachialis, and coracobrachialis	Flexion of the elbow	Craniomedial antebrachium and palmar aspect of the paw	Biceps reflex, withdrawal reflex (flexion of elbow)	Little gait abnormality and weakened flexion of the elbow Anesthesia of medial antebrachium
Axillary	C6, C7, C8	Deltoid and teres major and minor	Flexion of the shoulder	None	None	Little gait abnormality Decreased shoulder flexion during withdrawal reflex Anesthesia of lateral brachium
Radial	C6, C7, C8, T1, T2	Triceps brachii and extensors of carpus and digits	Extension of the elbow, the carpus, and the digits	Cranial aspect of antebrachium and dorsal aspect of paw	Triceps reflex (proximal) and extensor carpi radialis (distal)	Loss of weight-bearing Knuckling of paw Decreased extensor carpi radialis and triceps reflexes Anesthesia of cranial surface distal to elbow

Median and ulnar	C8, **T1**, T2	Flexors of carpus and digits	Flexion of the carpus and the digits	Caudal aspect of antebrachium, palmar aspect of paw, and lateral aspect of fifth digit	Withdrawal reflex (flexion of carpus and digits)	Little gait abnormality, slight sinking of the carpus Loss of carpal flexion on flexor reflex Partial loss of pain perception of the palmar surface of the foot and caudal medial antebrachium (distal third)
Lateral thoracic	**C8**, T1	Cutaneous trunci muscle	Cutaneous muscle of the trunk	Respective dermatome to each spinal nerve	Cutaneous trunci reflex	Absent ipsilateral cutaneous trunci reflex Normal sensory evaluation
Sympathetic[a]	T1, T2, T3	Dilator pupillae, orbitalis membrana nictitans, and ciliary muscle	Dilation of the pupil	None	Pupillary light reflex and presence of Horner syndrome	Miosis, ptosis, enophthalmos, and protrusion of third eyelid

The major spinal cord segments that contribute to the nerve are underlined.

[a] The sympathetic nerve is included since it travels along the roots of the brachial plexus, but it is not considered part of the brachial plexus.

two-engine gait. The presence of a two-engine gait is localizing to the cervical intumescence (C6–T2 spinal cord or caudal cervical myelopathy).

If only the C6–T2 nerve roots are injured (i.e. a radiculopathy), a thoracic limb root signature lameness and/or monoparesis usually results and the pelvic limbs will be normal. Whether lameness or monoparesis predominates in a radiculopathy depends on the pathologic involvement of the dorsal or ventral rootlets, respectively. This distinction is far less important than realizing that both lameness and/or monoparesis can occur with a radiculopathy.

Differential etiologic diagnoses causing caudal cervical myelopathies and radiculopathies are outlined below and summarized in Table 16.1. An etiologic diagnosis is established based on signalment, history, clinical signs, and results of diagnostic tests, where available. Advanced imaging modalities such as computed tomography (CT), or preferably magnetic resonance imaging (MRI) in most cases, combined with cerebrospinal fluid (CSF) analysis most accurately confirms the neurologic cause, establishes the anatomic diagnosis, and many times, determines an etiologic cause.

Treatment and prognosis are highly variable depending on severity and cause, ranging from emergency surgical intervention to conservative management. In general, conditions that are acute, severe, and/or progressive typically warrant more definitive therapy. For example, decompressive surgery for a Type I IVD extrusion and recovery may be more complete. Whereas, conditions that are chronic, mild, and/or slowly progressive can often be managed with conservative therapy. However, recovery tends to be incomplete with residual neurologic deficits. Judicious use of corticosteroids is important as they can falsely alter test results (e.g. MRI and CSF) and potentially affect future prognosis if an animal is being undertreated (e.g. meningomyelitis or lymphoma) or incorrectly treated (e.g. discospondylitis).

16.3.1.1 Degenerative Intervertebral Disc Disease and Herniation

Degenerative changes of the IVD and subsequent herniation is one of the most common neurologic disorders in dogs (Brisson 2010). IVD degeneration is known to predispose to intervertebral disc herniation (IVDH), as either extrusion or protrusion of disc material. However, IVD *degeneration* must not be thought of as synonymous with IVD *herniation*, as it is also a common incidental finding in dogs without clinical signs.

The pathophysiology of IVD degeneration can be divided into chondroid metaplasia causing a Hansen Type I IVD extrusion and fibrous metaplasia causing Hansen Type II IVD protrusion. *Chondroid metaplasia* describes the process of premature degeneration frequently seen in young chondrodystrophic breeds but medium- to large-breed dogs can also be affected. Type I IVD extrusion is a common cause for a root signature lameness or monoparesis. The extruded disc material can be lateralized in the vertebral canal and/or extend into the intervertebral foramen, causing unilateral compression of the C6–T2 spinal cord and/or nerve roots, respectively. Alternatively, a short-strided, choppy thoracic limb gait (i.e. LMN paresis) can occur with a midline IVD Type I extrusion or Type II protrusion. *Fibrous metaplasia* describes the process of natural degeneration frequently seen in middle-aged dogs; as such, symptoms are more likely to be slowly progressive.

Dogs with a Type I IVD extrusion tend to present more acutely and have more spinal hyperesthesia compared to dogs affected by Type II IVD protrusions. Dogs with Type I IVD more often show lateralized symptoms deficits although symmetrical symptoms are also common. A more insidious onset and slow progression (days to several months) with various degrees of spinal hyperesthesia is seen with Type II IVD protrusions and cervical spondylomyelopathy (CSM; see Section 16.3.1.4). However, Type II IVD protrusions can have sudden worsening of the otherwise slowly progressive signs.

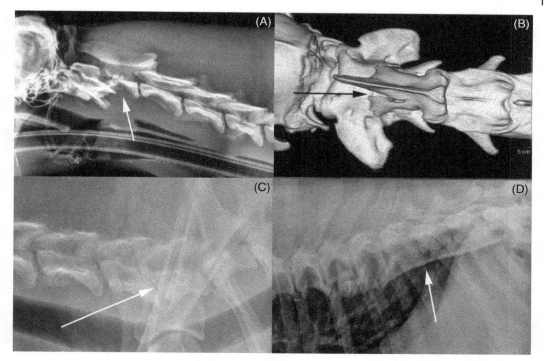

Figure 16.1 Imaging abnormalities illustrating a cervical fracture, radiographic changes of degenerative intervertebral disc disease, and diffuse idiopathic skeletal hyperostosis (DISH): (A) lateral survey radiograph illustrating a comminuted fracture of C2 with minimal displacement; (B) CT of same patient highlighting an incomplete fracture through the cranial to mid-aspect of the left lamina of C2; (C) narrowed disc space, sclerotic end plates, and spondylosis deformans at C6–C7 suggestive of degenerative disc disease; and (D) classic radiographic appearance of DISH; note this condition generally does not cause clinical symptoms.

The imaging modality of choice in patients with IVDH is MRI, given its superior anatomic detail, allowing determination of the affected disc space(s), the lateralization, and dispersion pattern (i.e. dispersed versus non-dispersed) of the herniated disc material. Comparably, CT has the advantage of being a faster imaging modality and can diagnose herniation of calcified discs in chondrodystrophic dogs. However, if there is no IVDH found on plain CT, CT myelography is necessary to diagnose compressive lesions. CT with contrast medium may be necessary to identify parenchymal lesions that contrast enhance, such as nerve sheath tumors or meningiomas. Radiographs can be used to evaluate for other diseases such as osseous neoplasia and signs that may be associated with IVDH (e.g. calcified disc material and narrowed disc spaces; Figure 16.1C). Unfortunately, such findings do not imply compression of the spinal cord making radiographs of limited use.

16.3.1.2 Acute Non-Compressive Nucleus Pulposus Extrusion

In recent years, another type of IVDH has been identified where there is acute extrusion of well-hydrated disc material that does not cause a compressive myelopathy: acute non-compressive nucleus pulposus extrusion (ANNPE; De Decker and Fenn 2018). Other terms to describe this condition include traumatic disc extrusion, high-velocity low-volume disc extrusion, and Hansen Type III disc extrusion. ANNPE is hypothesized to occur when supraphysiologic forces cause a small tear in the annulus fibrosus (e.g. during intense exercise or trauma, allowing sudden extrusion of gelatinous disc material). The force of extrusion into the vertebral canal causes focal contusive injury to the spinal cord. Unlike Type I and II IVDH, the disc material herniated during an ANNPE is nondegenerated, highly hydrated, and gelatinous so it rapidly dissipates leaving minimal to no spinal cord compression. For a visual, this can be likened to a water pistol being discharged towards a person's soft abdomen, leaving a bruise.

Affected patients are frequently older, large-breed dogs. Typically, vocalization during intense activity is reported along with a characteristic clinical presentation: peracute onset of often severe, asymmetric neurologic deficits that are nonprogressive after the initial 24–48 hours. The clinical signs in most cases are lateralized and while a monoparesis can occur, other limbs are commonly affected to a lesser severity. Approximately 40% will have moderate spinal hyperesthesia on examination. Most dogs will regain complete or near-complete neurologic function with conservative therapy. Since these are non-compressive lesions, surgery is typically not indicated.

The imaging modality of choice to diagnose ANNPE is MRI, with the following criteria used: focal spinal cord signal changes (indicating pathology like inflammation and edema), a lesion that is located over the IVD space and is often lateralized, reduction in size of the well-hydrated nucleus pulposus, mild narrowing of the IVD space, and a small volume of IVD material with minimal to no spinal cord compression.

16.3.1.3 Fibrocartilaginous Embolism

Infarction from an FCE or other vascular-related diseases (e.g. arterial embolism causing ischemic neuromyopathy) are common causes for hemiparesis but can also produce a thoracic limb monoparesis if the cervical intumesce gray matter is involved. Histologically, the embolus is identical to the nucleus pulposus of the IVD, indicating that penetration of this material into spinal vessels causes the embolism and associated ischemia of the spinal cord (Nakamoto et al. 2008). The clinical presentation, diagnostic steps, and treatment of dogs with FCE and ANNPE are very similar; however, dogs with FCE are generally non-painful after 24 hours and therefore show spinal hyperesthesia less frequently on examination. Other differentiating features of ANNPE and FCE include the following clinical features: dogs with ANNPE are significantly older and are more likely to have history of vocalization at the onset of clinical signs. While any age and breed can be affected, large and giant breeds seem overrepresented with FCE. Additionally, dogs with ANNPE had lesions affecting the C1–C5 spinal cord segments more often than FCE (Fenn et al. 2016). Differentiating these two is not necessarily of clinical importance; however, ruling out other diseases (such as acute bleeding from a tumor or compressive lesion) can be important. Since it can be difficult to differentiate lesions on CT that do not contrast enhance, MRI is the modality of choice to diagnose both FCE and ANNPE (De Risio and Platt 2010).

16.3.1.4 Cervical Spondylomyelopathy

CSM ("Wobbler Syndrome") is a common cause of cervical myelopathy in medium- to giant-breed dogs, where dynamic and static compressive factors leading to a chronic progressive (typically over weeks to months) proprioceptive ataxia, with varying degrees of cervical hyperesthesia and paresis (Da Costa 2010). Two pathophysiologic processes have been described, with some amount of overlap. *Osseous-associated compression* is more common in young adult giant-breed dogs (e.g. Great Danes). It typically affects the C1–C5 spinal cord region, therefore resulting in symmetric, UMN clinical signs. *Disc-associated compression* commonly affects the C6–T2 spinal cord region. Middle-aged large-breed dogs, especially Doberman Pinschers are overrepresented. Classically, these dogs will have ventral compression from encroachment of Type II IVDH resulting in the classic symmetric tetraparesis with a stiff short-strided, LMN thoracic limb gait and GP/UMN pelvic limb gait. However, rarely CSM may cause asymmetric clinical signs that could be confused with lameness.

16.3.1.5 Other Causes of Cervical Myelopathies and Radiculopathies

Other conditions that can cause cervical myelopathies include trauma, discospondylitis, inflammatory conditions, extradural synovial cysts, spinal arachnoid diverticulum, and neoplasia (Chapter 17).

If there is witnessed severe external trauma, *vertebral fracture and luxation (VFL)* is considered, with supportive clinical evidence (e.g. severe pain and radiographic confirmation). However, the cervical spine is an uncommon region for VFL, apart from those affecting the axis. ANNPE should also be a differential, particularly if diagnostic imaging does not show osseous abnormalities. Traumatic injuries resulting in fractures can frequently be diagnosed with radiography, but if they are minimally displaced, advanced imaging may be necessary (Figure 16.1A, B). Advanced imaging also allows for less manipulation and 3D reconstruction potentially required for surgical planning.

Discospondylitis is more likely to affect gait in the pelvic limbs (Chapter 21); however, it should be considered as a differential diagnosis for any patient presenting with spinal pain as part of the presenting history, particularly if neurologic deficits are absent or mild.

Inflammatory conditions involving the brain (meningoencephalitis) and/or spinal cord (myelitis, meningomyelitis, and steroid-responsive meningitis–arteritis [SRMA]) can have infectious, or more commonly, idiopathic (likely immune-mediated) etiologies (Coates and Jeffery 2014). Idiopathic inflammatory conditions occur most frequently in young adult, small-breed dogs, causing CNS dysfunction that is usually multifocal. If the cervical intumescence is involved, thoracic limb gait dysfunction could be recognized. Infectious etiologies typically have progressive signs that are also multifocal but focal infections, for example tetanus, are reported.

Extradural cystic abnormalities are reported in the spinal column of dogs (Da Costa and Cook 2016). While many times these are incidental findings, they can cause lameness or monoparesis. Extradural synovial cysts arising from the periarticular joint tissue are commonly associated with osteoarthritic changes as well as CSM. Spinal arachnoid diverticulum (previously known as cysts) is focal, fluid-filled dilation of the subarachnoid space, and is common in the cervical regions of the spinal cord, especially in large-breed dogs. Collectively, these conditions have a progressive clinical course with variable spinal hyperesthesia.

16.3.2 Neuropathies (Nerves and Brachial Plexus)

While disorders of the peripheral nervous system (PNS) are less common than those affecting the brain or spinal cord, they are by no means rare as a group. As such, the clinician should be able to readily recognize the characteristic neurologic presentation localizing to PNS disease. Many of these disorders are diffuse diseases (e.g. polyradiculoneuritis), but they can present with lameness or monoparesis prior to generalizing; other conditions remain focal (e.g. brachial plexus neuritis).

Unique to this level in the spinal column is the brachial plexus, where injury or disease can have severe consequences on mobility of the limb, many of which present an LMN paresis and/or an apparent lameness. Cutaneous sensation will aid in mapping which nerves are affected (Chapter 4).

The list of causes of neuropathies is extensive, continues to grow, and many causes remain unknown. Common causes of acute mononeuropathies include nerve root tumors (Chapter 17 and Video 4.1), traumatic neuropathies, and neuritis. Other causes such as degenerative, paraneoplastic, or metabolic usually have a chronic insidious onset history and usually cause generalized, symmetric clinical signs.

16.3.2.1 Neoplasia

Tumors affecting the nervous system of the thoracic limb, particularly neoplasia of spinal nerves (Video 4.1), occur commonly and are an important differential diagnosis for thoracic limb lameness. These are discussed in Chapters 11 and 17.

16.3.2.2 Traumatic Neuropathies

16.3.2.2.1 Brachial Plexus Injuries Brachial plexus injuries are the most common traumatic neuropathies in veterinary medicine (Gemmill and Mckee 2012). The term *brachial plexus avulsion* is often used to describe these injuries, but the term *brachial plexus injury* is more appropriate as there is not always a true avulsion (i.e. physical separation). They are most often due to severe traction of the thoracic limb or abduction of the scapula as the result of severe trauma, for example vehicular, falls from a height, gunshot, and bite wounds. These injuries may result from compression, stretching, tearing, crushing, laceration (from fractures), or complete transection of the nerves or nerve roots. Most commonly the damage occurs at the level of the spinal nerve roots where there is less resistance to stretch than in more peripheral regions of nerves owing to the lack of epineurium. The ventral (motor) roots appear to be more susceptible to injury than the dorsal (sensory) root (Steinberg 1988; Platt and Da Costa 2012).

A clinical diagnosis is often made based on history of a traumatic injury, clinical presentation, and neurologic examination. Depending on the extent of the trauma, all or only part of the brachial plexus may be injured. Clinical signs will vary depending on which nerves are involved and the severity of the injury. The major motor and sensory distribution of the brachial plexus is outlined in Table 16.2.

Partial injuries most commonly involve the *caudal plexus*, originating from the ventral branches of C8, T1, and sometimes T2 spinal nerves. The muscles innervated by these nerves are involved in elbow extension which is essential for weight-bearing and locomotion, as well as the cutaneous trunci muscle. Clinically the animal cannot bear weight and stands with the elbow and shoulder flexed and dropped; the carpus is knuckled (Video 16.1). Cutaneous sensation may be lost distal to the elbow and over the caudolateral aspect of the antebrachium. If the avulsion is severe enough, it may damage spinal cord pathways causing ipsilateral pelvic limb deficits. A partial Horner syndrome, characterized by anisocoria due to ipsilateral sympathetic dysfunction and resulting miosis, can develop if the T1 nerve root is involved. Complete Horner syndrome is not commonly seen in brachial plexus injuries in dogs. If the C8 and T1 nerve roots supplying the lateral thoracic nerve are affected, there will be ipsilateral loss of the cutaneous trunci (panniculus) muscle reflex (Chapter 4).

Injury to the *cranial plexus* roots of C6 and C7 causes loss of elbow flexion and shoulder movement; however, the animal can still support weight since the elbow extensors are spared. Loss of cutaneous sensation may be appreciated cranially and medially. *Complete* injury to all brachial plexus roots (C6–T2 nerve roots) causes flaccid LMN paresis or paralysis, inability to support weight, and loss of cutaneous sensation over the entire limb.

Orthopedic injuries, particularly humeral fractures can cause nerve damage, and therefore radiographs are indicated to rule out osseous pathology. Electrodiagnostics may assist in identifying the affected nerves, although spontaneous electrical activity (indicating denervation) cannot be detected until five to seven days after the injury. An MRI may demonstrate the abnormalities in the nerves, intumescence, or surrounding soft tissues that are consistent with focal inflammation, edema, and/or hemorrhage, but this is not often performed when there is definite history of trauma since the treatment is unlikely to change. Nevertheless, MRI is recommended if there is no witnessed trauma nor any apparent cause to explain the clinical signs.

In general, the prognosis for brachial plexus injury is fair to be guarded. Nociception is the most important prognostic factor and, if absent, is associated with poor prognosis for recovery. The success of nerve regeneration is largely determined by the degree of disruption of the neuronal elements. Nerve injury can be classified into three broad categories, from least to most severe: neuropraxia, axonotmesis, and neurotmesis (Welch 1996). Neuropraxia is a transient nerve dysfunction (physiologic conduction block) with little to no structural damage. It may be due to transient ischemia or mild demyelination but typically resolves over one to two months. Sensation is often persevered because large diameter sensory axons are often spared. Axonotmesis is disruption of axons but the nerve sheath remains intact. Both motor and sensory deficits are common along with typical LMN signs. Spontaneous recovery occurs, although not as rapidly as neuropraxia. Lastly, neurotmesis is complete disruption and/or separation of the nerve (i.e. avulsion). Complete paralysis of the denervated muscle and absent nociception is expected. Spontaneous recovery only occurs rarely.

Treatment for brachial plexus injury most commonly consists of conservative treatment with a focus on rigorous physical therapy and general supportive care to prevent complications such as self-mutilation due to abnormal sensation, excoriation of the digits, neurotrophic ulcers, and muscle contracture.

16.3.2.2.2 *Radial Nerve Injury* Traumatic injury to the radial nerve is usually associated with first rib fractures causing proximal nerve injury or humeral fractures affecting the distal portion. Clinically, the elbow is dropped and the animal walks with the carpus and digits knuckled. If the nerve branches supplying the triceps muscle are not involved, elbow extensor function may be preserved. Clinical history (of trauma) usually aids in establishing the diagnosis. Appropriate therapy of the orthopedic injuries is essential. Treatment of the neurological injury is typically conservative as described for brachial plexus injury. Similarly, the prognosis varies depending on the severity of neuronal injury. Neuropraxia is more common in cases of radial nerve injury; thus, most animals recover in one to two months. Cutaneous sensation, including nociception, is the most significantly guiding factor where loss of sensation carries a poor prognosis.

16.3.2.3 Neuritis

Brachial plexus neuritis is a rare multiple mononeuropathy, meaning multiple nerves within the same limb are affected. This distinguishes this relatively focal disease from more generalized dysfunction of multiple nerves on different limbs and/or cranial nerves called polyneuropathies (e.g. idiopathic polyradiculoneuritis). The disease can be unilateral or bilateral but if it is bilateral, signs are usually asymmetric; less severe forms have been reported with a shifting leg lameness. The pathogenesis is unknown but, given the similarities to a disease described in humans called serum neuritis, a hypersensitivity reaction to an immunogen (e.g. rabies vaccine and feeding horse meat) leading to axon and myelin loss has been proposed (Dewey and Talarico 2016). A tentative diagnosis can be made based on history, especially if there is exposure to a possible immunogen, and clinical findings of acute unilateral or bilateral LMN paresis or plegia. Neuroimaging such as CT or MRI may show nerve pathology (e.g. enlargement, increased signal intensity, and contrast enhancement). Electrodiagnostic testing and muscle and/or nerve biopsies would support, and possibly confirm, the diagnosis further. With only a few reported cases, little is known about the prognosis, but recovery appears to be very protracted (Steinberg 1988; Summers et al. 1995). There is no specific treatment for this disorder, although glucocorticoid therapy has been used.

16.3.3 Myopathies and Junctionopathies

Myopathies include disorders of skeletal and smooth muscle that can be acquired, hereditary, and congenital (Taylor 2000). More commonly encountered conditions causing shifting lameness include polymyositis, endocrine myopathies, and infectious myopathies. Fibrotic myopathies such as infraspinatus contracture may also cause a unilateral lameness; this condition is commonly confused with neurologic origin (Chapter 15).

Junctionopathies refer to conditions altering the neuromuscular junction, with myasthenia gravis being the most reported and investigated. These are typified by generalized paresis, fatiguability, and stiff and stilted gait. Occasionally a shifting or unilateral leg lameness, particularly during the early stages, is reported but more commonly affects the pelvic limbs first (Chapter 21).

Diagnosis of myopathies and junctionopathies is supported by clinical presentation and examination and, in many cases, is confirmed by muscle and/or nerve biopsies. Serum muscle enzyme levels (creatine kinase, lactate dehydrogenase, and aspartate aminotransferase) are elevated in myositis while elevated titers of acetylcholine receptor antibodies confirm a diagnosis of myasthenia gravis (Chapter 21). Treatment and prognosis are highly variable and will depend on the specific condition present.

16.3.4 Other Spinal Diseases Affecting the Thoracic Limb

While not a neurologic condition, dogs with immune-mediated polyarthritis (IMPA) can first present with spinal hyperesthesia (Shaughnessy et al. 2016). Since affected animals may not show accompanying peripheral joint effusion or pain upon range of motion (Chapter 13), this disease can be confused with a neurologic problem. A shifting leg lameness and short-stilted gait may also first appear in a single limb prior to becoming more generalized. The neurologic exam is usually normal. Joint fluid analysis is necessary to establish a diagnosis (Chapter 9). Additionally, IMPA can occur concurrently with SRMA in some dogs, another cause of cervical spinal pain.

The following conditions rarely cause neurologic deficits and clinical signs unless nerve roots are involved, in which case a lameness or monoparesis may be seen:

Spondylosis deformans is a noninflammatory, degenerative disease of the vertebral column thought to be caused by degeneration of the annulus fibrosis and its bony attachments (Romatowski 1986). Typical radiographic features include focal new bone formation and osteophytes on the ventral and lateral aspects of the vertebrae (Figure 21.1F). Spondylosis deformans is a frequently encountered condition and while it may be associated with IVD protrusions and foraminal stenosis, almost always, it is an incidental finding. As such, a radiographic diagnosis of this condition should not be overinterpreted as a clinical problem. Importantly, while the term *spondylosis* sounds similar to *spondylitis* (i.e. disco*spondylitis*), these two conditions are entirely different and must be differentiated. Most readily, the vertebral end plates in spondylosis are radiographically smooth and regular in contrast to the lytic and irregular end plates of discospondylitis (Chapter 21).

Diffuse idiopathic skeletal hyperostosis (DISH) is a rare condition that affects the axial and appendicular skeleton of young dogs. It causes extensive ossification of soft tissues along the vertebral bodies, including the spinal ventral longitudinal ligament (Figure 16.1D). There is resulting bridging of the disc spaces without evidence of IVD degeneration (Kranenburg et al. 2011). DISH is rarely associated with clinical signs, but nerve root entrapment from foraminal stenosis has been described (Taylor-Brown and De Decker 2017).

Multiple cartilaginous exostosis (MCE), also termed osteochondromatosis, is a skeletal disorder of young dogs causing multifocal, benign, and proliferative lesions near sites of normal endochondral ossification (Franch et al. 2005). The vertebrae, ribs, and long bones are most frequently affected. Clinical signs are related to anatomic malformations, disfigurement, and compression of surrounding structures. Neurologic abnormalities can develop if bony tissue causes compression of neural structures (Figure 16.2). Treatment in dogs with subclinical disease is usually not necessary since MCE is usually self-limiting after skeletal maturity. Growth after maturity suggests neoplastic transformation.

Spinal dural ossification is a relatively common metaplastic and degenerative finding in dogs, especially those that are middle-aged or older (Morgan 1969). It rarely is associated with clinical signs but is commonly encountered on advanced imaging (Jones and Inzana 2000).

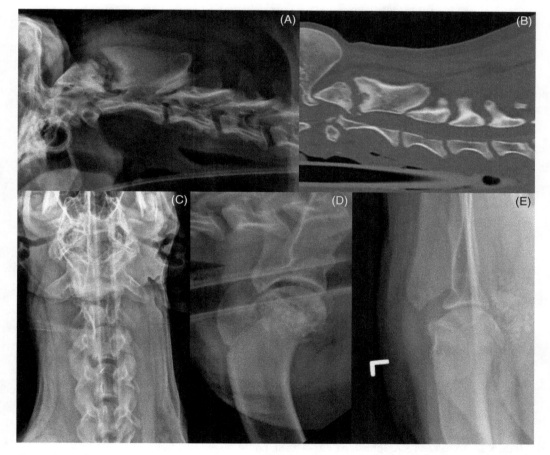

Figure 16.2 Images of a puppy diagnosed with multiple cartilaginous exostoses (MCE) affecting the shoulder and cervical vertebrae: (A) lateral survey radiograph showing multiple mineral opacities within interspinous soft tissue between C1–C2; (B) CT illustrating the mass causing compression of the spinal cord; (C) ventrodorsal survey radiograph of the cervical spine; and (D, E) lateral and craniocaudal shoulder radiographs showing a large, amorphous mineral opacity at the medial aspect of the shoulder joint.

References

Brisson, B.A. (2010). Intervertebral disc disease in dogs. *Vet Clin North Am Small Anim Pract* 40 (5): 829–858.

Coates, J.R. and Jeffery, N.D. (2014). Perspectives on meningoencephalomyelitis of unknown origin. *Vet Clin North Am Small Anim Pract* 44 (6): 1157–1185.

Da Costa, R.C. (2010). Cervical spondylomyelopathy (wobbler syndrome) in dogs. *Vet Clin North Am Small Anim Pract* 40 (5): 881–913.

Da Costa, R.C. and Cook, L.B. (2016). Cystic abnormalities of the spinal cord and vertebral column. *Vet Clin North Am Small Anim Pract* 46 (2): 277–293.

De Decker, S. and Fenn, J. (2018). Acute herniation of nondegenerate nucleus pulposus: acute noncompressive nucleus pulposus extrusion and compressive hydrated nucleus pulposus extrusion. *Vet Clin North Am Small Anim Pract* 48 (1): 95–109.

De Risio, L. and Platt, S.R. (2010). Fibrocartilaginous embolic myelopathy in small animals. *Vet Clin North Am Small Anim Pract* 40 (5): 859–869.

Dewey, C.W. and Talarico, L. (2016). Disorders of the peripheral nervous system: mononeuropathies and polyneuropathies. In: *Practical Guide to Canine and Feline Neurology*, 3e (eds. C.W. Dewey and R.C. Da Costa), 445–479. Ames: Wiley-Blackwell.

Fenn, J., Drees, R., Volk, H.A., and De Decker, S. (2016). Comparison of clinical signs and outcomes between dogs with presumptive ischemic myelopathy and dogs with acute noncompressive nucleus pulposus extrusion. *J Am Vet Med Assoc* 249 (7): 767–775.

Franch, J., Font, J., Ramis, A. et al. (2005). Multiple cartilaginous exostosis in a Golden Retriever cross-bred puppy. Clinical, radiographic and backscattered scanning microscopy findings. *Vet Comp Orthop Traumatol* 18 (3): 189–193.

Gemmill, T. and Mckee, M. (2012). Monoparesis and neurological causes of lameness. In: *Small Animal Neurological Emergencies* (eds. S.R. Platt and L.S. Garosi), 299–315. London: Manson/The Veterinary Press.

Hermanson, J.W. (2013). The muscular system. In: *Miller's Anatomy of the Dog*, 4e (eds. H.E. Evans, A. DeLahunta and M.E. Miller), 185–280. Philadelphia, PA: Saunders.

Jones, J.C. and Inzana, K.D. (2000). Subclinical CT abnormalities in the lumbosacral spine of older large-breed dogs. *Vet Radiol Ultrasound* 41 (1): 19–26.

Kranenburg, H.C., Voorhout, G., Grinwis, G.C. et al. (2011). Diffuse idiopathic skeletal hyperostosis (DISH) and spondylosis deformans in purebred dogs: a retrospective radiographic study. *Vet J* 190 (2): e84–e90.

Morgan, J.P. (1969). Spinal dural ossification in dog: incidence and distribution based on a radiographic study. *J Am Vet Radiol Soc* 10: 43–48.

Nakamoto, Y., Ozawa, T., Katakabe, K. et al. (2008). Usefulness of an early diagnosis for the favorable prognosis of fibrocartilaginous embolism diagnosed by magnetic resonance imaging in 10 small- to middle-sized dogs. *Vet Res Commun* 32 (8): 609–617.

Platt, K.B. and Da Costa, R.C. (2012). Brachial plexus trauma. In: *Veterinary Surgery: Small Animal* (eds. K.M. Tobias and S.A. Johnston), 424–430. St. Louis: Elsevier/Saunders.

Romatowski, J. (1986). Spondylosis deformans in the dog. *Compend Contin Educ Pract Vet* 8: 531–535.

Shaughnessy, M.L., Sample, S.J., Abicht, C. et al. (2016). Clinical features and pathological joint changes in dogs with erosive immune-mediated polyarthritis: 13 cases (2004-2012). *J Am Vet Med Assoc* 249 (10): 1156–1164.

Steinberg, H.S. (1988). Brachial-plexus injuries and dysfunctions. *Vet Clin North Am Small Anim Pract* 18 (3): 565–580.

Summers, B.A., Cummings, J.F., and DeLahunta, A. (1995). Diseases of the peripheral nervous system. In: *Veterinary Neuropathology* (eds. B.A. Summers, J.F. Cummings and A. DeLahunta), 402–501. St. Louis: Mosby.

Taylor, S.M. (2000). Selected disorders of muscle and the neuromuscular junction. *Vet Clin North Am Small Anim Pract* 30 (1): 59–75.

Taylor-Brown, F. and De Decker, S. (2017). Diffuse idiopathic skeletal hyperostosis causing L4 and L5 nerve root entrapment. *J Small Anim Pract* 58 (12): 724–724.

Welch, J.A. (1996). Peripheral nerve injury. *Semin Vet Med Surg (Small Anim)* 11 (4): 273–284.

17

Neoplastic Conditions of the Thoracic Limb

Bernard Séguin

Department of Clinical Sciences, College of Veterinary Medicine and Biomedical Sciences, Flint Animal Cancer Center, Colorado State University, Fort Collins, CO, USA

17.1 Introduction

One of the most important neoplastic differential diagnoses for thoracic limb lameness includes osteosarcoma of the distal radius and proximal humerus. However, other neoplastic conditions, such as brachial plexus tumors and soft tissue tumors affecting the triceps, should also be considered. Although these latter tumors are rare, establishing a diagnosis early during the course of progression is crucial to provide the best treatment and outcome possible. Please refer to Chapter 11 for details regarding the diagnostic workup of neoplasia.

17.2 Neoplasia of Specific Regions

17.2.1 Distal Limb Region

Tumors of the distal region of the limb commonly lead to visible swelling and/or palpable mass formation, thereby making them visible to owners. On the other hand, absence of swelling or a mass does not rule out neoplasia. Dogs may also present with lameness. Pain on palpation is a common finding but because some dogs do not tolerate palpation of their digits or manus/pes, interpretation of the physical exam findings in these dogs can sometimes be difficult. Radiographs should be considered whenever any subcutaneous tumors or non-movable masses or swellings are identified. Digital lesions causing bone lysis are more likely to be a malignant neoplasm (Marino et al. 1995); however, common differential diagnoses include osteoarthritis and osteomyelitis. To obtain a diagnosis, a fine-needle aspirate (FNA) can be performed for non-osseous tumors or osseous tumors with lysis. A biopsy is generally necessary for non-lytic osseous tumors or when a nondiagnostic sample is acquired from FNA. Once a diagnosis of neoplasia is suspected or confirmed, chest radiographs and FNA of the regional lymph node(s) should be considered.

Neoplasia of the distal limb can be arbitrarily divided into tumors that affect the digits and those that affect other tissues (i.e. non-digital tumors). Regarding the latter, the most common non-digital tumors include mast cell tumor and soft tissue sarcoma, and the diagnostic approach to these tumors is consistent with other regions. Of tumors affecting the digits, the majority are malignant, with squamous cell carcinoma being the most common type followed by malignant melanoma (Marino et al. 1995; Henry et al. 2005; Wobeser et al. 2007). Secondary infections may accompany digital tumors and lead to increased pain and lameness. On examination, the digit may be swollen or malformed or may have been sloughed, and discharge may be present. These signs are easily mistaken for a primary infectious paronychia.

Digital squamous cell carcinoma affects the thoracic limb twice as often as the pelvic limb. Most squamous cell carcinomas arise from the subungual epithelium, which typically will cause bone lysis of the third phalanx (Figure 17.1), whereas only 5% of melanomas cause radiographically evident bone lysis (Marino et al. 1995). Squamous cell carcinoma arising from the subungual epithelium has a better prognosis than other locations on the digit. Dogs with multiple squamous cell carcinomas of the digits are typically large-breeds with black skin and haircoat. Breeds at higher risk to get squamous cell carcinoma are standard Poodles, Labradors, Giant Schnauzers, Gordon Setters, Rottweilers, Dachshunds, Flat-Coated Retrievers, Beaucerons, and Briards. Dogs with digital malignant melanoma are overrepresented by Scottish Terriers, and in females more often than males. Both digital squamous cell carcinoma and malignant melanoma can affect multiple digits; however, this is uncommon.

Osteosarcoma accounts for 2–6% of digital tumors (Henry et al. 2005; Wobeser et al. 2007). Other malignant tumors of the digit include mast cell tumor, undifferentiated sarcoma, fibrosarcoma, synovial cell sarcoma, plasma cell tumor, hemangiosarcoma, adenocarcinoma, and

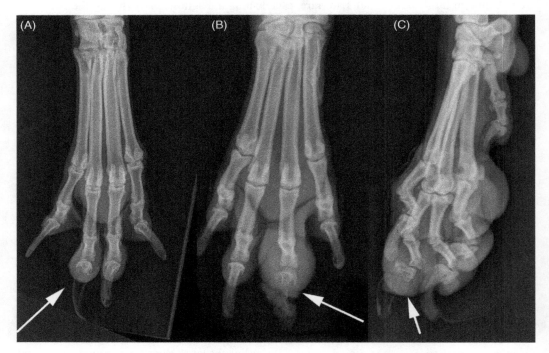

Figure 17.1 Digital neoplasia: (A–C) radiographs of the distal limb of three patients affected by digital neoplasia, and white arrows indicate the affected distal phalanx and evident bone lysis. The most likely differential diagnoses would be squamous cell carcinoma, although malignant melanoma and osteomyelitis should be considered as differential diagnoses (but are less likely to cause the depicted degree of bone lysis). (C) Oblique views can be helpful to clearly outline radiographic abnormalities.

chondrosarcoma. Benign tumors and lesions include epithelial inclusion cyst, histiocytoma, hemangiopericytoma, fibroma, sebaceous gland adenoma, keratoacanthoma, adnexal dysplasia, follicular cyst, keratoma, hamartoma, plasmacytoma, trichoblastoma apocrine gland cyst, basal cell epithelioma, fibroma, hemangioma, and sebaceous hyperplasia.

Although osteosarcoma distal to the antebrachiocarpal and tarsocrural joint occurs, it appears to be rare (Gamblin et al. 1995). While the metacarpal or metatarsal bones are the most common sites, there does not appear to be a predilection for the thoracic or pelvic limb. Treatment options for malignant tumors of the pes and manus include digit amputation, partial foot amputation, partial limb amputation with prosthesis, and full limb amputation. The type of surgery will depend on size and location of the tumor. Non-osseous malignant tumors can be treated with marginal excision and adjuvant radiation therapy when amputation is not possible or allowed.

17.2.2   Carpal Region

The carpal region, and more specifically the distal radius, is one of the two most common anatomic sites for osteosarcoma (Section 11.3.3). Osteosarcoma of the distal radius remains the most frequent neoplastic cause of lameness in this region for large- and Giant-breed dogs. Because of the paucity of soft tissues around the distal aspect of the radius, particularly on the cranial surface, it is common for owners and veterinarians to see a "swelling" or mass effect in that region when neoplasia is present. This holds true for osseous (i.e. osteosarcoma; Figure 13.13) or soft tissue (such as soft tissue or joint capsule tumors) swelling. Tumors of the joint capsule are uncommon in the carpal area, nonetheless villonodular synovitis (Section 11.3.4), histiocytic sarcoma, and synovial cell sarcoma should all be considered as differential diagnoses. Treatment of carpal region neoplasia depends on the specific diagnosis and extent. Options include local excision, radiation therapy, full or partial limb amputation, as well as a variety of limb-sparing surgeries for primary bone tumors specific to the distal radius.

17.2.3   Elbow Region

Although osteosarcoma of the distal humerus, as well as of the proximal radius and ulna, occurs, it is rare (Liptak et al. 2004) and the maxim, "osteosarcoma occurs away from the elbow" generally holds true. Several other rare neoplastic conditions have been described for this region: primary osteosarcoma of the synovium of the elbow has been reported in a Labrador Retriever and should be differentiated from calcinosis circumscripta (Section 14.14.1). While tumors of the synovium typically display lytic changes in the bones on "both sides" of the joint, radiographs of this case of osteosarcoma of the joint capsule did not reveal periarticular bone lysis (Thamm et al. 2000). Additionally, the elbow is one of the three most common joints to develop periarticular histiocytic sarcoma. Other reported types of sarcomas originating from the synovium in canines include malignant fibrous histiocytoma, fibrosarcoma, and undifferentiated sarcoma (Craig et al. 2002). Synovial osteochondromatosis with malignant transformation to chondrosarcoma has also been reported in another Labrador Retriever (Aeffner et al. 2012). Treatment of tumors of the elbow region is challenging due to the limited soft tissues and therefore frequently requires full limb amputation for malignant tumors.

17.2.4   Shoulder Region

The shoulder region, and more specifically the proximal humerus, is one of the two most common anatomic sites for osteosarcoma, making it a frequent cause of lameness in large- and Giant-breed dogs. In general, scapular tumors are uncommon but, when they do occur, they are most often malignant due to osteosarcoma. Other tumor types include chondrosarcoma, fibrosarcoma, soft tissue sarcoma, hemangiosarcoma, and histiocytic sarcoma. In fact, the shoulder is one of the three most common joints to develop periarticular histiocytic sarcoma. Villonodular synovitis of the shoulder has also been described in four dogs. Although an infrequent cause of lameness, lipomas in the axillary area can become large enough to interfere with normal range of motion.

Palpation of this region must include the proximal humerus and scapula, which can reveal a mass effect or pain in the presence of a tumor. The axillary region needs to be carefully palpated, by sliding a hand in between the body wall and scapula from caudal to the scapula. Deep palpation of the area may reveal a mass effect or pain, which is suggestive of tumors of the brachial plexus (Section 17.2.5).

Compared to lesions of the distal radius, subtle lesions of the bones of the shoulder region can be more easily missed on radiographs (Figure 17.2). This is due to the larger muscles surrounding the area and greater difficulty positioning the dog to take radiographs, which often leads to super-imposition of the shoulder region over the chest. As such, sedation to allow for appropriate positioning or advanced imaging such as CT should be considered if osseous neoplasia is a differential diagnosis. Similarly, if a mass (suspected primary bone tumor) cannot be confidently palpated, FNAs of the bone may require ultrasound guidance to direct the needle through the large muscle coverage into the bone. Minimally invasive biopsy procedures of the bone performed with a Jamshidi needle are best performed with image guidance via fluoroscopy, radiographs, or CT.

Given the proximal location, osseous neoplasia of the region is most frequently treated with either radiation therapy or full limb amputation. Scapulectomy is a treatment option for scapular tumors (Montinaro et al. 2013).

17.2.5 Nervous System

Tumors affecting the nervous system can be divided into those affecting the intracranial nervous tissues, the spinal cord, or peripheral nerves. The latter two may cause unilateral symptoms and are therefore important differential diagnoses for patients with lameness.

17.2.5.1 Spinal Cord Tumors

Spinal tumors are uncommon in dogs (McEntee and Dewey 2013). The clinical signs can be insidious, chronic, and progressive (e.g. slow growing tumors), but can also be acute (e.g. acute hemorrhage of a chronic tumor). The neurologic signs vary according to the location of the tumor and their severity depends on the degree of compression, neural tissue destruction, edema, and hemorrhage, as well as the degree of compensation of the spinal cord. Similarly, neurologic signs attributed to the presence of spinal neoplasia can be unilateral, bilateral symmetrical, or asymmetrical. Spinal hyperesthesia is common in instances where the tumor is found in the extradural or intradural-extramedullary location (see below) and may be the only abnormal finding. Animals with intramedullary tumors may not have spinal hyperesthesia as there are no nociceptors within the spinal parenchyma. If the mass expands to the point of stretching the meninges, or nerve roots, focal spinal hyperesthesia may result.

Advanced imaging (most frequently MRI) is generally required to detect tumors affecting the function of the spinal cord. The only exception is tumors that cause significant lytic or proliferative changes to the vertebrae, which can be seen on radiographs. FNAs and biopsies can be challenging to acquire depending on the location of the lesion with respect to the nervous tissue. Cerebrospinal fluid (CSF) analysis is typically abnormal (e.g. increased protein concentration, with or without elevated cell count) but usually does not provide specific information about the tumor type since neoplastic cells are rarely found unless the tumor is intradural or involves the meninges. Lymphoma

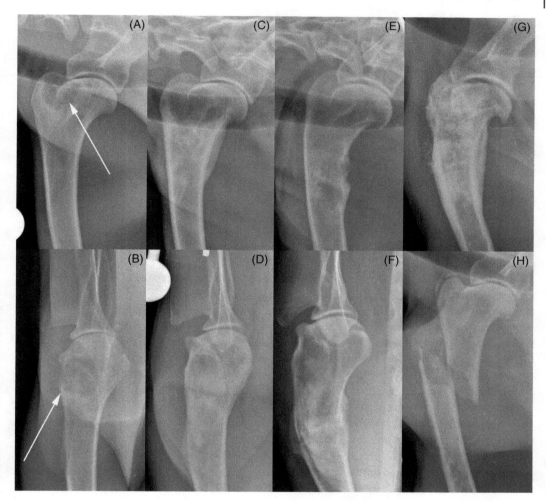

Figure 17.2 Proximal humeral osteosarcoma: (A) lateral and (B) craniocaudal radiographs display a subtle lesion (white arrows) that may be missed without performing orthogonal views; (C, D) predominant osteolytic changes extending throughout the proximal one-quarter of the humerus are visible; (E, F) osteolytic and proliferative changes extend throughout the proximal one half of the humerus; (G) osteolytic and osteoproductive changes, irregular osseous production along the cranial aspect of the proximal humerus, as well as a smooth periosteal reaction along the caudal aspect of the humerus; and (H) pathologic fracture due to osteosarcoma. Note the periosteal reaction, punctate lysis of the cortices and patchy, heterogenous, and moth-eaten appearance to the medullary cavity of the humerus.

is the one tumor type where tumor cells are most likely to be seen in the CSF. A sample collected from the lumbar cistern has been reported to be more likely to be diagnostic than one collected from the cerebellomedullary cistern (Thomson et al. 1990).

Tumors of the spinal cord are categorized into intramedullary, intradural-extramedullary, and extradural based on their location with respect to the spinal cord tissue itself and meninges: *Intramedullary neoplasms* are located within the spinal cord substance and can be primary spinal parenchymal tumors or metastatic. Primary tumors are more common in the C6–T2 segment and are predominantly of glial cell origin; astrocytoma and ependymoma are the most frequent but other types reported include oligodendroglioma, undifferentiated sarcoma, choroid plexus papilloma, and meningeal sarcoma. Tumors reported to metastasize to the substance of the spinal cord are hemangiosarcoma, mammary gland carcinoma, malignant melanoma, and thyroid carcinoma. Antemortem confirmation of a diagnosis of an intramedullary tumor can be challenging and carries risks of worsening the neurologic status. For these reasons, it is rarely attempted. Nonetheless when it is attempted, it may be done with a needle aspirate or biopsy. A small gauge needle is preferred but it limits the diagnostic ability of the procedure. A biopsy can be obtained through a laminectomy or hemilaminectomy approach followed by a durotomy.

Intradural-extramedullary neoplasms arise outside the spinal cord but are within the subdural space. The most common tumors are nerve sheath tumor, meningioma, and hemangioma. Antemortem diagnosis is possible with a needle aspirate or biopsy; minimally invasive CT-guided techniques may be feasible in selected cases. A biopsy also requires a laminectomy or hemilaminectomy approach to the lesion.

Extradural neoplasms originate outside the dura mater and include osseous and soft tissue neoplasia. Lymphoma is the most common soft tissue extradural tumor. Other soft tissue tumors found in this location include meningioma, nerve sheath tumors, myxoma, myxosarcoma, plasma cell tumor, and lipoma.

Osseous tumors include osteosarcoma, fibrosarcoma, hemangiosarcoma, multiple myeloma, and chondrosarcoma. Osteosarcoma, fibrosarcoma, and hemangiosarcoma of the vertebrae may also be a metastasis and therefore evaluation for a primary neoplasm should be performed. Other tumors may metastasize to soft tissues adjacent to the vertebrae and cause secondary spinal invasion and eventually compression. Malignancies can also metastasize directly to the vertebrae via the hematogenous route. An example of the former would be metastasis from prostatic adenocarcinoma to the sublumbar lymph nodes and eventually invasion into the lumbar vertebrae. Numerous other neoplasms can metastasize to vertebrae and include mammary carcinoma, perianal gland adenocarcinoma, transitional cell carcinoma, Sertoli cell carcinoma, thyroid carcinoma, and pheochromocytoma. The lumbar area is the most common site for spinal metastasis, but the cervical and thoracic segments can also be affected.

Extradural spinal cord tumors can generally be diagnosed with a needle aspirate or biopsy. Either procedure can be performed with a surgical approach to the lesion or image guidance with either CT or ultrasound.

17.2.5.2 Peripheral Nerve Tumors

Tumors originating from the peripheral nervous system are termed peripheral nerve sheath tumors. These include schwannoma, neurofibroma, perineurioma, and malignant peripheral nerve sheath tumors (MPNST). The majority of tumors are MPNST and are biologically aggressive by exhibiting local invasion but rarely metastasize. Being that MPNST are soft tissue sarcomas, grade is prognostic for local recurrence and metastatic potential. These tumors can be affecting a nerve root, spinal nerve, or the brachial plexus or be distal to the brachial plexus. The location relative to the brachial plexus (distal, within, or proximal) has prognostic value with tumors distal to the plexus having the best prognosis (Brehm et al. 1995).

Diagnosing these tumors can be challenging, since the only clinical sign can be lameness, which can be mild or severe. Some dogs will show a lack of weight-bearing while standing (i.e. lift their leg, Video 4.1), yet the lameness improves during ambulation. This has been termed "nerve root signature lameness" and is thought to be due to compression of inflammation of a nerve root. Pain while manipulating the neck can be detected if the tumor is present in the spinal canal and causing cord compression. Presence of a partial Horner syndrome or loss of panniculus reflex will raise the suspicion of a lesion proximal to the brachial plexus (Chapter 4) but their absence does not rule it out. Muscle atrophy is usually significant (neurogenic atrophy), in fact moderate-to-severe muscle atrophy was the most common physical exam finding (>90% of cases) in one study (Brehm et al. 1995). The muscles affected will depend on which nerve root or nerve is affected by the tumor. Deep palpation of the axillary area can elicit pain or the observer may be able to palpate a mass effect if the tumor involves the distal aspect of the brachial plexus. In the latter cases, ultrasound can be helpful to establish a diagnosis; however, MRI is the imaging modality of choice, with CT being a less desirable alternative. Early tumors can cause visible lameness with no pain detected on physical exam and in some dogs, no changes may be observed on MRI. These cases require sequential MRIs to accomplish a diagnosis (i.e. initially the tumor is too small to see on MRI). FNA or biopsy is needed to provide a definitive diagnosis. Yet, since these tumors are mesenchymal in origin, an FNA may yield a nondiagnostic sample (which does not rule out a malignant tumor). A biopsy will be needed in these instances to provide an accurate diagnosis.

Early diagnosis of these tumors is critical since cases with distal tumors can be cured with amputation if treated prior to developing metastatic disease. The location and extent of the tumor with respect to the plexus will influence the treatment options. Tumors in or distal to the plexus can be treated with amputation alone, while tumors invading the spinal canal should be treated with a hemilaminectomy, and radiation therapy in addition to amputation. Local excision can be possible in some cases and stereotactic radiation therapy is an alternative treatment.

References

Aeffner, F., Weeren, R., Morrison, S. et al. (2012). Synovial osteochondromatosis with malignant transformation to chondrosarcoma in a dog. *Vet Pathol* 49 (6): 1036–1039.

Brehm, D., Vite, C., Steinberg, H. et al. (1995). A retrospective evaluation of 51 cases of peripheral nerve sheath tumors in the dog. *J Am Anim Hosp Assoc* 31 (4): 349–359.

Craig, L.E., Julian, M.E., and Ferracone, J.D. (2002). The diagnosis and prognosis of synovial tumors in dogs: 35 cases. *Vet Pathol* 39 (1): 66–73.

Gamblin, R., Straw, R., Powers, B. et al. (1995). Primary osteosarcoma distal to the antebrachiocarpal and tarsocrural joints in nine dogs (1980–1992). *J Am Anim Hosp Assoc* 31 (1): 86–91.

Henry, C.J., Brewer, W.G. Jr., Whitley, E.M. et al. (2005). Canine digital tumors: a veterinary cooperative oncology group retrospective study of 64 dogs. *J Vet Intern Med* 19 (5): 720–724.

Liptak, J.M., Dernell, W.S., Ehrhart, N., and Withrow, S. (2004). Canine appendicular osteosarcoma: diagnosis and palliative treatment. *Compend Contin Educ Vet* 26 (3): 172–182.

Marino, D.J., Matthiesen, D.T., Stefanacci, J.D., and Moroff, S.D. (1995). Evaluation of dogs with digit masses: 117 cases (1981–1991). *J Am Vet Med Assoc* 207 (6): 726–728.

Mcentee, M.C. and Dewey, C.W. (2013). Tumors of the nervous system. In: *Withrow and MacEwen's Small Animal Clinical Oncology*, 5e (eds. S. Withrow, D. Vail and R. Page), 583–596. St-Louis: Elsevier.

Montinaro, V., Boston, S.E., Buracco, P. et al. (2013). Clinical outcome of 42 dogs with scapular tumors treated by scapulectomy: a Veterinary Society of Surgical Oncology (VSSO) retrospective study (1995–2010). *Vet Surg* 42 (8): 943–950.

Thamm, D.H., Mauldin, E.A., Edinger, D.T., and Lustgarten, C. (2000). Primary osteosarcoma of the synovium in a dog. *J Am Anim Hosp Assoc* 36 (4): 326–331.

Thomson, C.E., Kornegay, J.N., and Stevens, J.B. (1990). Analysis of cerebrospinal fluid from the cerebellomedullary and lumbar cisterns of dogs with focal neurologic disease: 145 cases (1985–1987). *J Am Vet Med Assoc* 196 (11): 1841–1844.

Wobeser, B.K., Kidney, B.A., Powers, B.E. et al. (2007). Diagnoses and clinical outcomes associated with surgically amputated canine digits submitted to multiple veterinary diagnostic laboratories. *Vet Pathol* 44 (3): 355–361.

Part V

Pelvic Limb Lameness

18

Tarsal Region

Kathleen Linn[1] and Felix Michael Duerr[2]

[1] *Department of Small Animal Clinical Sciences, Western College of Veterinary Medicine, University of Saskatchewan, Saskatoon, Saskatchewan, Canada*
[2] *Department of Clinical Sciences, College of Veterinary Medicine and Biomedical Sciences, Colorado State University, Fort Collins, CO, USA*

18.1   Introduction and Common Differential Diagnoses

The tarsus is a joint with minimal soft tissue covering, making the bones and ligaments susceptible to traumatic injuries such as fractures and ligament disruption. This lack of soft tissue covering is a boon for diagnosis of lameness, because even subtle swellings, bone displacements, or instabilities are readily palpable. Injuries to components of the common calcanean tendon (CCT) comprise the other major cause of lameness attributable to the tarsal region. As dogs walk with a degree of tarsal flexion through most of each stride, this extensor apparatus is critical in preventing collapse when the limb is weight-bearing. Extensor tendon injuries are rare and seldom a cause of more than transient lameness as they do not have to counteract the same magnitude of force.

Since there is no "tarsal dysplasia," *osteoarthritis* (OA) of the tarsus is less often encountered than, for example, hip or elbow OA. The only developmental disease of the region that is associated with the development of OA is osteochondritis dissecans (OCD), which is rarely encountered. Other causes for tarsal OA include traumatic injury and instability. Being a distal joint, immune-mediated polyarthritis (IMPA; Chapter 13) also needs to be considered as a differential diagnosis. Therefore, arthrocentesis and synovial fluid evaluation should be considered in cases where inflammatory arthritis is possible.

The most commonly employed tests include radiographs and computed tomography (CT) for the diagnosis of osseous disease and ultrasound for the diagnosis of pathology involving the CCT. Figure 18.1 and Table 18.1 outline common differential diagnoses and diagnostic steps for the tarsal region.

18.2   Normal Anatomy

The tarsus is a complex joint that works largely as a hinge, with 90% of its motion occurring at the junction of the talus with the tibia and fibula (tarsocrural joint). A normal canine tarsus can move from approximately 35° in full flexion to 155° in full extension, although the gastrocnemius apparatus

Table 18.1 Key features for selected diseases affecting the tarsal region.

Disease	Common signalment	Diagnostic test of choice	Exam findings	Treatment	Clinical pearls	Terminology
Fractures	Any dog with trauma; Greyhounds and Border Collies prone to stress fractures of the central and fourth tarsal bones during exertion	Radiographs: (orthogonal and often oblique views needed); CT can be helpful	Pain, swelling over injured bone; sometimes tarsal deformity; non-weight-bearing lameness	Depends on location	Central and fourth tarsal bones commonly fracture together. Malleolar fractures are often accompanied by mediolateral tarsocrural instability	
Luxations and subluxations	Any dog with *trauma* but may also occur secondary to *immune-mediated disease* or *idiopathic* (Shetland Sheepdogs and Collies)	Radiographs: orthogonal and stressed views	Moderate to non-weight-bearing lameness, deformity, and sometimes palpable instability	Collateral ligament repair or replacement; partial or pantarsal arthrodesis may be needed	Luxations may happen at any of the tarsal joints. Both medial and lateral collateral ligaments may be injured with tarsocrural luxation. Evaluation of plantar and dorsal instability as well as mediolateral instability should be performed. Carpal hyperextension may also be present in dogs with idiopathic hyperflexion	Idiopathic tarsal hyperflexion describes subluxation without an underlying cause. The term "dorsiflexion" is sometimes used for hyperflexion
Tarsal hyperextension	Young dogs, with concurrent pelvic limb abnormalities or idiopathic	Orthogonal radiographs generally normal (unless tarsal OCD is present); plantaro-dorsal stress view show hyperextension	Tarsus can be extended to or beyond 180° but is usually non-painful. Ipsilateral hip or stifle abnormalities are frequently evident	Generally no treatment needed unless tarsal OCD present	Treatment of concurrent orthopedic problems relieves pain, but tarsal hyperextension generally persists	Subluxation of the tarsus due to dorsal instability; "slipped hock"; sometimes referred to as tarsal "plantarflexion"
Immune-mediated polyarthritis	Large-breed (nonerosive) and small-breed (erosive)	Radiographs and arthrocentesis	Effusion, pain, and hyperflexion	Immunosuppressive drugs and partial or pantarsal arthrodesis	Instability suggests that polyarthritis is erosive; pain or effusion may not always be present	

Condition	Signalment	Diagnosis	Clinical signs	Treatment	Comments	Related terms
Talar osteochondrosis/osteochondritis dissecans	Labrador Retrievers, Rottweilers, Bullmastiffs; young dogs >4.5 months; females predisposed	Radiographs; CT helpful	Short-strided gait in affected limb(s); tarsocrural joint is effusive, especially medially and caudolaterally	Fragment removal; advantage of surgery over conservative management remains controversial	This condition is often bilateral. Tarsal hyperextension may be present	Talar ridge OCD
Common calcanean tendon laceration	Dogs of any age or breed	Physical exam findings generally sufficient for diagnosis	Plantigrade stance; with stifle held in extension tarsus can be fully flexed	Suturing of tendon combined with external coaptation or rigid external fixation	With this injury, the affected limb is generally *fully* plantigrade; an obvious skin laceration may not be present	Achilles tendon laceration; traumatic rupture; Type I common calcanean tendon lesion
Gastrocnemius tendinopathy	Middle-aged medium- to large-breed dogs, Dobermans and Labradors predisposed	Radiographs: soft tissue swelling and often mineralization; ultrasonography helpful	Excessive tarsal flexion and crab-claw appearance of digits when weight-bearing	Surgical re-apposition with external support; orthosis	Stance is rarely fully plantigrade; excessively flexed digits imply presence of intact superficial digital flexor tendon	Type IIc common calcanean tendon lesion; Partial avulsion or strain of the gastrocnemius tendon
Superficial digital flexor tendon displacement	Shelties and Collies overrepresented; young adults	Ultrasonography; radiography	Soft tissue swelling over tuber calcanei; tendon can be luxated and replaced	Suturing of retinacular tear	Luxation can be either lateral or medial. In chronic cases, the displaced tendon may not be mobile	Superficial digital flexor tendon luxation
Tarsal osteoarthritis	Middle-aged medium- and large-breed dogs	Radiographs	Firm tarsal swelling, decreased range of motion; crepitus may be present	Management as for osteoarthritis in other locations; tarsal arthrodesis if response to treatment is inadequate	Osteoarthritis is a common sequela to talar OCD	Degenerative joint disease

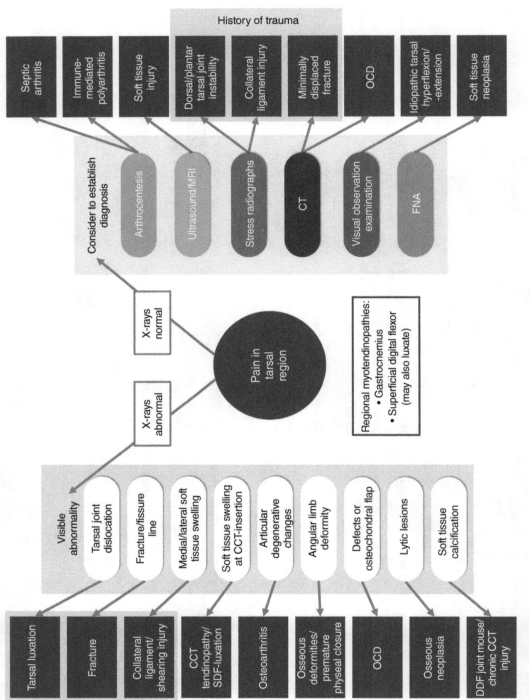

Figure 18.1 Schematic of common diseases affecting the tarsal region and the steps necessary to establish a diagnosis.

limits its ability to flex when the stifle is extended (Chapter 5). The mean tarsal standing angle for dogs is around 137°, but there is considerable variation due to breed, with an average angle of 116° for German Shepherds and 140–147° for other large-breed dogs (Sabanci and Ocal 2018). Tarsal extension is maintained by the CCT.

When the angle between the cranial aspect of the tibia and the dorsal aspect of the pes decreases, the tarsocrural joint (and thus the tarsus as a whole) is in flexion. There is no consensus on terminology for dorsoplantar movement of the joint levels distal to the tarsocrural joint, since normally the tarsal bones remain in a straight line and move very little relative to each other. In this chapter, movement of the tarsus (regardless of joint level) and pes towards the cranial aspect of the tibia will be called flexion (or hyperflexion if the angulation at that level is excessive). When the pes angles away from the cranial aspect of the tibia, the tarsus will be said to be extended (or hyperextended if degree of angulation is abnormal).

The tarsus is composed of seven *bones* that are stacked to form *joints* at four levels on the medial side and two on the lateral side (Figure 18.2). Two small, variably present sesamoids have been described in Greyhounds (Wood and McCarthy 1984). These sesamoids are located on the lateral (termed lateral plantar tarsometatarsal sesamoid bone) and medial (termed intra-articular tarsometatarsal sesamoid bone) side of the tarsometatarsal joint. These sesamoids are rarely described in the current literature and generally not visible on radiographs; however, with the increased use of advanced imaging, they are more frequently observed in other breeds as well (Deruddere et al. 2014). The tarsocrural joint, which is responsible for almost all of the motion in the tarsus, is formed by the junction of the trochlea of the talus with the tibia and the fibula. The malleoli of these bones overhang the talus to provide mediolateral stability. The talar trochlea has two nearly circular ridges that correspond with two recesses in the tibial articular surface that are divided by an intermediate ridge. The calcaneus does not participate in the tarsocrural joint but instead has a long proximal projection, the tuber calcanei, that serves as an attachment point for the powerful CCT. The sustentaculum tali of the calcaneus is a shelf on the plantar aspect of the tarsus that hosts the lateral digital flexor muscle and is closely bound to the talus. Both bones end distally at the proximal intertarsal joint, which is a collective joint formed by the junction of the talus with the central tarsal bone (the talocalcaneal central joint) on the medial side and the junction of the calcaneus and the fourth tarsal bone (the calcaneoquartal joint) on the lateral side (Figure 18.2). The proximal intertarsal joint allows for a small amount of flexion/extension as well as motion in the mediolateral plane.

The medially located central tarsal bone has a small articulation with the calcaneus, but it is most broadly mated with the head of the talus proximally, the fourth tarsal bone laterally, and the first, second, and third tarsal bones distally. Its junction with tarsal bones I–III is called the centrodistal or the distal intertarsal joint. Unlike the proximal intertarsal joint, the distal intertarsal joint is only present on the medial side, since the long fourth tarsal bone spans this level on the lateral side. All of the bones of the tarsus are bound to their neighbors on either side with short, strong ligaments in what are termed vertical intertarsal joints. Finally, the numbered tarsal bones articulate with corresponding metatarsal bones at the collective tarsometatarsal joint.

Each tarsal bone forms from a single ossification center except for the calcaneus, which also has an apophysis, the tuber calcanei. Ossification centers of the talus and the body of the calcaneus are present at birth, with the central and numbered tarsal bones (along with the ossification center of the tuber calcanei) appearing between 3 and 6 weeks of age on radiographs (Thrall and Robertson 2016). There are several growth plates around the tarsus that can complicate radiographic interpretation in young animals. The distal tibia has a physis that closes between 5 and 15 months of age, while its attached medial malleolus has its own growth plate that closes by

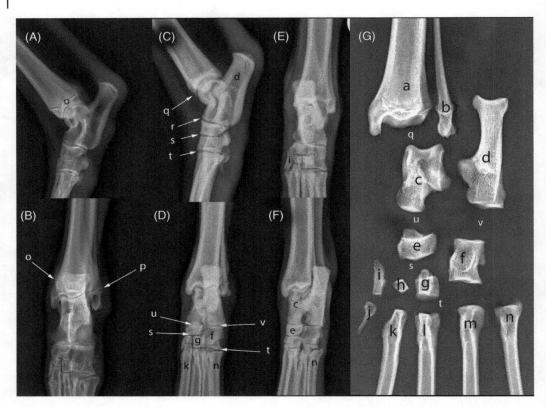

Figure 18.2 (A–G) Normal radiographic anatomy of the tarsal region (Note: for all dorsoplantar images lateral is on the right): (A, B) lateral and dorsoplantar views of the tarsus of an immature dog; note that the physes of the tuber calcanei and medial malleolus have already closed in this dog; (C) lateral; (D) dorsoplantar; (E) dorsomedial plantaro-lateral oblique (DMPLO); and (F) dorsolateral plantaro-medial oblique (DLPMO) views of an adult dog; (a) tibia; (b) fibula; (c) talus; (d) calcaneus; (e) central tarsal bone; (f) fourth tarsal bone; (g) third tarsal bone; (h) second tarsal bone; (i) first tarsal bone; (j) first metatarsal bone; (k) second metatarsal bone; (l) third metatarsal bone; (m) fourth metatarsal bone; (n) fifth metatarsal bone; (o) distal tibial physis; (p) distal fibular (lateral malleolar) physis; (q) tarsocrural joint; (r) proximal intertarsal joint (formed by joints u, and v); (s) centrodistal (or distal intertarsal) joint; (t) tarsometatarsal joint; (u) talocalcaneal central joint; and (v) calcaneoquartal joint.

5 months of age. The fibular lateral malleolar growth plate closes by 11 months, and the growth plate of the apophysis of the tuber calcanei closes by 8 months after birth. The only metatarsal bone with a proximal physis is the first; growth plate closure here happens by 7 months of age (von Pfeil and Decamp 2009; Thrall and Robertson 2016).

The tarsal joint capsule originates on the distal tibia and fibula and inserts on the proximal extents of the metatarsal bones, with fibrous attachments to each of the tarsal bones. There are three lateral and four medial joint sacs. The proximal (tarsocrural, talocalcaneocentral, and calcaneoquartal) joints communicate with each other and with the sheath of the lateral digital flexor tendon, but they are separate from the conjoined centrodistal and tarsometatarsal joints. Although intra-articular anesthesia (Chapter 8) is rarely used for diagnosis of tarsal lameness in dogs, these joint divisions should be considered when performing injections in the tarsal region.

The medial collateral ligament limits valgus and the lateral collateral ligament limits varus angulation of the tarsus. Both medial and lateral collateral *ligaments* have a superficially located long

TARSAL REGION

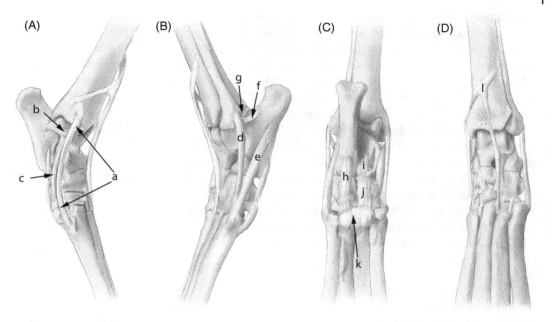

Figure 18.3 Ligaments of the tarsal joint: (A) *medial* aspect illustrating the (a) *medial long* collateral and the (b, c) *medial short collateral complex* which includes the (b) tibiotalar short collateral and (c) tibiocentral short collateral; (B) *lateral* aspect illustrating the (d) *lateral long* collateral, (e) calcaneoquartal ligament and the (f, g) *lateral short collateral complex* which includes the (f) calcaneofibular short collateral, and (g) talofibular short collateral; (C) *plantar* aspect illustrating the (h) long plantar ligament, (i) calcaneocentral ligament, (j) plantar centrodistal ligament, and (k) tarsal fibrocartilage; and (D) *dorsal* aspect illustrating the (l) crural extensor retinaculum.

component that runs from the appropriate malleolus to the base of metatarsals I and II on the medial side and V on the lateral side, attaching to each tarsal bone the ligament passes on the way (Figure 18.3). This long component is taut when the tarsocrural joint is extended. On both sides, there are two short components located deep to the long component (Aron and Purinton 1985); these are taut when the tarsocrural joint is flexed. As most dogs walk with a few degrees of valgus angulation that places tensile stress on the medial aspect of the tarsus, medial collateral injuries are more likely to result in persistent lameness than lateral collateral injuries (Decamp et al. 2016).

The tarsocrural joint flexes to varying degrees during gait, but the rest of the tarsus remains straight because of the support provided by the strong plantar ligaments. The middle (or long) plantar ligament originates on the body of the calcaneus and attaches to the fourth tarsal bone before inserting on the fourth and fifth metatarsal bones. The medial plantar ligament runs from the sustentaculum tali to the central tarsal bone to attach to the first through third metatarsal bones. Before reaching their metatarsal insertions, both of these ligaments attach to a thickened portion of the joint capsule called the tarsal fibrocartilage. The lateral (or calcaneoquartal) plantar ligament originates on the plantarolateral surface of the calcaneal body and joins the long part of the lateral collateral ligament before inserting on the fifth metatarsal bone (Carmichael and Marshall 2018).

Dorsal support of the tarsus is provided by a slender band running from the crural extensor retinaculum to the talus, where it joins with a shorter, denser ligament (the dorsal centrodistal) running from the talar neck to the second, third, and fourth tarsal bones. This ligament system, along with the action of the fibularis and cranial tibial tendons, helps to limit tarsal extension.

A number of *tendons* insert on or (in the case of digital flexors and extensors) pass over the tarsal region. The major flexors of the tarsus include the cranial tibial tendon, which passes obliquely from lateral to medial over the central tarsal bone to insert on the first and second metatarsal bones, and the fibularis (peroneus) longus and brevis tendons, which insert on the fourth tarsal bone and plantar surfaces of the metatarsals (longus) or the fifth metatarsal bone alone (brevis). The major extensor of the tarsus is the common calcanean (Achilles) tendon, which is composed of three major components: the gastrocnemius tendon (GT), which inserts on the tuber calcanei; the conjoined tendon, formed from portions of the biceps femoris, semitendinosus, and gracilis tendons, which also inserts on the tuber calcanei; and the superficial digital flexor tendon (SDFT), which passes over the tuber calcanei on its way to the pes. The CCT will be discussed in greater depth later in Section 18.5.

Seven tendons have synovial sheaths as they pass the tarsus: the cranial tibial tendon and long extensor of the first digit; the fibularis (peroneus) longus and brevis; the long and lateral digital extensors; and the deep digital extensor tendon. The sheath of the deep digital extensor communicates with the tarsocrural joint. The cranial tibial tendon, the fibularis longus and fibularis brevis tendons, and the SDFT have bursae near their insertions in the tarsal region (Johnson 1985).

18.3   Fractures of the Tarsal Region

Pain in the tarsal region may originate from fractures of the metatarsi (discussed in Chapter 12), fractures of the tarsal bones and fractures of the distal tibia and fibula (lateral malleolus). In immature animals, Type I and II Salter-Harris fractures (Chapter 13) are most commonly observed. In mature animals, malleolar fractures or fractures of the distal tibial metaphysis are the most common types. Fractures of the malleoli may result in tarsocrural luxations because the collateral ligaments originate there.

Because the tarsal bones are held together so tightly by ligaments, these fractures often involve more than one bone and may be accompanied by intertarsal luxations. Displaced fractures or luxations of the central tarsal bone, which acts a medial strut, cause angular deformity of the tarsus.

A wide variety of fractures of the specific tarsal bones have been described and treatment varies based on the fracture specifics (Carmichael and Marshall 2018). Simple fractures and single-bone luxations are generally treated with internal fixation, while partial tarsal arthrodesis (i.e. fusion of joints distal to the tarsocrural joint) is used to treat injuries (including many calcaneal fractures) distal to the tarsocrural joint. Pantarsal arthrodesis (i.e. fusion of all tarsal joints including the tarsocrural joint) may be needed to treat articular fractures of the talus or tibia and other severe injuries.

18.3.1   Signalment and History

As for any fracture, trauma is the main cause which can happen to dogs of any age/signalment. Nevertheless, tarsal fractures and luxations are predominantly seen in medium-to-large, active adult dogs. Bone fractures of the tarsal region are most commonly the result of a single traumatic event. However, in racing Greyhounds, repetitive stress can cause fatigue fractures of the central tarsal bone, and Dalmatians have been reported to suffer from atraumatic fractures of this bone (Armstrong et al. 2019). Racing Greyhounds develop central tarsal bone fractures (and related injuries, especially to the calcaneus and fourth tarsal bone) in the pelvic limb opposite to the direction of turn on an oval racetrack. Sighthounds and Dalmatians seem to be particularly susceptible to central tarsal bone injuries (Armstrong et al. 2019). In most cases, there is a history of acute onset of non-weight-bearing lameness. Avulsions of the tuber calcanei are occasionally seen in immature dogs following falls or jumps.

18.3.2 Physical Exam

When the injury is recent, the affected limb is usually carried. There may be an angular deformity evident at or distal to the tarsocrural joint. Because of the acute nature of the injury, physical exam findings usually show severe pain upon tarsal manipulation requiring sedation to perform a full examination and diagnostics of the limb. Examination of the limb should include placing the tarsus through full range of motion, evaluation for joint effusion, and stress testing of the limb in varus and valgus stress as well as applying dorsal and plantar stress (Figure 18.4). If the distal tibia is held in position while the metatarsus is manipulated, excessive flexion, extension, or mediolateral motion may be elicited.

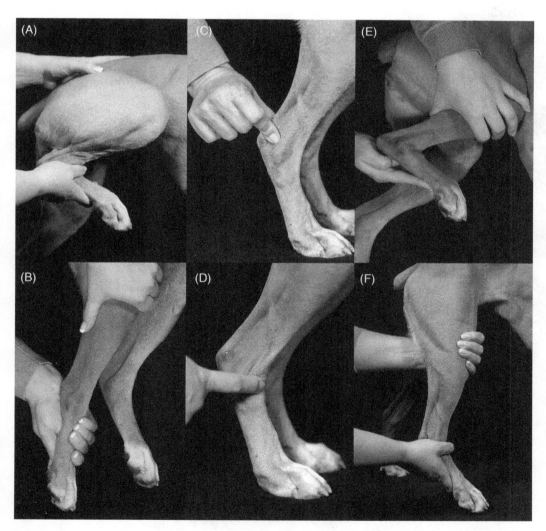

Figure 18.4   Physical examination steps to detect tarsal joint pathology: (A) to fully flex the tarsal joint, the hip and stifle joint also have to be flexed; (B) isolated tarsal hyperextension can be performed by grasping the tibia below the stifle and extending the tarsus with the lower hand – this allows the observer to differentiate stifle from tarsal pathology; joint effusion is palpable (C) caudal and (D) cranial to the lateral malleolus; (E) applying upward pressure from plantar while flexing the stifle stresses the distal tarsal joints and may show instability; (F) the common calcanean tendon can be stretched by holding the stifle in extension from cranially while flexing the tarsus.

Fractures of the proximal aspect of the tuber calcanei are usually associated with lameness that features excessive tarsal flexion and sometimes the curled digits (crab-claw appearance), that is more commonly associated with gastrocnemius insertion disruption (Figure 18.5).

Swelling is easy to detect, since there is very little soft tissue covering the bones of the tarsus. It is usually limited to the site of the injury. Displacement of the central tarsal bone produces a palpable and sometimes slightly mobile projection on the craniomedial aspect of the tarsus.

18.3.3 Diagnostics

Diagnosis of tarsal fractures (and associated luxations) is generally made on the basis of physical and radiographic findings. Standard dorsoplantar and mediolateral projections are often sufficient,

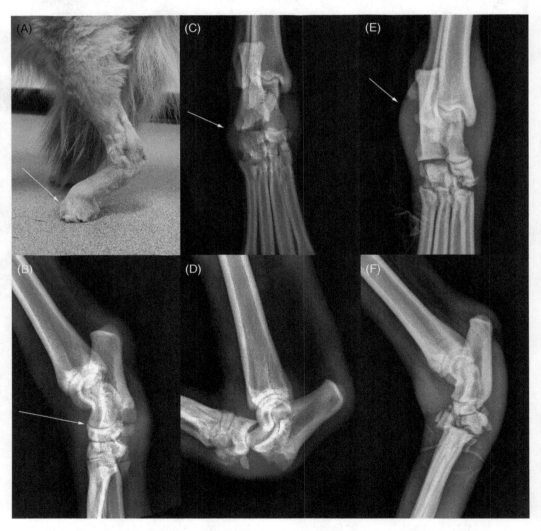

Figure 18.5 Examples of traumatic tarsal joint injuries: *Patient I* (A–D) was diagnosed with proximal intertarsal joint luxation due to disruption of the plantar ligaments. The patient shows (A) hyperflexion of the tarsus with flexed digits, a similar appearance to patients presenting with Type IIc Achilles tendinopathy. Standard (B) lateral views do not show obvious evidence of the (white arrow) fracture luxation; however, it can be visualized on the (C) dorsoplantar view and the degree of disruption becomes obvious when performing (D) flexed stress views; *Patient II* (E, F) was diagnosed with comminuted fractures of the central, second, third, and fourth tarsal bones and proximal second metatarsal bones with associated (white arrow) soft tissue swelling.

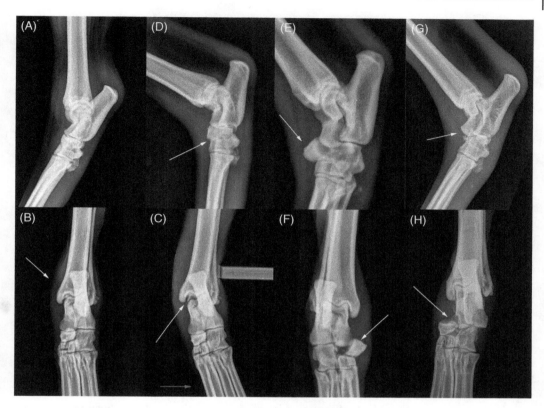

Figure 18.6 Examples of traumatic tarsal joint injuries: *Patient I* (A–C) was diagnosed with a medial collateral and talar ridge fracture; (A) lateral radiographs were nondiagnostic, (B) dorsoplantar radiographs show (white arrow) soft tissue swelling on the medial side, (C) stress radiographs confirm disruption of the medial collateral ligament as indicated by the (white arrow) opening of the joint and also illustrate the talar ridge fracture. Stress views were performed by applying (blue arrows) medial pressure proximal to the tarsus and lateral pressure distal to the tarsus (valgus stress view). *Patient II* (D–F) was diagnosed with a central tarsal bone fracture that could be missed on the (D) standard lateral view since it only shows (white arrow) mild displacement of the fracture; however, (E) with gentle flexion, the (white arrow) displacement becomes more evident and (F) dorsoplantar views also clearly show the (white arrow) displaced fragment. Radiographs of *Patient III* (G, H) show severely displaced (white arrows) fracture luxation of the proximal intertarsal joint.

but oblique views can be useful. Images taken with the tarsus in flexion, extension, and mediolateral stress (with a fulcrum placed on the tarsus to lever the metatarsus against; Figure 18.6) can help define the level and direction of instability. CT is the most sensitive modality, but it is seldom needed for detecting the presence of tarsal fractures; it can, however, help to define the nature of the fracture and guide its repair (Butler et al. 2018).

18.4 Tarsal Joint Luxations

Tarsal joint luxations can occur at any level and may be due to ligament disruption or fractures of the associated bones. Injuries to the collateral ligaments cause instability at the level of the *tarsocrural* joint. The two other reasons for tarsocrural joint luxations are shearing injuries or fractures of the medial and or lateral malleoli, which are the origins of the collateral ligaments. These injuries result in *medio-lateral* instability. Luxations or instability of the *distal tarsal joints* may involve the plantar or dorsal intertarsal ligaments and the resulting instability may be *dorso-plantar* and/or *medio-lateral*. The majority of these injuries are traumatic, but they may be due to immune-mediated or (uncommonly) idiopathic disease. The *proximal intertarsal* joint (i.e. calca-neoquartal and talocalcaneocentral joints) is the level most commonly involved but *tarsometatar-sal* luxations are also encountered.

Treatment of these injuries may include nonsurgical approaches for mild injuries, but surgery is generally recommended for complete (grade 3) sprains. Surgical treatment may include recon-struction of the collateral ligaments, fracture fixation (e.g. for malleolar fractures), or partial and pantarsal arthrodesis depending on the location and severity of the injury.

18.4.1 Signalment and History

Dogs of all breeds and ages can be affected by traumatic tarsal luxations, although medium-to-large, active dogs seem to be most often affected. Motor vehicle accidents are the most common cause, but collateral injuries can also follow falls, running mishaps, and lower limb entrapment. Collisions with vehicles can cause shearing injuries, which almost always happen on the medial side of the tarsus. When the medial malleolus is ground away, medial collateral instability results. Herding dogs can incur tarsometatarsal luxations when a foot is caught in the rungs of a gate dur-ing a jump. When trauma is involved, the limb is initially carried. With time weight-bearing is resumed, but severe (and apparently painful) lameness persists. With disruption of the dorsal liga-ments, this lameness may be less severe compared to plantar ligament or collateral ligament pathology. Please refer to Section 18.7.2 regarding idiopathic tarsal luxation and tarsal luxation caused by immune-mediated disease.

Isolated rupture of one or both of the short lateral collateral ligaments has been reported in 6 young (3–40 month old) dogs, most of which were Retrievers (Sjöström and Håkanson 1994). This injury was associated with fracture or fragmentation of the lateral trochlear ridge in three of these dogs. It is not known if the talar injuries were strictly traumatic in origin or if osteochondrosis of the lateral talar ridge was a predisposing factor.

18.4.2 Physical Exam

Diagnosis is straightforward when both the short and long *collateral* ligaments of one side are completely ruptured. The affected limb is usually carried right after the ligament has been injured, but as time passes most dogs begin using it again. When the limb is bearing weight, medial collat-eral insufficiency allows valgus angulation and lateral collateral insufficiency allows varus angula-tion of the foot. There may be a wound present over the medial (most common) or lateral aspect of the tarsus; sometimes this wound is small compared to the extent of the injury beneath. The tarsus will be swollen, with the swelling usually centered on the tarsocrural joint and more severe on the injured side. Crepitus and luxation may be felt when the joint is manipulated. Testing the collateral ligament integrity is done with the tarsus both in extension and in moderate flexion. This allows for testing of the short and long collateral ligaments. The distal tibia is held steady, and varus and valgus stress is applied to the pes. If the lower limb deviates laterally with the tarsus in extension and flexion, complete disruption of the medial collateral ligaments is present. Similarly, if medial deviation of the pes happens in both tarsal positions, the lateral collateral ligaments are completely torn. If deviation only happens with the tarsus in extension, just the long part of the collateral liga-ment is torn; instability only in flexion suggests injury to the short collateral ligaments. Isolated damage to the short lateral collateral ligament can produce just a subtle rotational instability that can only be detected with the dog under heavy sedation. Testing is done with the tarsus in 60–90° of flexion; the tibia is stabilized, and the foot is rotated in both directions. When the short lateral collateral ligaments are torn, a click may be felt on the lateral side as the pes is supinated (Sjöström and Håkanson 1994).

Dogs walk with the tarsocrural joint in some degree of flexion throughout the weight-bearing phase of the gait. Below the tarsocrural joint, the rest of the tarsus resists this bending tendency and normally remains straight, but disruption of the plantar tarsal ligaments or their attachments allows flexion (and often subluxation) here. With acute *distal tarsal joint* injuries, the affected limb may be held up throughout the gait, but most patients return to a severe but weight-bearing lameness. In animals with *proximal intertarsal* luxation due to disruption of the *plantar* ligaments, the tarsus can be seen to flex distal to the tarsocrural joint (i.e. at two levels rather than just at the tarsocrural joint), when the dog is bearing weight (Video 18.1). There is usually some firm swelling on the plantar aspect of the tarsus, at or distal to the base of the calcaneus. To demonstrate this instability, the examiner holds the calcaneus in position and applies pressure on the pes through the metatarsal pad as a dog would do while walking (Figure 18.4). Normally the distal pes will remain aligned with the long axis of the calcaneus, but in dogs with tarsal injuries the pes will angle cranially. In contrast, disruption of the *dorsal* ligaments does not cause these obvious instabilities, since weight-bearing does not stress the dorsal ligaments. Instability may be visible during liftoff/swing phase or during palpation, which is performed by reversing the palpation performed for plantar ligament pathology. These injuries are encountered less frequently and cause less severe signs and pain. Depending on the plane of instability, dogs with *tarsometatarsal* luxations may show similar exam findings to dogs with proximal intertarsal luxation. If severe displacement is present (Figure 18.6), obvious instability, pain, and deviation of the bones will be palpable, but with less severe injuries exam findings can be subtle.

Video 18.1

Achilles tendinopathy gaits.

18.4.3 Diagnostics

Orthogonal radiographs are part of the database, but diagnosis of the specific condition is usually made through stress radiography. Stress radiographs can be done in any direction and are performed in the same fashion as palpation during the physical exam. For example, for detection of *collateral ligament* disruption, dorsoplantar radiographs should be taken both with the tarsus in neutral position and with varus and valgus stress applied using a radiolucent fulcrum such as a wooden spoon placed slightly above the tarsocrural level to lever against; the tarsocrural joint will open up on the side of the collateral disruption (Mauragis and Berry 2012). There is also almost always marked soft tissue swelling evident at the tarsocrural joint at the side of the collateral ligament that is affected. With shearing injuries, the medial malleolus may be ground flat. Malleolar fractures may be apparent, or small bone fragments may suggest avulsion of the origin of the collateral ligament. Oblique views may show other injuries accompanying the ligament tear.

For detection of *plantar ligament* instability, a lateral view is made with the stifle held in moderate extension while upward pressure is placed on the metatarsal pad and plantar aspect of the metatarsus to stress the lower part of the tarsus in flexion (Figure 18.5). Dorsal angulation will be evident at the level of instability. And vice versa, for detection of dorsal ligament instability, the pressure to the distal pes would be applied in a plantar fashion during extension of the tarsal joint.

18.5 Pathology of the Common Calcanean Tendon

The CCT (also referred to as "Achilles tendon") includes all structures that attach to the tuber calcanei. It is formed by the (i) GT, (ii) the SDFT, (iii) and the conjoined tendon (also referred to as "accessory" or "combined" tendon) of the following three muscles: biceps femoris, gracilis, and semitendinosus. The gastrocnemius muscle originates from the distal, caudal femur and forms the GT approximately at the level of mid-tibia. This tendon is the main component of the CCT and the major muscle responsible for tarsal extension. The superficial digital flexor (SDF) muscle originates together with the lateral head of the gastrocnemius muscle on the distal, caudal femur and continues cranially to the gastrocnemius muscle proximally but then the SDFT wraps around the GT medially to become the most caudal attachment to the tuber calcanei (Figure 18.7). This attachment is accomplished by a broad, fibrocartilaginous "caplike"-structure attaching collaterally to the calcaneus, which allows the SDFT to continue distally to its distal attachment at the plantar surface of the proximal base of phalanges II–V, thereby providing stifle flexion, tarsal extension,

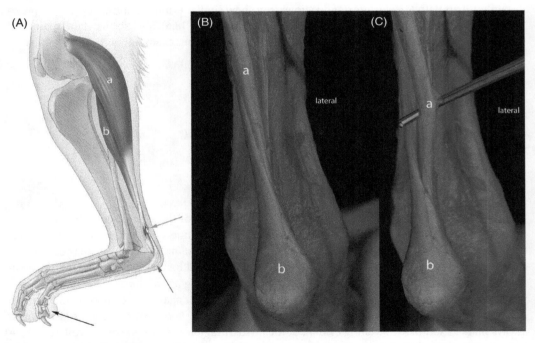

Figure 18.7 Type IIc Achilles tendinopathy: (A) the (a) gastrocnemius tendon is (red arrow) partially disrupted, resulting in slight hyperflexion (plantigrade) stance. Since the (b) superficial digital flexor tendon is (blue arrow) intact, the increased flexion angle forces the digits into (black arrow) flexion, which results in the typical "crab-claw" stance. (B, C) The superficial digital flexor tendon wraps around the gastrocnemius tendon medially to form a cap that attaches caudally to the tuber calcanei. When palpating the tendons above the calcaneus, isolation of the tendons is possible if the tendons are not affected by pathology.

Box 18.1   Grading of Pathology of the CCT (Meutstege 1993)

1) Type I = complete rupture
   (a) Stance = plantigrade

2) Type II = partial rupture
   (a) Stance = slightly increased hock flexion
      i) Type IIa affects the musculotendinous junction
      ii) Type IIb is similar to Type I but has an intact paratenon and therefore dogs are not completely plantigrade
      iii) Type IIc affects the GT only (with intact SDFT) resulting in increased flexor tension on the digits ("crab claw")

3) Type III = tendinosis only
   (a) Stance = normal

---

and digit flexion. The conjoined tendon inserts medially on the tuber calcanei and plays a minor role in tarsal extension.

A classification system (Box 18.1) that differentiates conditions causing structural changes of the CCT based on location and severity of injury has been described (Meutstege 1993). An important distinction should be made between acute, traumatic (e.g. Type I) rupture and a chronic, degenerative (e.g. Type IIc) process, since the treatment differs substantially (Figure 18.8). Another rarely encountered condition is luxation of the SDFT. Pathology affecting the origin of the gastrocnemius muscle (e.g. avulsion and myotendinopathy) is also rare and discussed in Chapter 19.

18.5.1   Traumatic Rupture

Traumatic rupture may occur at any level of the CCT, with the musculotendinous junction and insertion most commonly affected. Disruption may involve any of the five structures of the CCT but most commonly affects all tendons (i.e. Type I or Type IIb injuries). Border Collies frequently sustain these injuries (Corr et al. 2010), but obviously any dog may suffer from trauma. Lacerations may be due to external trauma (e.g. sharp lacerations) or occur during exercising; the injury may be open or closed. While open injuries simplify establishing a diagnosis based on the visible disruption of the skin (and visibly disrupted tendon in some cases), closed injuries are diagnosed based on palpation of the tendon and the associated plantigrade stance (i.e. the entire pes touching the ground; Figure 18.8). However, recent literature (Corr et al. 2010; Gamble et al. 2017) has shown that plantigrade stance (note that plantigrade stance was defined more loosely as an increased flexion angle by these authors) does not always predict the specific tendons affected but is more likely to be present in patients with injury at the musculotendinous junction. Palpation of a gap between the ruptured ends of the tendon is facilitated by stretching the CCT, which is accomplished by extending the stifle and flexing the tarsus (Figure 18.4). The entire CCT should be palpated, since diffuse injuries or injuries at multiple sites have been reported. Radiographs should be performed to rule out any fractures or other osseous abnormalities. Ultrasonography can be utilized to determine the exact location and extent of CCT disruption, and a grading system for this has been reported (Gamble et al. 2017). As with palpation of the tendon, dynamic evaluation while the CCT is stretched can help identify pathology. Treatment of acute injuries generally involves surgical apposition of the tendon ends followed by some form of external or internal support while the tendon is healing.

TARSAL REGION

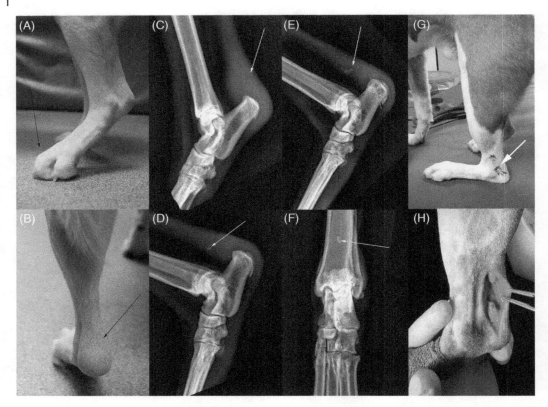

Figure 18.8 Examples of dogs with pathology of the Achilles tendon: (A) typical stance with Type IIc Achilles tendinopathy caused by an intact SDF with a partially disrupted gastrocnemius muscle resulting in the typical "crab-claw" stance with the (black arrow) digits flexed and the tarsus slightly hyperflexed; (B) typical (black arrow) swelling associated with Type IIc Achilles tendinopathy; (C) early stages of Achilles tendinopathy as illustrated by the (white arrow) soft tissue swelling of the tendon; (D–F) chronic Achilles tendinopathy is frequently associated with (white arrows) calcification and (blue arrow) enthesopathy at the insertion at the tuber calcanei; (G, H) typical stance and intra-operative appearance with acute, traumatic Type I Achilles injury.

18.5.2   Chronic Gastrocnemius Tendinopathy

Type IIc common calcanean tendinopathy (CCT2c) is a degenerative condition of the GT with an intact SDFT (Meutstege 1993; Gamble et al. 2017). It is well recognized in medium- and large-breed dogs and especially in middle-aged Doberman Pinschers and Labrador Retrievers (Corr et al. 2010; Gamble et al. 2017). The degeneration leads to elongation of the GT, thereby causing the increased flexion of the tarsus. Since the SDF is not affected and the GT is only elongated, animals are not presented with a completely plantigrade stance but rather with the typical "crab-claw" appearance from increased tension on the SDF that results in flexion of the digits (Figure 18.7, Video 18.1). This condition has also been described as an avulsion injury of the GT; however, this is somewhat confusing since the soft tissue opacities visible on radiographs proximal to the calcaneus likely represent dystrophic calcification rather than avulsion fragments. A chronic tendinitis (Type III) has also been described in the literature. This condition may be a precursor to Type IIc injuries, but little information about this is available.

The etiology of this condition is unclear, but a degenerative process is suspected given the atraumatic, chronic, and frequently bilateral presentation (Meutstege 1993; Gamble et al. 2017). As with cruciate ligament pathology, once the tendon is weakened, minor trauma may cause acute exacerbation of lameness, which may be the first time that owners notice the abnormality.

Palpation of the entire CCT should be performed as described for cases with traumatic rupture. It is essential to evaluate the other pelvic limb, since approximately 50% of cases are bilaterally affected (Gamble et al. 2017). Underlying conditions such as Cushing's disease and long-term steroid and perhaps enrofloxacin (Lim et al. 2008) administration should be excluded.

Radiographs may show soft tissue swelling of the affected region (most commonly at the insertion at the tuber calcanei), avulsion fragments, enthesopathy, or dystrophic calcification of the tendon (Figure 18.8). The latter can be difficult to differentiate from an avulsion fragment, but with dystrophic calcification, the tuber calcanei does not show a defect, and multiple foci of calcification are often present. Ultrasonography is more sensitive than palpation or radiography and facilitates the identification of the specific tendons involved as well as the severity of the disruption (Gamble et al. 2017). Ultrasonography therefore provides a simple, noninvasive, and cost-effective method to evaluate the CCT.

There is a lack of peer-reviewed literature comparing available treatment options for this disease. Surgical repair is generally recommended (Corr et al. 2010), but treatment with orthotics combined with surgery or as a sole treatment has also been reported (Wallace 2012; Mich 2014).

18.5.3 Luxation of the Superficial Digital Flexor Tendon

Luxation of the SDFT is an infrequent condition that results in pelvic limb lameness due to displacement of the tendon at the level of the calcaneus. The tendon generally luxates laterally due to disruption of the medial retinaculum. The condition may be triggered by mild trauma, although a traumatic event is not always observed. While osseous abnormalities of the calcaneus have been proposed as the underlying etiology (Reinke and Mughannam 1994), a weaker attachment on the medial side has been suggested as the main cause by Kara (1998). Shetland Sheepdogs appear to be predisposed (Solanti et al. 2002) but other breeds are also affected.

Patients show varying degrees of lameness depending on the acuity of the condition. Initially dogs may be non-weight-bearing on the limb, but most dogs have a low-grade lameness at the time of presentation. Some dogs show a skipping gait as is observed with patellar luxations. Swelling will be palpable and sometimes visible over the tip of the calcaneus. In some cases, bursitis is severe, causing the swelling to be fluctuant. In relatively acute cases, the diagnosis is made by a popping sensation as the tendon displaces (Video 18.2). The SDF may become fixed in its displaced condition when the condition is chronic. In this case, there is no palpable popping, but the focal swelling remains. Radiographs should be taken to rule out other osseous pathology. Luxation of the SDFT may be confused with Type IIc Achilles tendinopathy, and ultrasonography can be used to confirm the integrity of the CCT, which differentiates this condition from all other CCT pathologies. Ultrasonography is also useful for identifying chronic SDF luxations. Surgical imbrication of the torn or stretched retinaculum usually gives good results, except in some chronically affected dogs.

Video 18.2

Superficial digital flexor tendon luxation.

18.6 Osteochondrosis Dissecans

Osteochondrosis/osteochondritis dissecans (OCD) of the tarsal joint is an uncommon disease of young, mostly large-breed dogs that affects the talus. Either talar ridge can be affected, although OCD is most common on the medial side. It is not unusual for both tarsi to be affected, so both tarsi should be carefully assessed for pathology.

OCD fragments can damage adjacent cartilage surfaces, especially if they displace or break into smaller pieces. If they migrate or are removed, the resultant defect causes joint incongruity. Because of this, talar OCD reliably leads to OA of the tarsocrural joint. The osteochondrosis fragments can contain a substantial amount of subchondral bone. Unsurprisingly, as fragment size increases, prognosis for good limb use decreases. Reattachment of fragments can be difficult, and healing is unpredictable. Surgical removal of talar ridge OCD remains controversial. Fragment removal brings about clinical improvement in about half of treated dogs, but some degree of lameness persists in most and OA progresses regardless of treatment (Van Der Peijl et al. 2012). Dogs with significant lameness due to OA later in life may benefit from pantarsal arthrodesis. Migration of osteochondrosis fragments into the synovial sheath surrounding the DDF tendon is a rare consequence of OCD (Section 18.7.4).

18.6.1 Signalment and History

Talar ridge OCD is generally a disease of young large-breed dogs and particularly of Labrador Retrievers. Other predisposed breeds include Rottweilers, Pit Bulls, and Australian Cattle Dogs. The majority of affected dogs are female.

Lameness develops during the first year of life and can be seen as early as 4½ months of age. However, some dogs are presented for evaluation later in life, when tarsal OA begins to affect quality of life.

18.6.2 Physical Exam

Talar OCD typically produces a weight-bearing lameness that is evident at both the walk and the trot. A shorter stride is taken on the affected limb, and range of motion in the tarsus during each step is reduced. The limb may be held abducted, especially when the dog rises from a sitting position. These dogs may also display a positive "sit-test," making talar OCD a differential diagnosis for cranial cruciate ligament disease (Video 18.3). In the author's experience, tarsal hyperextension may be present, but in a recent study this was not found to be a common feature (Van Der Peijl et al. 2012).

Video 18.3

Typical gait with tarsal OCD.

Effusion is usually present on the cranial as well as on the plantaro-medial or plantaro-lateral aspect of the tarsocrural joint, depending on the location of the osteochondral fragment. The degree of swelling that is present gives an indication of the size of the fragment; larger fragments (and thus poorer prognoses) tend to be associated with more impressive effusions. Crepitus may be felt on joint manipulation, and the dog usually objects to joint flexion and full extension. Occasionally a displaced osteochondral fragment can be felt just caudal to the malleolus and medial or lateral to the trochlear ridge, but palpation for such fragments is usually prompted by radiographic findings.

18.6.3   Diagnostics

Orthogonal radiographs can be diagnostic for OCD; however, smaller lesions are easily missed due to the complexity of the joint. In normal tarsi, both talar ridges are circular on the lateral radiographic view, but when OCD is present flattening of one of the ridges will be evident (Figure 18.9). On the dorsoplantar projection, a gap between the talus and the tibia – normally a close fit – can be seen, sometimes with osteochondral fragments visible within the defect. A dorsoplantar skyline view of the caudal aspect of the talar trochlea taken with the tarsus in slightly

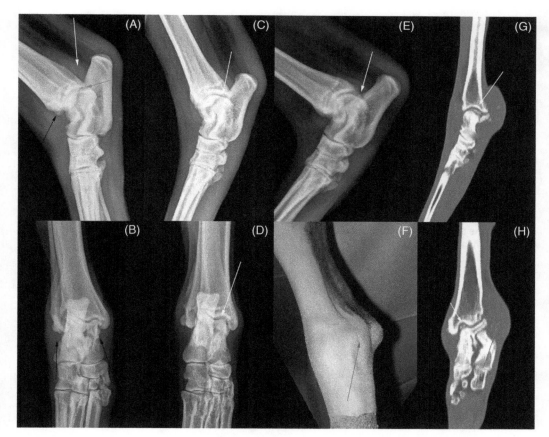

Figure 18.9   Examples of surgically confirmed tarsal OCD: *Patient I* (A, B) was diagnosed with OCD of the lateral talar ridge. Radiographs show only subtle changes including (A) mild periarticular osteophytosis (black arrow) on the lateral view mild, joint effusion (white arrow), and very subtle flattening of the proximo-plantar aspect of the trochlea (red arrow). *Patient II* (C–H) showed more obvious changes including the (C) extended lateral view shows flattening (white arrow) of the trochlea; (D) the dorsoplantar view shows (white arrow) an increased joint space indicating a medial trochlear ridge defect; (E) the flexed lateral view makes the (white arrow) trochlear ridge flattening more easily visible; (F) typical location for (blue arrow) joint effusion in patients with OCD; (G, H) CT illustrating the (white arrow) OCD lesion and (blue arrow) joint effusion.

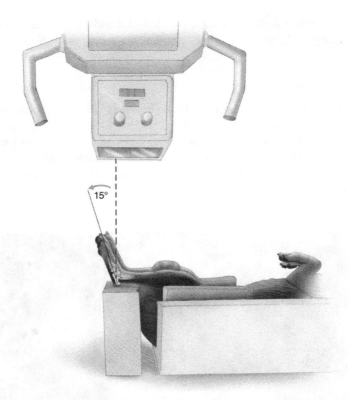

Figure 18.10 Radiographic positioning for dorsoplantar skyline radiographic evaluation of tarsal OCD in canine patients is performed by placing the dog in dorsal recumbency. The legs should be elevated on a foam pad and the tarsus should be angled slightly caudally to avoid superimposition. This skyline view highlights the trochlear ridges and should be performed if a definitive diagnosis cannot be accomplished with the standard views.

less than 90° flexion (to avoid superimposition) is occasionally helpful for highlighting ridge defects (Mauragis and Berry 2012; Figure 18.10).

Small defects and fragments can be difficult to see on plain radiographs, especially on the lateral side, where superimposition of the calcaneal shadow can obscure the trochlear ridge. CT is a more sensitive modality (detecting 100% of OCD lesions in one study) and can be helpful in cementing the diagnosis (Gielen et al. 2002).

18.7 Other Diseases Affecting the Tarsal Region

Although *panosteitis* more commonly affects the long bones of the thoracic limb, it can also affect the femur and tibia and should therefore be considered a differential diagnosis in juvenile patients with shifting limb lameness and pain on long bone palpation (Chapter 14).

Immune-mediated polyarthritis (IMPA) commonly affects the carpal and tarsal joints and is therefore an important differential diagnosis when joint effusion and/or pain in the tarsal joint is present. Affected dogs show a wide variation in clinical signs and examination findings, ranging from crying in pain with palpable joint effusion to no apparent gait abnormality, pain, or palpable

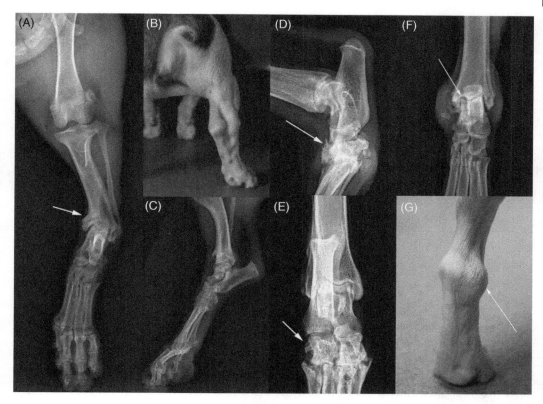

Figure 18.11 Other diseases affecting the tarsal region: (A–C) pes varus deformity in a miniature Dachshund; note the marked varus of the distal limb, (white arrow) shortening of the medial cortex of the tibial diaphysis compared to the lateral cortex, and widening of the medial aspect of the tibiotarsal joint. (D, E) Erosive immune-mediated polyarthritis in an adult dog that resulted in bilateral tarsal hyperflexion and carpal hyperextension; note that the (white arrow) lytic changes are limited to the distal tarsal joints resulting in instability at the tarsometatarsal joint. (F, G) Patient with chronic OCD and chronic enthesopathy of the medial collateral ligament; (F) the dorsoplantar view shows (white arrow) flattening of the medial trochlear ridge consistent with OCD; and (G) image of the patient illustrating (white arrow) severe periarticular swelling.

joint effusion. Dogs with advanced erosive arthritis may experience joint luxations (Figure 18.11) and walk plantigrade or have other joint deformities. Please refer to Chapters 9 and 13 for further details regarding joint fluid analysis and the classification of IMPA, respectively.

Septic arthritis should also be considered as a differential diagnosis, but in the tarsus it is much less frequent than immune-mediated disease.

18.7.1 Tarsal Deformities

Pes varus is a deformity of the distal tibia caused by premature closure of the medial distal tibial physis (Radasch et al. 2008). The asymmetric closure results in varus angulation of the distal tibia. It may be unilateral or bilateral. Since the majority of affected dogs are Dachshunds, the disease is thought to have a genetic component, but it may be caused by trauma in other dogs. Affected dogs have a "bow-legged" appearance (Figure 18.11) and variable clinical signs. The deformity may be limited to the distal limb but may clinically affect. Depending on the severity of the deformity, surgical correction may be considered.

18.7.2 Idiopathic Tarsal Hyperflexion

Luxation or subluxation of the distal tarsal joints is usually of traumatic origin, but it can also develop in the later stages of erosive immune-mediated arthropathies (Figure 18.11). Some dogs (especially Shetland Sheepdogs and Collies) without history of trauma or evidence of immune disease develop the instability gradually, and it may happen in both tarsi, sometimes in concert with carpal hyperextension. If arthrocentesis and testing for antinuclear antibody and rheumatoid factors speak against underlying immune-mediated disease, either inherent connective tissue weakness or degeneration of the plantar support structures is suspected but not proven (Carmichael and Marshall 2018). Dogs with this idiopathic, atraumatic presentation gradually develop a gait abnormality that often appears to be more mechanical than painful in nature. Treatment is challenging due to the number of joints affected but generally involves partial tarsal arthrodesis, although orthotic support can be considered.

18.7.3 Idiopathic Tarsal Hyperextension

Tarsal hyperextension can occur at multiple levels but most prominently involves the tarsocrural joint. This condition may accompany talar OCD and is a feature of some myopathies (Marioni-Henry et al. 2014). Additionally, tarsal hyperextension may be due to painful conditions more proximal in the limb, such as cranial cruciate ligament rupture, hip dysplasia, or lumbosacral stenosis. In cases with more proximal pathology, tarsal hyperextension is thought to develop as a compensation mechanism in which the associated weight shifting towards the thoracic limbs results in tarsal hyperextension to gain pelvic limb length. Alternatively, pain in a more proximal joint may result in a changed stance angle (i.e. a dog with stifle pathology may prefer to stand with increased flexion of the stifle and therefore the tarsus is hyperextended to compensate). The presence of tarsal hyperextension should therefore alert the diagnostician to the possibility of pathology located more proximally, even though the tarsal abnormality may be the most noticeable clinical sign.

In some cases, no other pathology can be identified. A congenital laxity of the fibularis musculotendinous region has been implicated in calves (Kilic et al. 2015), but tarsal hyperextension is seldom evident during the first few months of life in dogs. The hyperextension typically develops gradually, usually during the first year of life. Dogs of any breed, age, or sex can be affected. The degree of hyperextension varies between cases and in some dogs, the abnormality may be intermittent. The tarsus extends up to or beyond 180° by the end of the stance phase of the gait. The tarsocrural joint may abruptly flip forward just before the foot is lifted. The affected tarsus may rock into and out of hyperextension when the dog is standing (Figure 18.12). Affected tarsi seldom appear to be painful on manipulation. Range of motion in flexion is unaffected, but the abnormal tarsus can be extended at least to 180°. Effusion or crepitus is usually absent unless there is concurrent talar OCD.

Radiographs of the tarsus are also usually normal unless talar OCD is present. If the tarsus is stressed in extension, a lateral view will document the abnormally high tarsocrural angle without other pathology (Figure 18.12). Degenerative changes may be seen, although they are observed infrequently and may be secondary to other pathology in some cases. Radiography of the stifle and the hip in the affected limb should be considered to evaluate for concurrent orthopedic abnormalities. Since lumbosacral stenosis is occasionally associated with tarsal hyperextension, radiographs and possibly MRI of this region may be indicated if lower back pain is evident.

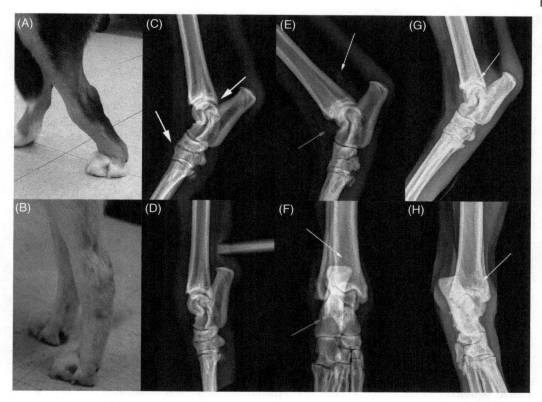

Figure 18.12 Other diseases affecting the tarsal region: (A, C, D) idiopathic tarsal hyperextension without identifiable underlying pathology; (B) tarsal hyperextension secondary to severe stifle disease; (C) standard lateral radiograph of patient depicted in image (A), note that there are (white arrows) degenerative changes several joints of the tarsus; (D) stressed image illustrating the hyperextension visualized in image (A); (E, F) calcification in the (white arrow) deep digital flexor tendon sheath likely representing a migrated OCD flap; there is another (blue arrow) calcification in the dorsal joint space of unknown origin; and (G, H) tarsal synovial cell sarcoma not the (white arrows) subtle lysis of the talus and distal tibia.

Tarsal hyperextension does not typically seem to be painful, so it is usually treated conservatively. Orthoses that allow tarsal flexion while limiting extension may be considered. In calves, shortening of the fibularis longus tendon seems to be effective in preventing hyperextension (Kilic et al. 2015), but specific surgical therapy has not been reported for dogs. Once tarsal hyperextension has developed, it persists even if concurrent orthopedic conditions have been successfully addressed.

18.7.4 Osteochondrosis Fragment Migration into the DDF Tendon Sheath

An unusual manifestation of talar OCD is the migration of osteochondrosis fragments into the synovial sheath surrounding the DDF tendon. This sheath communicates with the tarsocrural joint just caudal to the medial malleolus and near the plantar aspect of the talus, making it possible for free fragments from the medial (and occasionally lateral) talar ridge to become trapped around the tendon.

These osteochondral fragments can irritate the DDF and restrict its motion within the sheath (Post et al. 2008). Lameness is intermittent (resembling patellar luxation by causing a "skipping" pelvic limb lameness) to continuous (particularly if severe arthritis is present due to the primary

OCD lesions), with decreased range of motion in the tarsus in both flexion and extension. Tarsocrural joint effusion is present. The DDF tendon sheath may be palpable as a distended and painful vertical swelling on the plantaro-medial aspect of the tarsus and distal tibia.

Orthogonal radiographs may show swelling of the DDF tendon sheath and opacities in the region of the tendon caudal to the tibia (Figure 18.12). Oblique views can be useful for highlighting additional fragments. CT is the most sensitive test for showing all of the fragments within the sheath, which is useful for guiding fragment removal surgery but generally not necessary for diagnosis of this condition. Ultrasonography of the tendon sheath can also be used to localize swelling to the DDF tendon sheath and find fragments.

Lameness attributed to irritation of the DDF can be treated with removal of the osteochondral fragments from around the tendon. However, lameness due to the secondary degenerative changes may persist following treatment.

18.7.5 Tarsal Region Neoplasia

Neoplasia is much less frequently observed in the tarsal region than in the carpal region, but tumors of the synovium (Figure 18.12) and osteosarcoma should be considered as differential diagnoses. Further details about neoplastic conditions are provided in Chapters 11 and 22.

18.7.6 Miscellaneous Other Conditions

While degenerative changes of the distal tarsal joints are frequently identified as an incidental finding, lameness associated with centrodistal OA has been described in Greyhounds and Border Collies (Guilliard 2005). Affected dogs show a pain response if the metatarsus is supinated while the limb is extended behind the dog and the calcaneus is fixed in place.

The authors have diagnosed rupture of the tarsal extensor retinaculum as a cause of lameness, but this has not been reported in the peer-reviewed literature.

Dee (2015) has reported lameness (often bilateral) in working German Shepherds associated with thickening and presumed repetitive trauma to the cranial tibial tendon of insertion.

Fragmentation of the medial malleolus has been reported in a small number of young large-breed (mostly Rottweiler) dogs; about half of the affected dogs had concurrent talar ridge OCD (Newell et al. 1994). The association of this condition with lameness is unclear.

References

Armstrong, A.J., Bruce, M., Adams, R. et al. (2019). Injuries involving the central tarsal bone in nonracing dogs: short-term outcomes and prognostic factors. *Vet Surg* 48 (4): 524–536.

Aron, D.N. and Purinton, P. (1985). Collateral ligaments of the tarsocrural joint an anatomic and functional study. *Vet Surg* 14 (3): 173–177.

Butler, D., Nemanic, S., and Warnock, J.J. (2018). Comparison of radiography and computed tomography to evaluate fractures of the canine tarsus. *Vet Radiol Ultrasound* 59 (1): 43–53.

Carmichael, S. and Marshall, W.G. (2018). Tarsus and metatarsus. In: *Veterinary Surgery: Small Animal*, 2e (eds. S.A. Johnston and K.M. Tobias), 1193–1209. St. Louis: Elsevier.

Corr, S.A., Draffan, D., Kulendra, E. et al. (2010). Retrospective study of Achilles mechanism disruption in 45 dogs. *Vet Rec* 167 (11): 407–411.

Decamp, C.E., Johnston, S.A., Déjardin, L.M., and Schaefer, S.L. (2016). Fractures and other orthopedic injuries of the tarsus, metatarsus, and phalanges. In: *Brinker, Piermattei, and Flo's Handbook of Small Animal Orthopedics and Fracture Repair*, 5e (eds. C.E. Decamp, S.A. Johnston, L.M. Déjardin and S.L. Schaefer), 707–758. St. Louis: Elsevier.

Dee, J. (2015). Management of distal limb injuries in Greyhounds and other working breeds. *Proceedings of the North American Veterinary Conference 2015*, Orlando, FL (17–21 January 2015).

Deruddere, K.J., Milne, M.E., Wilson, K.M., and Snelling, S.R. (2014). Magnetic resonance imaging, computed tomography, and gross anatomy of the canine tarsus. *Vet Surg* 43 (8): 912–919.

Gamble, L.-J., Canapp, D.A., and Canapp, S.O. (2017). Evaluation of Achilles tendon injuries with findings from diagnostic musculoskeletal ultrasound in canines—43 cases. *Vet Evid* 2 (3).

Gielen, I., Van Bree, H., Van Ryssen, B. et al. (2002). Radiographic, computed tomographic and arthroscopic findings in 23 dogs with osteochondrosis of the tarsocrural joint. *Vet Rec* 150 (14): 442–447.

Guilliard, M.J. (2005). Centrodistal joint lameness in dogs. *J Small Anim Pract* 46 (4): 199–202.

Johnson, D.E. (1985). Bursitis/tendinitis. In: *Textbook of Small Animal Orthopedics* (eds. C.D. Newton and D.M. Nunamaker). Philadelphia: J.B. Lippincott Company.

Kara, M.E. (1998). Anatomical factors in displacement of the superficial digital flexor tendon in dogs. *Dtsch Tierarztl Wochenschr* 105 (7): 278–279.

Kilic, E., Ozaydin, I., Aksoy, O., and Yayla, S. (2015). Diagnosis and surgical management of congenital laxity of the fibularis musculotendinous unit resulting in hyperextension of the tarsus in 14 calves. *Vet Surg* 44 (7): 825–828.

Lim, S., Hossain, M.A., Park, J. et al. (2008). The effects of enrofloxacin on canine tendon cells and chondrocytes proliferation in vitro. *Vet Res Commun* 32 (3): 243–253.

Marioni-Henry, K., Haworth, P., Scott, H. et al. (2014). Sarcolemmal specific collagen VI deficient myopathy in a Labrador Retriever. *J Vet Intern Med* 28 (1): 243–249.

Mauragis, D. and Berry, C.R. (2012). Small animal tarsus and pes radiography. *Todays Vet Pract* 2 (6): 47–55. https://todaysveterinarypractice.com/wp-content/uploads/sites/4/2016/05/T1211C03.pdf (accessed 16 June 2019).

Meutstege, F. (1993). The classification of canine Achilles tendon lesions. *Vet Comp Orthop Traumatol* 6: 53–55.

Mich, P.M. (2014). The emerging role of veterinary orthotics and prosthetics (V-OP) in small animal rehabilitation and pain management. *Top Companion Anim Med* 29 (1): 10–19.

Newell, S.M., Mahaffey, M.B., and Aron, D.N. (1994). Fragmentation of the medial malleolus of dogs with and without tarsal osteochondrosis. *Vet Radiol Ultrasound* 35 (1): 5–9.

Post, C., Guerrero, T., Ohlerth, S. et al. (2008). Joint mice migration into the deep digital flexor tendon sheath in dogs: clinical cases and anatomical study. *Vet Comp Orthop Traumatol* 21 (5): 440–445.

Radasch, R.M., Lewis, D.F., Mcdonald, D.E. et al. (2008). Pes varus correction in Dachshunds using a hybrid external fixator. *Vet Surg* 37 (1): 71–81.

Reinke, J.D. and Mughannam, A.J. (1994). Lateral luxation of the superficial digital flexor tendon in 12 dogs. *J Am Anim Hosp Assoc* 29: 303–309.

Sabanci, S.S. and Ocal, M.K. (2018). Categorization of the pelvic limb standing posture in nine breeds of dogs. *Anat Histol Embryol* 47 (1): 58–63.

Sjöström, L. and Håkanson, N. (1994). Traumatic injuries associated with the short lateral collateral ligaments of the talocrural joint of the dog. *J Small Anim Pract* 35 (3): 163–168.

Solanti, S., Laitinen, O., and Atroshi, F. (2002). Hereditary and clinical characteristics of lateral luxation of the superficial digital flexor tendon in Shetland Sheepdogs. *Vet Ther* 3 (1): 97–103.

Thrall, D.E. and Robertson, I.D. (2016). Basic imaging principles and physeal closure time. In: *Atlas of Normal Radiographic Anatomy and Anatomic Variants in the Dog and Cat*, 2e (eds. D.E. Thrall and I.D. Robertson), 1–19. St. Louis: Elsevier.

Van Der Peijl, G.J., Schaeffer, I.G., Theyse, L.F. et al. (2012). Osteochondrosis dissecans of the tarsus in Labrador Retrievers: clinical signs, radiological data and force plate gait evaluation after surgical treatment. *Vet Comp Orthop Traumatol* 25 (2): 126–134.

von Pfeil, D.J. and Decamp, C.E., 2009. The epiphyseal plate: physiology, anatomy, and trauma. Compend Contin Educ Vet, 31(8), pp.E1–E11.

Wallace, A.M. (2012). Assessment and treatment of diseases of the common calcanean tendon in dogs. *Companion Anim* 17 (4): 16–21.

Wood, A.K. and McCarthy, P.H. (1984). Radiologic and anatomic observations of plantar sesamoid bones at the tarsometatarsal articulations of Greyhounds. *Am J Vet Res* 45 (10): 2158–2161.

19

Stifle Region
Jennifer Warnock¹ and Felix Michael Duerr²

¹ *Carlson College of Veterinary Medicine, Oregon State University, Corvallis, OR, USA*
² *Department of Clinical Sciences, College of Veterinary Medicine and Biomedical Sciences, Colorado State University, Fort Collins, CO, USA*

19.1 Introduction and Common Differential Diagnoses

Pathology of the stifle joint is a common source of clinical pelvic limb lameness in dogs. While many conditions affect the stifle region, cranial cruciate ligament disease (CCLD) and patellar luxation are the two diseases responsible for the majority of clinical lameness seen in dogs. Fortunately, both of these conditions can be tentatively diagnosed based on physical exam and radiographs. Additional imaging modalities such as computed tomography (CT), ultrasound, magnetic resonance imaging (MRI), arthrocentesis, and arthroscopy can be used to confirm diagnoses, detect additional and less common injuries affecting the region, and allow for surgical planning.

Osteoarthritis of the stifle joint most frequently is the consequence of cranial cruciate ligament (CCL) deficiency. Other conditions such as patellar luxation and osteochondrosis dissecans (OCD) are less common primary causes of osteoarthritis. The stifle is one of the joints reported to be affected by immune-mediated as well as infectious arthritis and, therefore, arthrocentesis and synovial fluid evaluation should be considered in cases where establishing a diagnosis is difficult.

Figure 19.1 and Table 19.1 outline common differential diagnoses and diagnostic steps for the stifle region.

19.2 Normal Anatomy

19.2.1 The Stifle Joint

The stifle joint is a large complex condylar joint. Articulating joint surfaces are found between the femoral and tibial condyles (*femorotibial joint*), the patella and femur (*femoropatellar joint*), and the fabellae (sesamoid bones of the gastrocnemius muscle) and the femur. The joint surfaces of the tibial and femoral condyles are convex, and the plateau of the tibia is sloped, making the stifle a relatively incongruent and unstable joint without its soft tissue supporting structures. This is one of the main reasons, why injury to the stabilizing articular structures typically results in instability, dysfunction, and pain.

Table 19.1 Key features for selected diseases affecting the stifle region.

Disease	Common signalment	Diagnostic test of choice	Exam findings	Treatment	Clinical pearls	Terminology
Fractures	Any (physeal fractures in immature animals)	Radiographs (orthogonal views needed, particularly for minimally displaced physeal fractures), may require CT or stress views	Pain, crepitus, and non-weight-bearing lameness	Depends on location but frequently surgical fixation recommended	Comparison to other (normal) limb can help to diagnose minimally displaced physeal fractures	Minimally displaced tibial tuberosity avulsion fracture (MDTTAF) describes fractures of the tibial tuberosity with secondary remodeling of the physis but minimal displacement
Cranial cruciate ligament disease (CCLD)	Any breed but middle-aged medium-/large-breed dogs predisposed	Palpation with radiographs generally sufficient, may need arthroscopy to confirm partial tears	See Box 19.1	Surgical treatment (TPLO) or nonsurgical treatment	Early, partial tears do not show drawer or thrust instability, but radiographs easily detect joint effusion	"Rupture" is obsolete terminology given the degenerative, slowly progressive nature of the disease
Caudal cruciate ligament rupture	Any breed, athletes predisposed since the trauma requires caudal blow to tibia	Stress views, arthroscopy, or MRI	Caudal drawer instability	Generally nonsurgical	Difficult to differentiate from CCLD based on exam	
Stifle luxation	Any breed since traumatic	Radiographs, stress views, and ultrasound	Severe pain and obvious instability	Surgical treatment	Stifle radiographs lack chronic, degenerative changes	Also known as "deranged" stifle
Patellar luxation	Small-breed dogs predisposed to MPL; large-breed dogs may have MPL or LPL	Palpation, radiographs, or CT to determine degree of deformities	Patella instability graded 1–4 (Box 19.2)	Surgical and nonsurgical treatment	Small-breed dogs with history of MPL and acute worsening of lameness may suffer from concomitant CCLD	
Osteochondrosis dissecans (OCD)	Large- and giant-breed puppies	Radiographs but CT may be required for subtle lesions	Pain on stifle manipulation without instability	Surgical removal or medical management	Ideally diagnose and treat early, once arthritis is present treatment is more controversial	

Patellar ligament desmopathy	Any for traumatic; athletic dogs for nontraumatic	Radiographs and ultrasound	Obvious disruption to mild or no pain upon palpation	Traumatic generally surgical, nontraumatic generally nonsurgical	Common after TPLO and TTA but does not cause lameness in these patients	Patellar tendinopathy
Angular limb deformity	Large- and giant-breed puppies	Radiographs (CT if surgery is performed)	Lameness and pain variable	Surgical or nonsurgical management depending on severity	Secondary patellar luxation or CCLD may be present	Tibial valgus and Genu varum/valgus
Panosteitis	Frequently seen in German Shepherd Dogs between 5 and 19 months of age	Radiographs (but may require CT during early stages) show intramedullary radiodensities	Pain on long bone palpation (more common in thoracic limb), shifting leg lameness	Rest and pain management	Disease should be self-limiting, if clinical symptoms continue in the same leg, further imaging should be considered	Other terms include eosinophilic panosteitis, juvenile osteomyelitis, and enostosis or medullary fibrosis
Septic arthritis	Postsurgical dogs most common but can happen in dogs with preexisting arthritis	Joint fluid analysis, culture, and physical exam findings	Moderate-to-severe pain on ROM, periarticular swelling, and pitting limb edema	Antibiotics and consider joint lavage; removal of implants once bone healing complete	Dogs with preexisting joint disease (such as arthritis) are predisposed. A lack of fever or negative culture results do not rule out septic arthritis	
Gastrocnemius myotendinopathy	Athletic dogs but described in pets as well	Radiographs may show calcification, enthesopathy, and displacement; however, ultrasound or MRI is needed if no radiographic changes are present	Variable degree of lameness and pain upon palpation and stretching of the muscle	Nonsurgical management unless acute, traumatic avulsion	To stretch the muscle, extend the stifle and flex the tarsus	Gastrocnemius avulsion is likely initial stage of the more chronic myotendinopathy
Long digital extensor tendinopathy	Athletic dogs but described as complication after TPLO	Palpation for luxation; radiographs may show calcification	Skipping lameness with luxation, asymptomatic with calcification	Nonsurgical most common	To stretch the muscle, flex the stifle, extend the tarsus, and flex the digits	

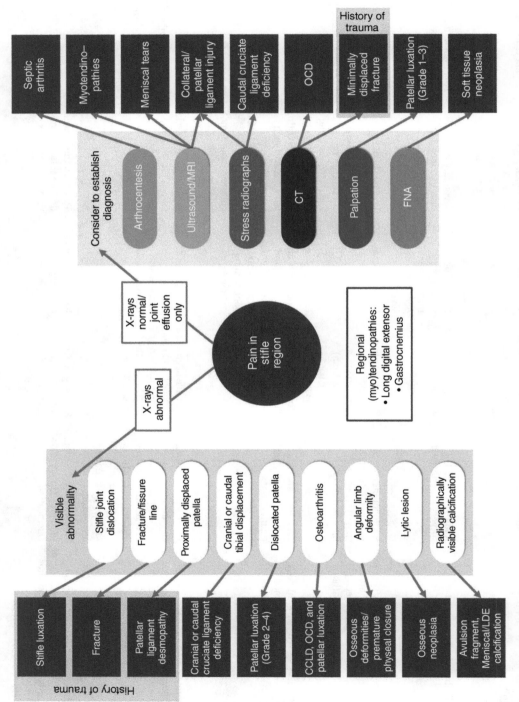

Figure 19.1 Schematic of common diseases affecting the stifle region and the steps necessary to establish a diagnosis.

The *joint capsule* volume is large, extending proximally under the quadriceps femoris by approximately one patella's length, laterally and medially to the margin of the femoral epicondyles, caudally to the femoral articulation of the fabellae, and distally following the course of the long digital extensor (LDE) tendon. There is a small joint sub-pouch extending around the tibial condyle and fibular head, as well as the axial surface of the origin of the popliteus. The infrapatellar fat pad is located just caudal to the patellar ligament but is extracapsular (i.e. located extra-articular). This becomes important when evaluating lateral view radiographs of the stifle joint to diagnose effusion of the joint. Understanding the location and volume of the stifle joint space also allows multiple entry points for therapeutic joint injections and arthrocentesis and also prevents accidental injections into the infrapatellar fat pad.

The cruciate ligaments of the stifle joint are located intracapsular but are covered by a thin synovial layer. The *cranial cruciate ligament* originates from the caudomedial aspect of the lateral femoral condyle (i.e. intra-articularly from the caudal aspect of the lateral femoral condyle) and courses diagonally, cranially, and medially to insert around the cranial intercondyloid area of the tibial plateau. The CCL serves to limit craniocaudal translation, hyperextension, as well as excessive internal rotation. The canine stifle joint is highly dependent on the CCL for stability during standing as well as the stance phase of weight-bearing; loss of this ligament causes profound instability of the stifle joint (Korvick et al. 1994). The CCL has two functional bands: the craniomedial band and the caudolateral band (named based on their tibial attachment sites). The craniomedial band is taut in extension and flexion, and the caudolateral band is taut in extension, but loose in flexion. This is important to keep in mind when palpating for pathology that exclusively affects the craniomedial band, as it may be difficult to detect instability unless the stifle is placed in flexion.

The *caudal cruciate ligament* (CaCL) originates from the craniolateral aspect of the medial femoral condyle (i.e. intra-articular from the cranial aspect of the medial femoral condyle), courses caudodistally, and inserts on the caudal tibia (lateral edge of the popliteal notch). Its principle function is to prevent caudal displacement of the tibia relative to the femur. It is larger than the CCL and, as the name implies, crosses the CCL.

There are two intra-articular tendons in the stifle joint. The *tendon of the long digital extensor* muscle originates in the extensor fossa of the femur and courses through the muscular groove of the tibial plateau located just cranial to the lateral tibial condyle. Its origin on the proximal femoral condyle can be confused for a stifle OCD lesion (Figure 19.2); this can be distinguished by the proximal location away from the joint surface, as well as by the small semilunar shape of the extensor fossa. The *popliteal tendon* is located in the caudal aspect of the joint, runs caudolaterally and serves to limit external rotation of the stifle in flexion, and has a small attachment to the fibula (Griffith et al. 2007).

The *collateral ligaments* serve to prevent varus/valgus joint instability, in addition to limiting rotational instability. They are principally taut and especially important to joint stability when the stifle is in extension. With increasing flexion of the stifle, the collateral ligaments, especially the lateral collateral ligament (LCL), become more lax, and the CCL and CaCL take on additional varus/valgus stabilization role (Vasseur and Arnoczky 1981).

The *menisci* (lateral and medial meniscus of the stifle joint) are concave, are semilunar-shaped fibrocartilages, are wedge-shaped in cross section, and have a thin synovial intimal covering. These meniscal fibrocartilages provide the majority of the weight-bearing surface of the stifle joint between the incongruent, unstable, convex surface of the femoral and tibial condyles, making them a crucial component of stifle joint stability. In the body of the meniscus, collagen bundles are arranged in a circumferential orientation and bound by perpendicularly oriented radial fibers, an arrangement that allows to mitigate compressive weight-bearing forces (Fithian et al. 1990). The

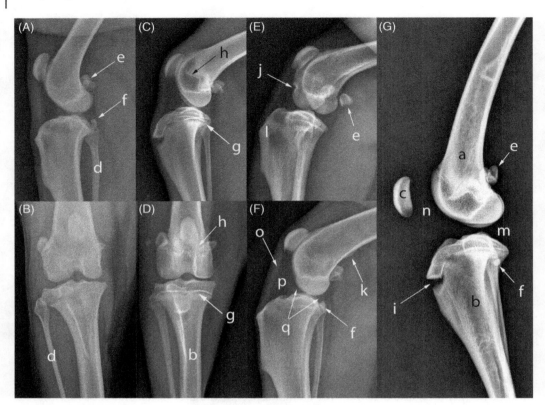

Figure 19.2 Normal radiographic anatomy of the stifle joint (Note: for images B, D lateral is on the left): (A, B, E, F) lateral and craniocaudal views of the stifle of adult dogs; (C, D, G) lateral and craniocaudal views of the stifle of immature dogs; (a) femur; (b) tibia; (c) patella; (d) fibula; (e) fabella(e), i.e. lateral/medial gastrocnemius sesamoid bone; (f) popliteal sesamoid bone; (g) proximal tibial physis; (h) distal femur physis; (i) apophysis of tibial tuberosity; (j) extensor fossa, i.e. fossa of origin of the long digital extensor tendon; (k) medial and lateral supracondylar tuberosities (i.e. origin of the gastrocnemius muscle) and superficial digital flexor (lateral tuberosity); (l) tibial tuberosity; (m) femorotibial joint; (n) femoropatellar joint; (o) patellar ligament; (p) infrapatellar fat pad; and (q) cranial and caudal horn of the menisci/joint fluid.

meniscal horns and attachments are nerve and blood vessel rich and, therefore, have important sensory functions (O'Connor and Mcconnaughey 1978). Regionally, an individual meniscus consists of a body and a cranial and caudal horn. The cranial and caudal horns of the medial meniscus are attached to the tibial plateau via meniscotibial ligaments, which hold the meniscus in place while weight-bearing (Pagnani et al. 1991). The transverse (formerly described as intermeniscal) ligament connects the cranial menisco-tibial ligaments of the two menisci. The menisci are quite mobile through range of motion (ROM) and move to match the position of the femur and tibia through ROM (Park et al. 2018). However, there are two important differences between the attachments of the medial and the lateral meniscus. The body of the medial meniscus has a close association with the medial collateral ligament (MCL) and joint capsule, which tethers it more firmly to the tibia. The lateral meniscus, on the other hand, has a strong association with the femoral condyle via the menisco-femoral ligament that anchors the caudal meniscal horn to the femur (rather than the tibia since the caudal menisco-tibial ligament of the lateral meniscus is infinitesimal). This association allows the lateral meniscus to move with the femur, rather than being tethered to the tibia, which is the main reason why the medial meniscus is injured more frequently than the lateral meniscus when CCL deficiency is present.

The *patella* is the articular sesamoid bone of the quadriceps complex. It is held in place by congruent positioning within the trochlear groove and by its centralized attachment of the patellar ligament on the tibial tuberosity and soft tissue support. Tension from the quadriceps group, patellofemoral ligaments, joint capsule, and the alar fibrocartilages which glide over the trochlear ridges through ROM is also a critical stabilizer of the patella. Derangement or injury of any of these structures can predispose to patellar luxation.

19.2.2 Muscles of the Stifle Joint

The primary muscle stabilizers of the stifle joint are the *quadriceps* group, which perform stifle extension, and the stifle flexors, the gastrocnemius and hamstring group (Hayes et al. 2013). The quadriceps muscle is innervated by the femoral nerve and consists of the vastus medialis, vastus intermedius, vastus lateralis, and the rectus femoris. The vastus lateralis and intermedius originate on the vastus ridge of the proximal femur, while the vastus medialis originates on the craniomedial aspect of the proximal femur on the cranial intertrochanteric crest. The rectus femoris is the only member of the group to cross the hip joint, with its origin on the tuberosity of the rectus femoris and the iliopectineal eminence located on the ilium. These four muscles form the tendon of insertion of the quadriceps muscle that includes the patella itself and the portion from the patella to the tibial tuberosity, the patellar ligament (sometimes referred to as the patellar tendon). The patellar ligament is the terminal insertion of the quadriceps mechanism and therefore contributes to stifle extension. The dynamic tension of the quadriceps muscle helps to keep the patella tracking within the trochlear groove.

The main muscles of the hamstring group are the semimembranosus, semitendinosus, and biceps femoris muscles. The *hamstrings* originate from the ischial tuberosity and are innervated by the sciatic nerve. The semitendinosus muscle branches, and part of it attaches to the proximal medial tibial fascia as well as courses distally with the tendon of the gracilis muscle as part of the common calcanean tendon. The semimembranosus inserts as a distinct but short tendon near the origin of the gastrocnemius and just beneath the MCL on the medial tibial condyle. The biceps femoris attaches via an aponeurosis of the fascia lata to the tibial tuberosity laterally, continuing distally to become a part of the common calcanean tendon. The hamstring group works reflexively via the cruciate ligament mechanoreceptors to limit cranial tibial translation, hyperextension, and excessive internal rotation, hence protecting the CCL from damage during movements of the tibia relative to the femur (Hayes et al. 2013).

The *gastrocnemius* has a medial and a lateral head, which originate from the caudal femur at the supracondylar tuberosities and attach on the tuber calcanei. Each muscle head contains a sesamoid bone (fabella) just below its origin. The gastrocnemius is innervated by the tibial branch of the sciatic nerve and its action is to flex the stifle and extend the hock. In contrast to the action of the hamstrings, the pull of the gastrocnemius works to pull the femur caudal relative to the tibia (Hayes et al. 2013).

The *long digital extensor* muscle originates intra-articularly in the extensor fossa of the lateral femoral condyle and courses through the stifle joint and into the extensor groove of the tibia. The tendon is located deep into the tibialis cranialis muscle and just cranial to a palpable prominence on the lateral aspect of the tibia, called the Tubercle of Gerdy in humans. In most dogs, this protuberance is large enough to palpate. The muscle inserts on the dorsal surface of the distal phalanx of digits II–V.

19.3 Fractures of the Stifle Region

Fractures of the stifle joint region are common and include fractures of the distal femur, proximal tibia/fibula, and patella. Mature animals most commonly sustain fractures of the diaphyseal area. These fractures are easily identified radiographically, and treatment frequently requires surgical intervention, particularly if substantial displacement is present. Fractures involving the articular surface (Figure 19.3) are rare but are likely to result in osteoarthritis. These fractures also have the potential to cause meniscal and cruciate ligament damage. As the stifle joint has a voluminous outpouching at the distal femur, even distal femur fractures have the potential to affect the stifle joint. Patellar fractures and fractures of the tibial tuberosity affect the quadriceps mechanism and may make weight-bearing impossible. Inappropriate healing (e.g. malunion) of fractures affecting the stifle region (in particular tibial tuberosity and distal femur fractures) can affect the quadriceps-patellar mechanism and thereby may result in secondary patellar luxation. This should be considered when making treatment decisions during initial presentation.

Fractures of the stifle region are frequently caused by severe trauma including vehicular collisions, gunshot, kicks, etc. Therefore, careful evaluation of the entire patient for concomitant non-orthopedic

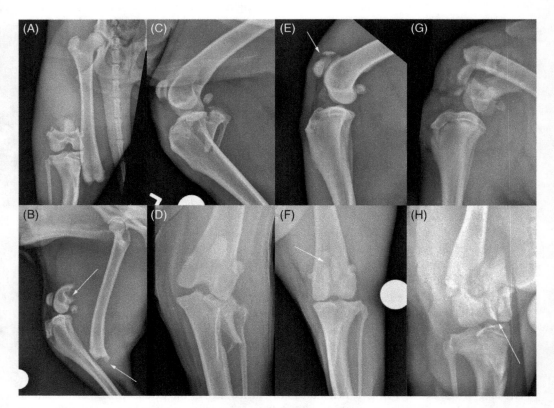

Figure 19.3 Examples of stifle region fractures in four patients. *Patient I* (A, B) severely displaced SH Type I fracture of the distal femur. Note the typical configuration of the distal femoral physis (white arrows). *Patient II* (C, D) moderately displaced articular fracture of the proximal tibia in a mature patient. These fractures are rare but require precise reconstruction since due to their disruption of the articular surface. *Patient III* (E, F) comminuted fracture of the patella (white arrows). *Patient IV* (G, H) comminuted, SH Type IV fracture of the distal femur. The white arrow indicates the articular component of the fracture, which is important to recognize per-operatively.

injuries is imperative. The patient will typically exhibit non-weight-bearing lameness, with variable amounts of swelling and crepitus around the fractured region. Examination of the area usually shows severe pain upon manipulation. Diagnosis of these fractures can generally be accomplished with orthogonal radiographs, although the diagnosis can be missed if only a single view is taken (Figure 19.4).

CT may be beneficial for complex fractures, to identify intra-articular components, bone fissures, and additional fragments that may be missed with radiographs.

19.3.1 Patellar Fractures

Traumatic patellar fractures are rarely encountered in dogs. They are the result of severe, direct trauma to the patella and can be diagnosed with standard radiography (Figure 19.3). Because of the extreme tension by the quadriceps muscle, treatment is challenging. Surgical fixation and partial patellectomy are potential treatment options. These fractures may also be associated with disruption of the patellar ligament and other soft tissue pathologies (e.g. cruciate and collateral ligaments, and menisci), which need to be carefully investigated (either at the time of surgery or

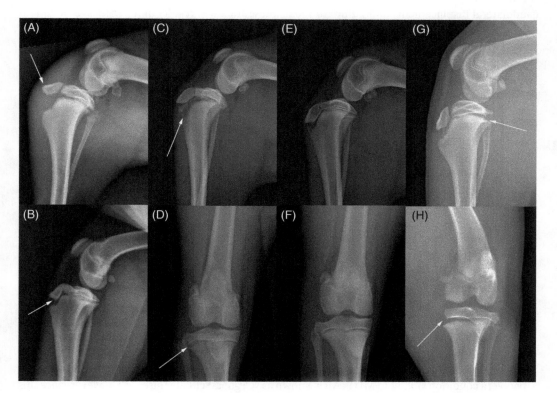

Figure 19.4 Examples of physeal fractures in four patients. *Patient I* (A) severely displaced avulsion fracture of the tibial tuberosity apophysis without disruption of the proximal tibial epiphysis. These fractures generally require surgical reconstruction. *Patient II* (B) minimally displaced tibial tuberosity avulsion fracture (MDTTAF). These patients are generally treated nonsurgically. *Patient III* (C–F) mildly displaced fracture (C, D) of the proximal tibial apophysis and epiphysis. The small fragment (white arrow image (C)) indicates that this is a Type II SH fracture. Note that the fracture is difficult to identify on the craniocaudal view. The only abnormality is a (white arrow) slight widening of the lateral aspect of the proximal tibial physis. Images (E, F) are of the normal leg and provided for comparison. *Patient IV* (G, H) mildly displaced SH Type I fracture. Note the subtle (white arrows) widening of the medial and caudal aspect of the proximal tibial physis.

with diagnostic imaging). Patellar fractures have also been reported to occur in up to 2% of dogs after tibial plateau leveling osteotomy (TPLO); however, these fractures generally do not require surgical treatment (Rutherford et al. 2012).

19.3.2 Salter-Harris Fractures

Proximal tibia and distal femur fractures most frequently affect the physes and therefore are most commonly observed in immature animals. Dogs of any breed with open physes may be affected. Physes of domestic dogs are fragile and very little trauma can result in a Salter-Harris (SH) fracture. Typical causes of these fractures include collision with humans or bigger dogs during play, falls off furniture or down stairs, and jump-down injuries out of an owner's arms, out of vehicles, or other mild-to-moderate heights.

SH fractures of the proximal tibia and distal femur are most commonly Type I or II and therefore do not involve the articular surface (see Chapter 13 for description of SH fractures). The proximal tibial growth plate rarely fractures on its own and, more commonly, fractures in conjunction with the tibial apophyseal growth plate (Figure 19.4C, D). The epiphysis generally rocks back (i.e. caudolateral displacement) and failure to repair these fractures results in an excessive tibial plateau which can cause CCL strain and tearing in the long term. The distal physis of the femur consists of four pyramidal grooves and corresponding pegs that result in the classis "W-shape" seen radiographically (Figure 19.3). Similar to proximal tibial physeal fractures, the distal femoral epiphysis commonly rocks back (i.e. caudolateral displacement) but failure to repair these fractures results in excessive distal femoral procurvatum. Type III and IV fractures are rare and can be challenging to identify radiographically if displacement is minimal (Figure 19.4). Oblique radiographs in addition to flexed and extended views can be used to identify minimal displacement.

Tibial tuberosity avulsion fractures may present in various degrees of severity ranging from a severely displaced, palpable fracture with non-weight-bearing lameness to a minimally displaced fracture with only mild clinical signs. Severely displaced fractures are best treated with surgical fixation that ideally permits continued growth of the physis, if the patient has significant growth potential left. Radiographs while fully flexing the stifle can exacerbate the displacement of these fractures and aid in decision-making if displacement is minimal. It is important to note that the growth plate of the tibial tuberosity apophysis (i.e. the site of the patellar ligament attachment) closes late during development and the ossification may be irregular (von Pfeil et al. 2009). As such, interpretation of radiographic changes to the area should be made with caution. Comparison to the non-affected limb is advised before making a diagnosis. Based on these observations, a condition termed minimally displaced tibial tuberosity avulsion fractures (MDTTAF) has been described (von Pfeil et al. 2012). Dogs affected with MDTTAF show secondary remodeling of the physis with no or mild displacement of the tibial tuberosity, while the most caudoproximal aspect of the tibial tuberosity always remains attached to the proximal tibial epiphysis. Patients present with mild-moderate lameness and pain when pressure is applied to the tibial tuberosity. Nonsurgical treatment is generally successful. In people, a condition similar to MDTTAF is known as "Osgood-Schlatter disease"; however, since this condition does not involve the physis, this terminology should not be used for dogs with MDTTAF.

19.4 Cranial Cruciate Ligament Disease

CCLD is the term used to describe any disruption of the CCL. This includes rare conditions such as *avulsion fractures* and *traumatic ruptures* but generally CCLD refers to *chronic degeneration* of the ligament. The latter is by far most commonly encountered and represents one of the most frequent reasons for pelvic limb lameness in the dog. The condition has a complex multifactorial etiology that is still incompletely understood (Griffon 2010; Comerford et al. 2011). Many factors have been shown to play a role including genetics, environmental (e.g. obesity, timing of sterilization, and poor physical condition), and conformational (e.g. tibial plateau angle [TPA]). Immune-mediated disease has also been suggested as an underlying cause.

While more research is needed to understand the etiopathology of CCLD, the clinical progression is well described – degenerative CCLD results in osteoarthritis of the stifle joint, in many cases bilaterally. The progressive inflammation and degradation of intra-articular structures eventually lead to gross joint instability and patient disability. As the CCL degenerates and global joint inflammation worsens, traumatic and degenerative meniscal tears occur secondarily.

Successful treatment of degenerative CCLD has been reported with both surgical and nonsurgical strategies (Wucherer et al. 2013). However, surgical treatment has been suggested to be superior and TPLO is the preferred surgical technique (Wucherer et al. 2013; Bergh et al. 2014; Beer et al. 2018). Treatment decisions should be made on an individual basis considering owner and patient factors including the severity of clinical symptoms, age, size, systemic health, and activity level of the patient. Meniscal tears frequently lead to more severe clinical symptoms. These tears can be successfully addressed surgically with partial meniscectomy. Avulsion fractures can be treated by reattachment of the avulsed bone or with proximal tibial epiphysiodesis (Vezzoni et al. 2008). The treatment of traumatic CCLD is similar to the treatment of degenerative CCLD.

19.4.1 Signalment and History

Degenerative CCLD most frequently affects dogs of approximately 3–7 years of age (Baker and Muir 2018). Commonly affected breeds include large-breeds such as Labrador Retrievers, Pit Bulls, Rottweilers, Golden Retrievers, Chesapeake Bay Retrievers, Queensland Heelers, Akitas, Australian Shepherds, Doodles, Bernese Mountain Dogs, Boxers, German Shepherds, and giant-breed dogs, such as English Mastiffs, Newfoundlands, Landseers, Great Pyrenees, and St. Bernards (Duval et al. 1999; Witsberger et al. 2008). *Avulsion fractures* are only observed in immature animals. Since the attachment of the ligament to the bone is stronger than the immature bone in these patients, the bone rather than the ligament itself "gives." *Traumatic CCLD* is not well described in adult patients, although the authors have observed this condition in agility and other sporting dogs. This condition has to be differentiated from more severe traumatic injuries (e.g. stifle luxations) that also cause disruption of other soft tissue structures (e.g. collateral ligaments and CaCL).

Patient history varies widely, from acute onset of severe lameness to insidious progressive lameness which worsens with exercise or activity. Dogs may experience difficulty in rising or morning stiffness consistent with stifle osteoarthritis as reported by owners. In dogs with patellar luxation, CCLD may cause sudden worsening of the preexisting lameness. Waxing and waning of the lameness severity may also be reported. This can be due to an initial, partial ligament tear and hemarthrosis, with further tearing of the ligament until the entire ligament is disrupted in addition to meniscal tears later in the disease stage. The progression through the disease stages varies greatly in timeline with some dogs having an insidious, slowly worsening lameness that can progress over years. Many of these cases maintain a partially intact CCL and meniscus and symptoms are due to the osteoarthritic changes, rather than instability. A recent study showed that Boxers have higher osteoarthritis scores compared to other commonly affected breeds (Gilbert et al. 2019), indicating that they may have a longer duration of joint inflammation before presentation for diagnosis. Other dogs progress rapidly from partial tears to complete tears, at which time the lameness frequently becomes non-weight-bearing. Owners often perceive the condition as an acute, traumatic event associated with a bout of activity or event (such as a dog park collision, stepping into a hole, etc.). However, as stated above, traumatic CCLD is extremely rare; therefore, the traumatic event perceived to coincide with the onset of injury is generally minor and only able to disrupt the ligament because of previous weakening and degeneration. This is confirmed by the presence of radiographic changes that indicate chronicity observed in these cases.

19.4.2 Physical Exam

A tentative diagnosis of CCLD can be established based on the specific physical exam findings associated with the progression of CCLD outlined in Box 19.1. Although early in the disease stage only some of these features may be present (e.g. joint effusion and pain on hyperextension), with complete ruptures all features can be observed solidifying the diagnosis.

19.4.2.1 Postural and Gait Changes

Observation can be used to identify postural and gait changes associated with CCLD. Patients will show varying degrees of *lameness* resulting in the classic features associated with pelvic limb lameness (Videos 1.1. and 1.3). The lameness can be a subtle weight-bearing lameness at the trot that worsens with exercise in the case of early stable disease or partial tears. Alternatively, it can also be a severe weight-bearing lameness easily observable at the walk and trot. The lameness typically is caused by an unwillingness to completely extend the stifle, which can help differentiate it from hip, hock, or foot causes of lameness. Some dogs may avoid full ROM of the stifle by externally rotating the stifle rather than flexing it. Dogs with meniscal tears or severe instability may be completely non-weight-bearing.

Typically, patients will also *offload* the affected leg *while standing*, or offload the more acutely painful side in bilaterally affected cases. This may be more obvious to observe than lameness during motion in some cases (Video 1.1).

Lastly, several postural changes are observed with CCLD. The stifle may be kept flexed while standing or during motion (Korvick et al. 1994) in an attempt to level the angle of the tibial plateau, and the hock may be hyperextended to compensate for reduced stifle ROM and reduce the caudal pull of the gastrocnemius muscle unit, which exacerbates tibial subluxation. Dogs with cranially displaced meniscal tears may be unable to extend the stifle into a normal weight-bearing position. When sitting, dogs with CCLD will sit with the affected stifle in extension due to the discomfort

---

Box 19.1   Progressive Physical Exam Findings Indicative of CCLD

1) Postural and gait changes
   (a) Lameness and offloading of affected limb during stance
   (b) Positive "Sit-test"

2) Palpation
   (a) Stifle joint effusion
   (b) Pain on hyperextension of the stifle joint
   (c) Pain on flexion and loss of range of motion of the stifle joint
   (d) Muscle atrophy
   (e) Medial buttress
   (f) Positive cranial drawer/tibial compression test
   (g) Meniscal click

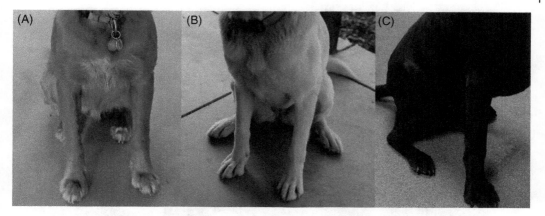

Figure 19.5   A positive "sit-test" is one of the hallmark features indicative of CCLD (A) normal patient illustrating a "square" sit with both stifles fully flexed; (B) bilaterally positive sit-test showing the limbs placed on each side of the body; (C) unilaterally positive sit-test indicative of right-sided CCLD.

associated with full flexion of the stifle. This is known as the positive "sit test." Dogs with unilateral CCLD may sit with only one stifle extended (and one stifle flexed and positioned normally under their body); whereas, dogs with bilateral disease may extend both legs. Some dogs will extend both legs by placing each leg on one side of their body, while others place the less affected limb under their body (Figure 19.5 and Video 19.1). A positive sit test is not pathognomonic for CCLD and may be observed in novrmal dogs (behavioral), or in dogs with hip or tarsal pathology.

Video 19.1

Positive "sit-test" examples in dogs with CCLD.

Bilaterally affected dogs will shift weight to the thoracic limbs by leaning forward and keeping the thoracic limbs placed more caudally under the body. These dogs may develop a bodybuilder appearance with hind end muscle atrophy and thoracic limb muscle hypertrophy. Bilateral disease severe enough to cause subluxation can result in a dog unable to get up and difficulty ambulating. This may be confused with neurologic disease. Performing a neurologic exam and looking for proprioception deficits will differentiate neurologic disease from severe bilateral CCLD.

19.4.2.2   Palpation

Degeneration of the CCL typically causes joint effusion, capsular and periarticular thickening, as well as muscle atrophy. These pathologic changes can be identified on palpation of CCL-deficient dogs. Standing behind the patient is the best way to detect asymmetries (Video 3.1). The examiner may appreciate atrophy of the quadriceps, hamstring muscle group, biceps femoris, and cranial tibialis muscle. In cases of severe stifle joint subluxation, careful palpation of the stifle may show a cranially displaced tibial tuberosity relative to the patella. Many of the palpable abnormalities can be identified in the awake patient; however, a sedated physical exam can be very helpful in testing for joint instability, particularly in large, energetic, tense, or unruly patients. The resulting

STIFLE REGION

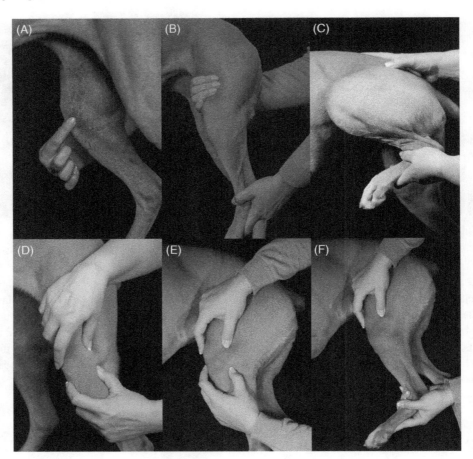

Figure 19.6   Physical examination procedures to detect CCLD include (A) palpation of joint effusion is best accomplished by palpating the indent just medial to the patellar ligament; (B) isolated hyperextension of the stifle while maintaining a standing angle of the hip and tarsus can be accomplished by reaching in between the dogs' pelvic limbs and placing the upper hand cranial to the stifle, while extending the stifle with the lower hand; (C) full stifle flexion can only be accomplished when simultaneously flexing the hip and tarsus; the cranial drawer (D, E; see also Figure 19.7) and tibial compression (F; see also Figure 19.8) tests can be performed while the patient is (D) standing or (E) in lateral recumbency.

muscle relaxation can allow for easier detection of subtle instability. Palpation of a meniscal click may also be more accurate with sedation/anesthesia (Neal et al. 2015).

Palpable *joint effusion* is a consistent hallmark of CCLD at any stage and can be detected by feeling for the medial and lateral borders of the patellar ligament. In the normal canine stifle, a divot representing the joint space can be detected medial and lateral to the patellar ligament (Figure 19.6). In the normal joint, the margins of the patellar ligament should be sharply apparent to the touch. The pad of the index finger should fit into the space located about halfway between the insertion of the patellar ligament at the tibial tuberosity (usually a distinct bony prominence) and the caudal aspect of the patella. The earliest sign of CCLD will be subtle joint effusion which is consistent with synovitis preceding ligament pathology. With joint effusion, this divot will fill in and the margins of the patellar ligament will be less distinct. Joint effusion in combination with intermittent lameness with exercise may be the only clinical signs detected in stable partial CCL tears. Initially this swelling may feel soft or water balloon-like, and over time as the disease progresses, swelling can be detected laterally and attains a harder thickening representative of joint capsule thickening.

Over time, a knob of thickened tissue can be felt on the proximal medial aspect of the medial tibial joint line, termed "medial buttress," which represents a buildup of scar tissue to counteract excessive internal tibial rotation with CCL deficiency. A challenge to the novice examiner is detection of CCL disease when present bilaterally, as the joint effusion and medial buttress can be fairly symmetrical.

Pain or resistance to stifle ROM is a hallmark sign of the painful inflammation accompanying CCL disease. Early on in the disease, pain on *stifle hyperextension* may be elicited, even when instability tests are negative. This is because the CCL counteracts hyperextension of the joint. Stifle hyperextension needs to be tested without hyperextension of other joints (e.g. hip/tarsus) and should therefore be performed with the hip and tarsus in a standing angle. The examiner can reach in between the back legs to place one hand cranially to the stifle while using the other hand to hyperextend the joint (Figure 19.6). As osteoarthritis and instability progress, the joint capsule thickening and joint effusion can make full stifle flexion physically impossible and quite uncomfortable.

In particular, patients with medial *meniscal tears* may have marked pain on flexion and in some cases, upon internal rotation of the stifle, in fact dogs with pain specifically of stifle flexion are 4.3 times more likely to have medial meniscal disease (Dillon et al. 2014). Meniscal tears most frequently involve the caudal aspect of the medial meniscus with various types of tears having been described (Kowaleski et al. 2018). Cranially displaced vertical ("bucket handle") or flap meniscal tears may make full stifle extension physically impossible. An additional finding on physical exam that supports the presence of a meniscal tear is a "meniscal click" – the popping or clunking sound emanating from torn or displaced meniscal tissue as the femur subluxates over the caudal medial meniscal horn, snapping into a subluxated position (Video 19.2). The sound can also emanate from a vertical longitudinal or flap meniscal tear as it displaces and reduces through ROM. When present, a meniscal click has been reported to be 75–96% specific for actual meniscal damage (McCready and Ness 2016). When combined with observation of pain on stifle flexion, the diagnostic accuracy (i.e. correctly identifying the presence or absence of a disease) of detecting a meniscal click is around 75% (Dillon et al. 2014; Neal et al. 2015). In other words, lack of a meniscal click does not mean that meniscal injury is not present, and surgical examination, ultrasound, CT, or MRI are necessary to definitively diagnose meniscal pathology. However, when a meniscal click and pain on stifle flexion are observed, there is high likelihood that meniscal damage is present. Performing ROM while placing the stifle in a stressed position (i.e. flexing the joint while performing tibial compression) can make it easier to detect a meniscal click in some patients. This test has been described as the "modified tibial compression test" and was associated with a sensitivity of up to 63% and specificity of up to 77% for detection of meniscal tears (Valen et al. 2017).

Video 19.2

Anatomy of meniscal tears.

Once osteoarthritis has developed, an additional noise that may be encountered during stifle ROM is *crepitus*. Caused by the rubbing of the joint capsule on periarticular osteophytes, crepitus has a higher pitched, light crackling sensation, that can be audible as well as palpable. Unlike a meniscal click which occurs only once during ROM, crepitus is most easily detected in the parapatellar region around the trochlear ridges and is observable throughout the whole ROM of the stifle joint.

The *cranial drawer* test elicits abnormal sagittal plane instability associated with CCLD and is highly specific for rupture of the CCL, with a sensitivity of 86% and specificity of 98% (De Rooster and Van Bree 1999c). The test can be performed with the patient standing or laying down. Particularly larger dogs that are off-weighting the limb at a stance generally allow palpation while standing. However, some dogs become tense, making it more difficult to assess for instability. To perform the test, the examiner stabilizes the distal femur with one hand by placing the tip of the index finger on the patella and the thumb on the lateral fabella. With the opposite hand, the proximal tibia is grasped with the thumb placed in the region of the fibular head and the tip of the index finger on the tibial tuberosity. The lower hand is used to first push the tibia caudally (to reduce any present cranial tibial subluxation); the thumb is then used to gently push the proximal tibia cranially (Figure 19.7). The lower hand also controls the angle of the tibia relative to the femur. Ideally the trajectory of the movement of the tibia relative to the femur is parallel to the slope of the tibial plateau, to maximize the drawer motion with minimal force or effort. If radiographs are unavailable (to estimate the tibial slope), the examiner can repeat the drawer test in flexion, increasing the angle of extension in 20° increments to find the position of maximal instability and elicit a positive test. The drawer test should always be performed in both flexion and mild extension. *Note that the collateral*

(A)   (B)

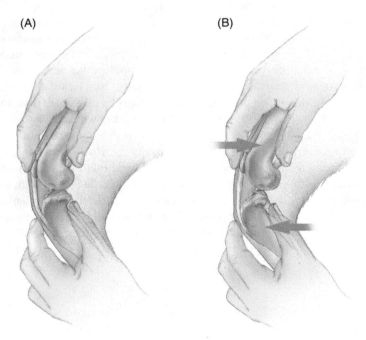

Figure 19.7   The cranial drawer test is performed by (A) placing the index finger on the patella and the thumb on the lateral fabella, with the opposite hand, the proximal tibia is grasped with the thumb placed caudal to the fibular head and the tip of the index finger on the tibial tuberosity. The lower hand is then used to (B) gently push the proximal tibia cranially, which indicates CCLD deficiency.

ligaments are taut during full extension, providing some additional stifle stability, which mini-
mizes the potential cranial drawer movement that can be elicited. Drawer testing should be performed in flexion, because if only the craniomedial band is torn, drawer will be absent in
extension but present in flexion (since the caudolateral band is lax in flexion). When performing cranial drawer testing in a CCL-deficient stifle, the tibia will translate cranially relative to
the distal femur with a subjectively loose/sloppy end-feel (i.e. capsular end-feel) when maximum, cranial tibial displacement is reached. This is in contrast to puppies that frequently
display cranial drawer movement with a hard stop (distinct end-feel) once the maximum, cranial displacement is reached (i.e. the intact CCL is engaged). This so-called "puppy drawer"
(Video 19.3) is normal and a similar finding can be observed in dogs with severe muscle atrophy. Dogs with tense pelvic limb muscles or chronic joint fibrosis on the other hand may have
diminished cranial drawer sign. The best way for the novice examiner to learn how to perform
the cranial drawer test is to learn on a dog under sedation. Technical pitfalls of this test include
eliciting normal tibial internal rotation and interpreting this as positive drawer.

Video 19.3

Puppy drawer.

The *cranial tibial compression* (or thrust) test is another test for detecting CCL tears. The test
mimics the craniocaudal instability which occurs during weight-bearing. This test is subjectively
easier to perform on awake, energetic, or tense dogs than the cranial drawer test. However, the
tibial compression test can be difficult to interpret for the novice examiner. This test can also be
done with the patient standing or recumbent. The limb is placed with the hock in a standing position and the stifle fully extended. One hand is placed over the cranial distal thigh with firm pressure to keep the knee in full extension. The index finger of this hand is placed on the tibial tuberosity
to palpate for abnormal movement and to allow replacing the tibia in a caudal position (in case any
tibial subluxation is present). The other hand is used to flex the hock only, while the stifle is maintained in extension (Figure 19.8). In a normal stifle, no movement should be observed; in a stifle
that is CCL deficient, the tibial tuberosity will displace cranially. With a partial tear, this movement
may only consist of a few millimeters, which can be easily missed by the untrained or inexperi-
enced examiner. Visualizing the movement can be difficult in obese, or dogs with long coats, which
is why simultaneous palpation of tibial movement should be performed with the index finger. In
dogs with complete tears, the movement may be as obvious as a complete buckling of the stifle and
gross cranial movement of the tibial tuberosity. Performing this test while the dog is sedated is very
helpful for learning, especially for visualizing subtle thrust in partial CCL tears. A technical pitfall
of the technique is failure to keep firm enough pressure on the femur, which simply results in stifle
flexion and is not a true positive tibial compression test.

In a minority of patients, particularly those that have more acute (i.e. lacking chronic fibrous
tissue that provides some stability) CCLD, a very obvious positive tibial compression test can be
observed when the tibia is rotated internally. This finding has been termed "pivot shift" and is
defined as abrupt, cranial tibial displacement of the joint when the tibia is internally rotated (Video
19.4). While this condition has been described as a "jerking lateral movement of the stifle" while
weight-bearing (Gatineau et al. 2011; Knight et al. 2017), pivot shift can also be detected during

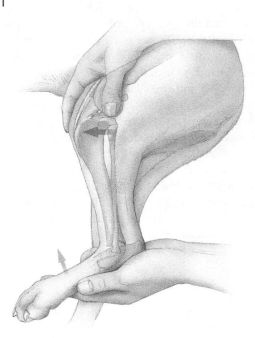

Figure 19.8   The cranial tibial compression test is performed by placing one hand over the cranial distal thigh with the index finger placed on the tibial tuberosity. The other hand is used to flex the tarsus, while the upper hand maintains the knee in extension (i.e. not allowing any flexion of the joint). Cranial tibial movement indicates CCLD deficiency and may be observed or detected with the index finger on the tibial tuberosity.

palpation. This is accomplished by internal rotation of the lower limb while performing the tibial compression test. This test can be performed before surgery to determine appropriate treatment strategies and after TPLO surgery, since pivot shift after this procedure may cause residual lameness. A significant additional rotational instability may require therapeutic intervention (Knight et al. 2017), most commonly with an anti-rotational suture. This rotation may be significant enough to also induce a low-grade medial patellar luxation (MPL) in predisposed patients.

Video 19.4

Pivot shift.

19.4.3   Diagnostics

While exam findings (such as positive cranial drawer) have shown a high specificity to detect CCLD, they are not pathognomonic for CCLD. Rare differential diagnoses (e.g. neoplasia such as synovial cell sarcoma and osteosarcoma, immune-mediated arthritis) need to be considered when establishing the diagnosis. Additional diagnostics, most often radiographs, are generally performed to rule out these differential diagnoses and to further confirm the tentative diagnosis. Surgical inspection (either via arthroscopy or arthrotomy) is most commonly used to confirm the diagnosis and further characterize the sequelae of osteoarthritis and meniscal degeneration seen with this disease. In case surgery is not performed, ultrasound or MRI can also be used to confirm the diagnosis and to evaluate the meniscal status.

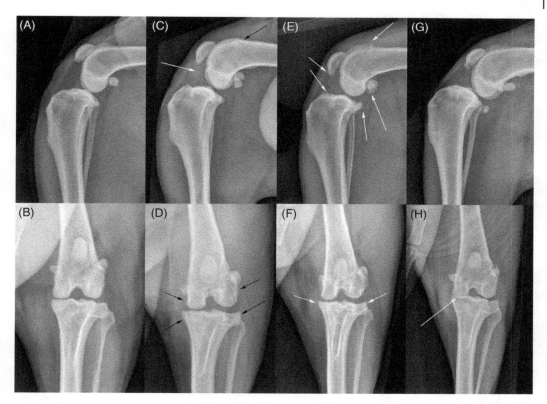

Figure 19.9   Cranial cruciate ligament disease (C–H) and normal radiographs for comparison (A, B): radiographic changes consistent with (C, D) early CCLD include (white arrow) joint effusion and (black arrows) early degenerative changes; (E, F) chronic CCLD include more (white arrows) advanced degenerative changes; (G, H) patient with complete rupture of the CCL resulting in cranial tibial subluxation. Note that although the craniocaudal view is frequently misinterpreted to show (white arrow) significant joint collapse, this is due to the subluxation and radiographic beam positioning, and not a true finding.

Stifle *radiographs* are helpful to assess the osseous anatomy, rule out other pathology, and evaluate for key features associated with CCLD (Figure 19.9). Specific radiographic views ("TPLO-views"; a craniocaudal view of the stifle including the entire tibia and hock joint, as well as a 90–90 flexed lateral view) are frequently performed if treatment with TPLO is considered as a treatment option. This radiographic technique allows to measure the TPA required for surgical planning (Figure 19.10). The degree of tibial sloping (i.e. TPA) may influence treatment decision-making. Classic radiographic features of CCLD include joint effusion and osteoarthritic changes. *Joint effusion* is easily identified with radiography because of the infrapatellar fat pad – effusion causes cranial displacement of the fat pad and caudal displacement of the gastrocnemius fascia (Figure 19.11). In the normal stifle, the cranial and caudal horns of the menisci can be seen as a small triangular radiopaque density, located cranially and caudally between the femur and tibial condyles (Figure 19.2). This should not be confused with early subtle joint effusion. *Osteophytes* form at the junction of synovium and articular cartilage and are most commonly seen at the pro distal pole of the patella, the joint capsule attachment on the femoral epicondyles, fabello-femoral articulation, origin of the LDE tendon on the femur, the extensor groove on the tibia, suprapatellar pouch, and the tibial condyles. In later stages of osteoarthritis, bone sclerosis can be seen in

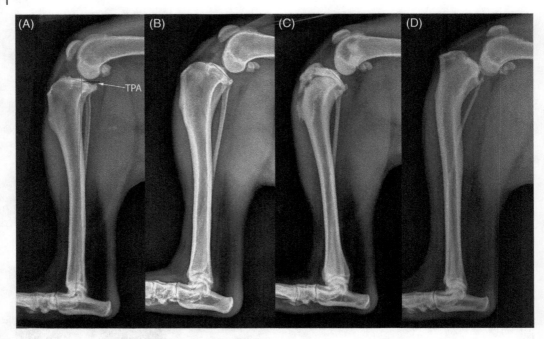

Figure 19.10 TPLO views of patients with varying degrees of tibial sloping: (A) red dots indicate landmarks for measurement of identification of the tibial slope (red line; i.e. the cranial and caudal articular margins of the tibial plateau); blue dots indicate landmarks for identification of the tibial axis (blue line; i.e. from the center of the talus to the intercondylar eminence); the tibial plateau angle (TPA) is defined as the angle formed by a line perpendicular to the tibial axis and the tibial plateau, in this case the TPA = 18°; (B) TPA = 33°; (C) this dog suffered from a proximal tibial SH fracture that resulted in caudal displacement of the proximal fragment resulting in a TPA = 43°, which is considered an "excessive TPA" requiring more careful surgical planning; (D) TPA = 62°, this patient is also displaying caudal bowing of the proximal tibia.

the subchondral bone plate of the femur and tibial condyles. Radiographic osteoarthritis has been shown to correlate with the degree of CrCL damage (Sample et al. 2017). If *cranial tibial displacement* (also described as caudal femoral displacement by some authors; Rey et al. 2014) is evident, disruption of the CCL can be confirmed radiographically. Several methods to objectively identify displacement have been described (Plesman et al. 2012; Fujita et al. 2017). Two simple methods that do not require any measurements include the evaluation of the intercondylar eminence in relationship to the femoral condyles and the caudal aspect of the femur in relationship to the caudal aspect of the tibia (Figure 19.12). In juvenile dogs, avulsion fractures may be visible (Figure 19.13). *Displacement of the popliteal sesamoid* is a less commonly observed (Figure 19.13), yet highly specific feature for diagnosis of CCLD with a reported accuracy of 99 and 100% specificity (De Rooster and Van Bree 1999a).

It should be noted that pathologic changes to the CCL and menisci will not necessarily induce radiographically visible laxity of stifle joints in dogs (De Rooster and Van Bree 1999b). For dogs with partial CCL tears, there may be minimal or no radiographic evidence of subluxation, but the radiographic signs of osteoarthritis will help add evidence towards a clinical diagnosis. While stress radiographs have been reported to have a 97% sensitivity and 100% specificity for CCL tears when subluxation is present (De Rooster and Van Bree 1999c), they are rarely necessary to diagnose

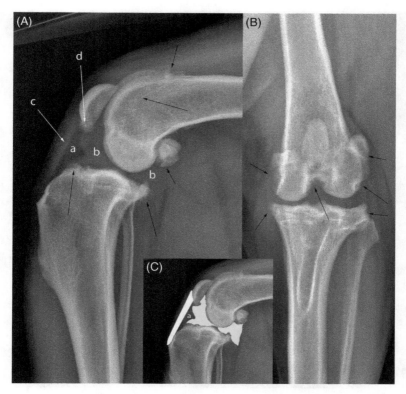

Figure 19.11 Frequent locations of (black arrows) degenerative changes associated with CCLD (A, B): (a) infrapatellar fat pad; (b) joint effusion – outlined in image (C) in yellow; (c) patellar ligament – outlined in image (C) in white; (d) degenerative changes at the distal tip of the patella.

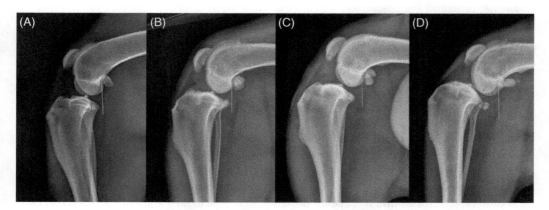

Figure 19.12 Cranial tibial displacement associated with CCLD (B–D) and normal radiographs for comparison: (A) the (green asterisk) intercondylar eminence is located in close proximity to the (red asterisk) center of the femoral condyles and a vertical line drawn tangential to the caudal aspect of the femoral condyles falls within close proximity of the proximal tibial margin (Note that the radiographic position will affect this measurement); (B) with mild and (C) moderate displacement, the distance between the intercondylar eminence and center of the femoral condyles increases; (D) with severe displacement, the line drawn from the condyles is distant from the proximal tibial margin.

STIFLE REGION

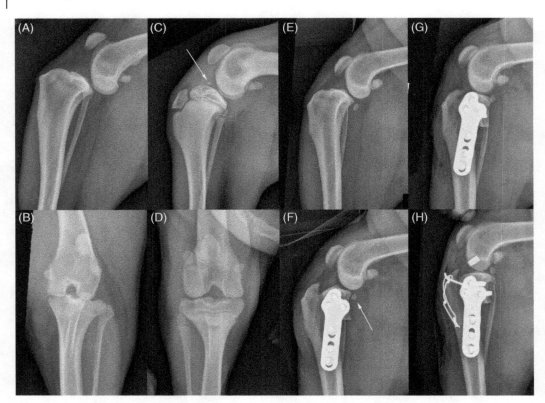

Figure 19.13   Examples of uncommon presentations of CCL disruption in three patients. *Patient I* (A, B) severe cranial tibial displacement in a dog with acute, traumatic rupture of the CCL. Note that the severe displacements make it difficult to evaluate the craniocaudal radiographs and give the (false) impression of a collateral ligament rupture. *Patient II* (C, D) avulsion fracture (white arrow) of the CCL in an immature patient. *Patient III* (E–H) this patient was diagnosed with a (E) complete rupture of the CCL and (F) TPLO surgery was performed. Postoperatively the tibia remained in cranial tibial displacement and "pivot shift" was present. When externally rotated, the tibia (G) reduced into a normal position. Application of an (H) anti-rotational suture was performed to eliminate internal rotation. Note the varying location of the (white arrow) popliteal sesamoid with subluxation and reduction of the tibia as a feature indicating appropriate position when located in a (G, H) normal position.

CCLD. These radiographs are performed by mimicking the cranial tibial compression test while taking the X-ray (De Rooster and Van Bree 1999c). This radiographic technique can also be utilized to demonstrate pivot shift instability after surgery (Figure 19.13).

Advanced imaging is rarely required to establish a diagnosis of CCLD. However, as outlined above, a definitive diagnosis of meniscal injury cannot be established based on physical exam and radiography. Ultrasound has been reported to diagnose meniscal tears with a correct classification rate of 84%, sensitivity of 86%, and specificity of 78%, while MRI has a correct classification rate of 77%, with a sensitivity of 68% and specificity 100% (Franklin et al. 2017). CT, with and without intra-articular contrast application (i.e. CT-arthrography), and ultrasound have also been reported for evaluation of the meniscus and parts of the CCL (Van Der Vekens et al. 2019).

19.5   Patellar Luxation

The patella is the largest sesamoid bone in the canine body. Its function is to redirect the forces of the quadriceps muscle during stifle ROM (i.e. to allow the quadriceps to act as the major stifle extensor). Patellar luxation is defined as dislocation of the patella outside (medial or lateral) of the trochlear groove. Contraction of the quadriceps muscle results in pulling the patella onto a straight line from the origin (proximal femur and ventral ilium for the rectus femoris muscle) to the insertion (tibial tuberosity) of the quadriceps muscle. As such, the location of the origin and insertion of this muscle determines whether the patella luxates.

Patellar luxation is one of the most commonly encountered orthopedic disease in dogs. It may be of congenital origin (i.e. present at birth) but in most cases, it is a developmental disease (i.e. develops after birth) that has frequently been described as having a congenital etiology because it is thought that abnormal skeletal development (with an underlying congenital etiology) results in dislocation of the patella during development. Although several hypotheses have been suggested (and been partially refuted), the etiology of patellar luxation remains somewhat unclear (Kowaleski et al. 2018). A prominent explanation is that MPL originates from primary hip skeletal abnormalities, including coxa vara (decreased femoral neck inclination) and relative retroversion of the femoral neck (i.e. a decreased anteversion angle). The resultant genu varus (i.e. bow-legged deformity, where the knees are too far apart while the hocks are too close together) may be accompanied by femoral deformities including distal external femoral torsion and femoral varus, hypoplastic or absent medial trochlear ridges, and a hypoplastic trochlear sulcus. Displacement of the patella medially draws the tibial apophysis medially, resulting in medial rotation of the entire joint, medial torsion of the proximal tibia, and medialization of the tibial apophysis. In the severest cases, the articular surfaces of the femoral and tibial condyles may be deformed and hypoplastic medially. The quadriceps muscle's resting tension causes it to follow the shortest possible path along the thigh, whereby acting like a bow string, it pulls the patella further out of the trochlear groove, exacerbating skeletal abnormalities in the growing dog. The joint capsule becomes adhered and contracted medially and stretched laterally, adding an overarching internal rotation of the entire stifle joint. Dogs with MPL may have a patella that rides proximally in the trochlear groove, termed "patella alta" (Mostafa et al. 2008).

Lateral patellar luxation (LPL) is associated with an opposing suite of skeletal abnormalities, including coxa valga, genu valgus (i.e. knock-knee deformity, where the knees are too close together while the hocks are too far apart), femoral valgus, an undersized lateral trochlear ridge, a laterally rotated joint, lateral tibial tuberosity torsion, lateral bowing of the proximal tibia, and medial torsion of the distal tibia. Dogs with LPL may have a patella that rides distally in the trochlear groove, termed "patella baja" (Mostafa et al. 2008).

Patellar luxation may occur concomitantly with CCLD in up to 25% of dogs with MPL (Campbell et al. 2010). It is of great importance to determine whether the CCL is also affected since dogs with the combination of CCLD and patellar luxation generally respond less favorably to nonsurgical treatment. The determination of patella alta or baja and the degree of skeletal deformities are particularly important to decide if surgical treatment should be considered. Various treatment options, including surgical and nonsurgical treatment options have been described (Di Dona et al. 2018). Most commonly employed surgical treatments include soft tissue reconstruction (e.g. release of the retinaculum on the side of luxation and imbrication of the opposing side), tibial tuberosity transposition (to realign the extensor mechanism), trochleoplasty (deepening of the trochlear groove), and corrective osteotomy of the distal femur (to correct underlying femoral varus or valgus for MPL or LPL, respectively). The decision on whether or not to pursue surgery is made on a case-by-case basis taking into consideration the age, breed, and clinical symptoms of the patient, the severity of luxation, as well as owner expectations. In general, lower-grade luxations in small-breed dogs are often treated nonsurgically, while large-breed dogs more frequently require surgical corrections including corrective osteotomies.

19.5.1 Signalment and History

Since patellar luxation is a developmental disease, the majority of dogs are diagnosed by 3 years of age. Neutered dogs are predisposed and by far the majority of patellar luxations are diagnosed in small-breed dogs (O'Neill et al. 2016). While previously thought that MPL is seen predominantly in small-breeds and LPL in large-breeds, this has been shown to be incorrect – medial luxation is by far the most common type of luxation, in both small- and large-breed dogs (Bosio et al. 2017). However, LPL is by far more common in large-breed dogs (Kalff et al. 2014; Di Dona et al. 2018) and rarely seen in small-breed dogs. MPL is commonly seen in toy and small-breed dogs such as Pomeranian and Yorkshire Terrier (O'Neill et al. 2016). Large-breed dogs commonly affected include Labrador and Golden Retrievers, Pit Bulls, Huskies, and Bull Dogs.

Dogs affected with patellar luxation may present with varying degrees of clinical symptoms ranging from nonclinical, to the typical symptoms of "skipping" pelvic limb lameness, to severe skeletal deformities and abnormal posture (Video 19.5). The symptoms depend on the severity of the deformities and degree of patellar luxation. Dogs with high-grade (Box 19.2) luxations are more likely to have angular limb deformities (ALDs), severe gait abnormalities, and postural disabilities. These severe abnormalities generally become apparent early in puppyhood. Dogs with Grade 2 luxations will show an intermittent non-weight-bearing lameness when the patella luxates and therefore are more likely to be presented to the veterinarian then dogs with Grade 3 luxations. The latter show a more consistent lameness that, particularly if bilaterally present, may not be recognized as an abnormality by owners. Dogs with Grade 1 luxations will generally not show any clinical signs. Similarly, they may present as puppies (when deformities are severe) or the diagnosis may be an incidental finding during routine examination.

Video 19.5

Patellar luxation gait.

Traumatic patellar luxation is poorly described in the veterinary literature. This condition is generally described as traumatic rupture of the retinaculum without any skeletal deformities. Onset of lameness is acute and moderate-severe pain is associated with the inciting cause.

19.5.2 Physical Exam

Patellar luxation is generally diagnosed based on physical exam findings and the degree of deformity is evaluated radiographically. The disease may affect both limbs, requiring careful examination of both stifles. However, most often one side is more severely affected clinically.

> **Box 19.2   Grading of Patellar Luxation**
>
> Grading of patellar luxation based on location of the patella with typical clinical symptoms and degree of skeletal deformities (*italicized*) known to occur:
>
> **Grade 1:** "In-In" (i.e. the patella is always located in the trochlear groove unless manually forced and held outside the groove):
>
> - Patella does not spontaneously luxate, but it can be manually luxated, however, it returns into the groove upon release of pressure
> - *No clinical symptoms and no skeletal deformities*
>
> **Grade 2:** "In-Out" (i.e. the patella is typically located in the trochlear groove but remains outside the groove at times even without manipulation):
>
> - Patella spontaneously luxates and reduces (*which causes the typical "skipping" pelvic limb lameness*)
> - Patella will readily luxate with manual pressure, but reduces on its own (i.e. returns back into the trochlear groove)
> - *Only mild skeletal deformities that may not be readily visible*
>
> **Grade 3:** "Out-In" (i.e. the patella is typically located outside of the trochlear groove but can be manually reduced back into the trochlear groove):
>
> - Patella is most often in a luxated position (*which causes more consistent low-grade lameness, but rare "skipping" pelvic limb lameness may be observed*)
> - Patella can be reduced with manual pressure, but it will reluxate spontaneously upon release of manual pressure
> - *Moderate skeletal deformities that may result in abnormal posture*
>
> **Grade 4:** "Out-Out" (i.e. the patella is always located outside of the trochlear groove and cannot be manually reduced):
>
> - Patella is always luxated (*which causes a consistent lameness of varying severity*)
> - *Severe, obvious skeletal deformities resulting in abnormal posture*

As noted above, the degree of lameness can vary but skipping pelvic limb lameness raises suspicion of a Grade 2 patellar luxation. There are other differential diagnoses for skipping pelvic limb lameness including luxation of the LDE tendon, superficial digital flexor, neurologic disease (e.g. lateralized disc), and "Happy Jack Skip." Patient conformation can indicate a propensity for patellar luxation. Dogs with genu varus may be more likely to have MPL; whereas, dogs with genu valgus may be more likely to have LPL.

Patellar luxation is graded 1–4 based on physical exam findings (Box 19.2). This categorization is important as it aids decision-making regarding the course of treatment and the need for surgical intervention. Some authors have also included the degree of skeletal deformities into this grading system (Kowaleski et al. 2018); however, this system is more difficult to apply if the degree of deformity does not match the palpation. Therefore, the grading should be primarily based on the location and ability to reduce the patella. However, higher-grade luxations are generally associated with more severe skeletal deformities, more severe clinical symptoms, and more obvious postural abnormalities. To assess the patella for luxation, the patella needs to be identified and the stifle should be moved through ROM. The direction of location should be noted, realizing that bidirectional luxation is possible. In normal dogs, identification of the patella is straight-forward, but in cases with substantial periarticular swelling or high-grade luxations it can be difficult. In these cases, the examiner should identify the tibial tuberosity and follow the patellar ligament proximally.

Some dogs will spontaneously luxate the patella as the stifle flexes and the quadriceps pulls the patella out of the trochlear groove. Luxation is generally associated with a popping sensation particularly in low-grade luxations. If the patella does not spontaneously luxate, the examiner must check to see if it can be manually luxated. Since dogs with MPL tend to have patella alta, the patella may luxate more easily when the stifle is in full extension (Mostafa et al. 2008). To luxate the patella medially, the examiner extends the stifle, rotates the distal limb internally, and pushes the patella medially. It is generally easiest to place the patella between the thumb and index finger of one hand while using the other hand to manipulate the distal limb. The opposite is performed for lateral luxation – partial flexion of the stifle, external rotation of the distal limb, and pushing the patella laterally. Applying pressure through ROM should be performed if the diagnosis is not obvious. Most animals will display patellar luxation in both standing and recumbent positions; however, in some patients, the muscle tension will mask a patellar luxation when standing. Therefore, evaluation should be performed in both positions if there is doubt about the diagnosis. Similarly, very tense animals may need to be sedated to diagnose mild patellar luxation. Placing the sedated dog in lateral recumbency with the affected leg down and "pulling" the patella medially can also be helpful for diagnosis. Depending on the degree and direction of dynamic patellar instability, removing the tension of the quadriceps may make patellar luxation easier, or more difficult. Therefore, in some animals, sedation or general anesthesia may make it actually more difficult to palpate the luxation. As noted above, the patella should be reduced (if possible) and the stifle evaluated for signs of CCLD (including drawer sign). In dogs with Grade 4 luxation, it can be difficult to differentiate whether mild drawer instability results from the abnormal anatomy or from CCLD.

19.5.3 Diagnostics

Radiographs are critical for surgical planning but are also helpful to document osseous anatomy, document secondary osteoarthritis, and evaluate for concomitant CCLD. However, they cannot be used to rule out patellar luxation since with Grade 2 and 3 luxations the patella may temporarily be located within the trochlear groove. In this capacity, radiographs can only be used to determine that a patient does not have radiographic evidence of patellar luxation (i.e. "not a Grade 4") or that there is radiographic evidence of patellar luxation (i.e. "not a Grade 1").

Standard *orthogonal radiographs* of the stifle should be obtained. The craniocaudal views are used to evaluate the position of the patella. A lateral, flexed radiograph is used to assess for evidence of joint effusion and degenerative changes. While both features are observed with patellar luxation, they are generally mild and substantial changes indicate CCLD (Figure 19.14). The lateral view can also be used to evaluate for patella alta or baja. This is accomplished by measuring the patellar length ("PL") and the distance from the distal apex of the patella to the tibial tuberosity (i.e. the length of the patellar ligament, "PLL"). Ratios of the PLL:PL that are greater than 2.06 indicate patella alta (Mostafa et al. 2008), predisposing the patient to MPL. Similarly, values lesser than 1.97 indicated patella baja, predisposing the patient to LPL.

If surgical correction is deliberated, particularly in large-breed dogs, additional radiographs of the femur should be considered. Craniocaudal radiographs of the femur should be performed to assess whether the degree of femoral varus (for MPL) or valgus (for LPL) requires surgical

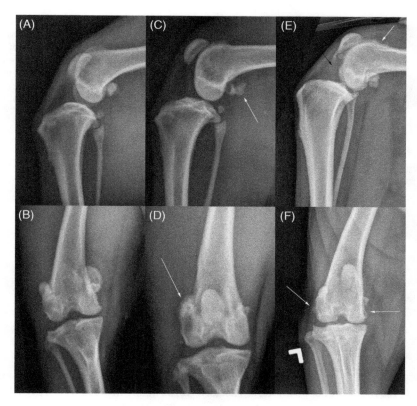

Figure 19.14   Examples of patients with MPL in two patients. *Patient I* (A–D) presented with bilateral Grade 2 MPL. Images (A, B) show a displaced patella, minimal joint effusion, and degenerative changes commonly seen with patellar luxation. Note that there is no radiographic evidence of MPL in images (C, D) since the patella was located within the trochlear groove at the time of the radiographs. The patient also had a chronic injury to the (white arrow) lateral head of the gastrocnemius muscle as indicated by degeneration of the lateral fabella. *Patient II* (E, F) was diagnosed with CCLD and MPL as indicated by the more advanced (white arrows) degenerative changes and (black arrow) moderate-severe amount of joint effusion. These features can be used to raise the index of suspicion for concurrent CCLD but are not diagnostic. The cranial tibial subluxation on the other hand (note the location of the femoral condyles in relation to the intercondylar eminence) indicates disruption of the CCL.

correction. Several techniques have been described to measure the *femoral varus angle* (FVA) (Dudley et al. 2006; Miles et al. 2015) and precise radiographic positioning is crucial to obtain accurate measurements. Several features have been suggested to determine appropriate positioning, namely that the patella should be centered within the trochlear groove, the fabellae should be bisected by the femoral cortices, the lesser trochanter should be partially visible, the proximal nutrient foramen should be visible in the center of the diaphysis, and the vertical walls of the intercondylar fossa should be visible as parallel lines (Jackson and Wendelburg 2012; Kowaleski et al. 2018). To accomplish a true craniocaudal view, the femur needs to be perpendicular to the radiographic beam and parallel to the detector. With modern X-ray equipment, this can be accomplished by angling the radiographic beam so that it is perpendicular to the femur or taking the radiograph in lateral recumbency with the beam horizontally. Alternatively, the patient's body may be elevated (Figure 19.15). Attempting to obtain a true craniocaudal view via traditional extended femur views will result in femoral foreshortening and inaccurate femoral varus measurements (Jackson and

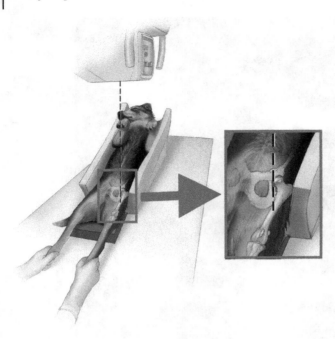

Figure 19.15 Illustration of technique used to obtain adequate positioned craniocaudal radiographs of the femur used to measure the degree of femoral varus. The patient's body is elevated of the table to allow parallel positioning of the femur to the detector.

Wendelburg 2012). If the limb is rotated, the normal anatomy of the femur (mild varus and procurvatum) will give the (false) appearance of excessive varus deformity (Figure 19.16). Alternatively, CT can be used to determine femoral varus and torsion (Dudley et al. 2006), as well to assess trochlear groove depth (Petazzoni et al. 2018). Therefore, in complex cases or for surgical planning, CT may be quicker and more accurate than radiographs.

19.6 Stifle Luxation

Stifle luxation, also known as "deranged stifle," happens secondary to severe trauma, especially trauma that involves traction or torsion of the joint. Stifle luxation results in injuries to the soft tissue stabilizers of the joint and can include disruption of one or both cruciate ligaments, one or both collateral ligaments, and the meniscotibial ligaments/menisci. Unlike the cruciate ligaments, the collateral ligaments of the stifle are very rarely individually injured in the dog. Therefore, any collateral ligament instability should raise the index of suspicion for additional injuries. Treatment of stifle luxation generally requires surgical reconstruction since the injuries are severe and result in substantial stifle instability in multiple planes.

19.6.1 Signalment and History

Any dog can suffer from stifle luxation since it is caused by trauma. However, the condition is more commonly seen in active medium- to large-breed dogs. Dogs that are free roaming or have the ability to escape to roam have an increased risk of vehicular trauma, a common cause of stifle luxations. Likewise, working dogs and hunting dogs are vulnerable to complex stifle injury from interaction with livestock or due to rough terrain.

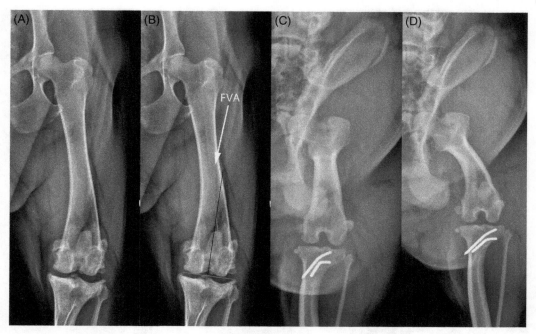

Figure 19.16 Measurement of the femoral varus angle (FVA) is performed on (A) accurately positioned craniocaudal radiographs of the entire femur. The (B) FVA is the angle formed between the (red line) proximal and (black line) distal femoral axis. The distal femoral axis is a line perpendicular to the (blue line) transcondylar axis, which is the line connecting the distal aspects of the lateral and medial femoral condyles. Note that inaccurate positioning can result in false measurements as illustrated by images (C, D) which are of the same patient that underwent surgical correction of MPL. Note that the femur appears straight in image (C), while image (D) gives the (false) impression of femoral varus.

19.6.2 Physical Exam

The patient with stifle luxation will likely be non-weight-bearing with swelling and joint effusion of the stifle. The source of lameness is generally obvious to identify. Palpation of the stifle typically shows severe pain and therefore should be done after pain medications are administered. Evaluation of the cruciate ligaments is performed by testing cranial and caudal drawer motion. The collateral ligaments are tested by applying varus and valgus stress to the stifle (Video 3.1). For testing the MCL, the examiner places one hand over the distal femur and one hand over the proximal tibia with the thumbs facing toward each other. Bracing the thumbs against the estimated position of the MCL, the examiner applies valgus (i.e. levering distal limb laterally) stress to the joint. If the joint opens up into valgus stress, the MCL has been compromised. The same is repeated with the thumbs aligned over the lateral collateral ligament. If the joint opens up into varus instability, the lateral collateral ligament has been compromised.

19.6.3 Diagnostics

Standard, orthogonal stifle radiographs in addition to stress radiographs are helpful to further define the extent of injuries and rule out any fractures. Radiographs will also show visible joint effusion, soft tissue swelling, and joint subluxation or complete luxation (Figure 19.17), as well as intra- or extra-articular avulsion fragments at ligamentous insertion sites.

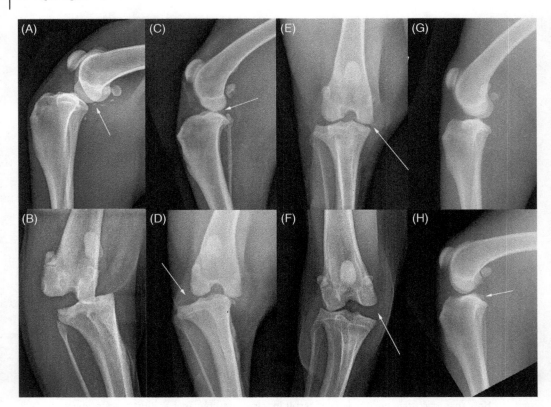

Figure 19.17 Examples of (A–F) stifle luxation and (G, H) caudal cruciate ligament rupture: (A) lateral view of a patient with stifle luxation. Note the multiple (white arrow) avulsion fragments indicative of severe trauma; (B) stress radiograph of patient with disruption of both, the medial collateral ligament (MCL) and lateral collateral ligament (LCL). Note the gapping of the lateral side and displacement that indicates disruption of both ligaments; (C–E) patient with disruption of the CCL and LCL. Note the (white arrow) avulsion fragment on the lateral view without evidence of displacement while the (D) varus-stress view shows disruption of the LCL as identified by the (white arrow) gapping of the lateral joint; the valgus-stress view shows that the MCL is functionally intact despite showing (white arrow) avulsion fragments indicating that a partial disruption of the MCL is present; (F) valgus-stress view showing gapping of the medial joint compartment indicating disruption of the MCL; (G, H) isolated caudal cruciate ligament rupture in an adult patient. Note that the standard lateral view does not show evidence of osteoarthritis; mild joint effusion is present. The stress view indicates caudal displacement of the tibia and also note the cranially displaced (white arrow) popliteal sesamoid bone.

A fractured fibular head or avulsed fibular head indicates lateral collateral ligament instability. On frontal view stress radiographs, the joint will gap open on the side with the torn collateral ligament. Although advanced imaging can be performed to further classify the injury, it is rarely needed.

19.7 Isolated Caudal Cruciate Ligament Rupture

Most CaCL injuries occur in conjunction with degeneration of the CCL. In fact, up to 88% of dogs with degenerative CCLD also have damage to the CaCL via the degenerative effects of synovitis and global joint inflammation (Sumner et al. 2010). The second most common cause of CaCL injury is due to stifle luxation, as part of multiple ligamentous injury or rupture. The CaCL is rarely injured on its own (Johnson and Olmstead 1987) but generally results from trauma such as a blow to the proximal tibia that stresses the integrity of the CaCL. However, since isolated CaCL disruption is easily mistaken for CCLD, it is important to be aware of this differential diagnosis. Since CaCL injury frequently does not require surgical intervention, preoperative identification is imperative to establish an appropriate treatment plan.

Isolated CaCL injury can be challenging to differentiate from CCL disruption. The mainstay of diagnosis involves physical examination and stress radiographs. To evaluate the integrity of the CaCL, the examiner performs the *caudal tibial drawer test*. This test is performed in the same fashion as the cranial drawer test; however, a positive test shows a tibia that translates caudally relative to the femur (rather than cranially as with CCLD). It is important to evaluate the end-feel when moving the tibia cranially and caudally – the intact CCL will create a hard stop (distinct end-feel) once the maximum, cranial displacement is reached (i.e. the intact CCL is engaged). When translating the tibia caudally relative to the distal femur, a subjectively loose/sloppy end-feel (i.e. capsular end-feel) will be encountered when maximum, caudal tibial displacement is reached (i.e. where in a normal dog the CaCL would be engaged). Unfortunately, even experienced evaluators are unable to reliably differentiate caudal, cranial, and combined injuries of the cruciate ligament(s) based on drawer testing (Might et al. 2013).

Stress radiographs can be used to confirm disruption of the CaCL. To perform these views, the observer levers the tibia caudally, requiring manipulation of the proximal tibia close to the joint; therefore, appropriate collimation is necessary. Caudal displacement of the tibia can be identified by evaluating the position of the intercondylar eminence in relation to the femoral condyles. Cranial displacement of the popliteal sesamoid may also be observed (Figure 19.17). Arthroscopy or advanced imaging can be used to definitely confirm the diagnosis.

19.8 Osteochondrosis Dissecans

Osteochondrosis/osteochondritis dissecans (OCD) is a rare disease of the canine stifle and overall the stifle joint is the least common joint to be affected by OCD (i.e. the shoulder, elbow, and tarsus are more common joints to be affected). It typically strikes large- or giant-breed puppies including Great Danes, Labrador Retrievers, Golden Retrievers, Newfoundlands, German Shepherds, Mastiffs, and Wolfhounds (Denny and Gibbs 1980; Fitzpatrick et al. 2012; Kowaleski et al. 2018). Male, rapidly growing puppies fed nutritionally inappropriate diets (e.g. excessive consumption or over supplementation of protein or calcium) are at greatest risk; clinical signs appear between 5 and 10 months of age. Stifle OCD can be bilateral or unilateral and is most commonly seen on the axial (medial) aspect of the lateral femoral condyle but can also be seen on the axial (lateral) aspect of the medial femoral condyle. Stifle OCD in the juvenile dog is treated similarly to other OCD lesions with simple removal of the flap or resurfacing techniques (Fitzpatrick et al. 2012). If OCD is diagnosed in older animals, secondary osteoarthritis is likely to be present. Additionally, concomitant CCLD needs to carefully be ruled out (and treated if present). In these cases, accomplishing a diagnosis can be challenging if there is only partial disruption of the CCL.

On physical exam, a mild-to-severe weight-bearing lameness can be observed unilaterally or bilaterally. In dogs with bilateral disease, there is generally one side more severely affected than the other. The dogs may stand with the stifles in extension, and in bilateral cases, may be shifting weight to the thoracic limbs. Patients may show significant pain and disability from this disease due to loss of a major weight-bearing surface of the stifle. Later in life, symptoms may be due to secondary osteoarthritis. Moderate to marked joint effusion without joint instability is a key feature of OCD yet does not allow differentiation from partial CCLD. OCD may also occur in combination with CCLD, particularly if OCD lesions are mild and not detected until later in life.

Standard orthogonal radiographs of the stifle joint are a reasonable first-line of diagnostics. However, identification of OCD of the stifle joint can be difficult since the femoral condyles normally display varying degrees of flattening radiographically. Therefore, advanced imaging may be preferable if the index of suspicion is high based on the patient's signalment and exam finding. Radiographic abnormalities range from subtle subchondral bone sclerosis, flattening of the condyles to easily visible cartilage flaps (Figure 19.18). Oblique views of the femoral condyles can help further visualize potential lesions. CT is more sensitive than radiography at detecting the location, size, and extent of OCD lesions. It is also more sensitive in detection of small osteochondrosis lesions or small displaced mineralized free bodies. Ultrasound has also been used to detect OCD

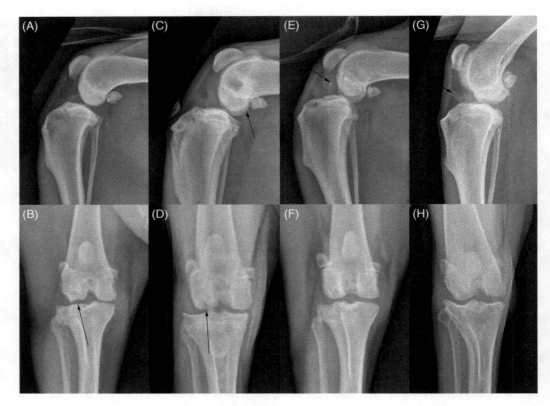

Figure 19.18 Examples of surgically confirmed stifle OCD in four patients. *Patient I* (A, B) adult patient with lateral femoral OCD lesion (white arrows) that was also diagnosed with partial CCLD at the time of surgery. Flattening and irregularity of the (black arrow) lateral condyle on the craniocaudal view indicate OCD; however, the lesion is not detectable on the lateral view and the diagnosis may therefore be missed/ confused with isolated CCLD. *Patient II* (C, D) OCD-lesion of the lateral femoral condyle in a juvenile patient that is visible as a (black arrow) flap on the lateral view and lucency in the condyle on the craniocaudal view. *Patient III* (E, F) juvenile patient with an OCD lesion of the medial femoral condyle, the fragment (black arrow) was found to be a displaced OCD fragment at the time of surgery. Note that neither view clearly establishes the diagnosis of OCD. *Patient IV* (G, H) adult patient with CCLD and chronic OCD of the lateral femoral condyle. Note the more severe osteoarthritis and the (black arrow) flap visible on the lateral view. However, the craniocaudal view does not show clear evidence of OCD.

lesions (Marino and Loughin 2010) and may offer a less costly and invasive method to establish a diagnosis. Arthroscopy allows direct assessment of cartilage health in the joint and may also be used to diagnose and immediately treat OCD.

19.9 Patellar Ligament Pathology

Pathology of the patellar ligament can be categorized into traumatic and nontraumatic etiologies. Nontraumatic patellar ligament desmopathy most commonly occurs in patients with a history of corrective osteotomies for CCLD (Figure 19.19) and generally does not require surgical intervention. Traumatic injury may be iatrogenic or due to sharp trauma and generally requires surgical apposition and external support. Patellar ligament rupture secondary to administration of steroids (Smith et al. 2000) and fluoroquinolones (Cabassu et al. 2001) have also been reported.

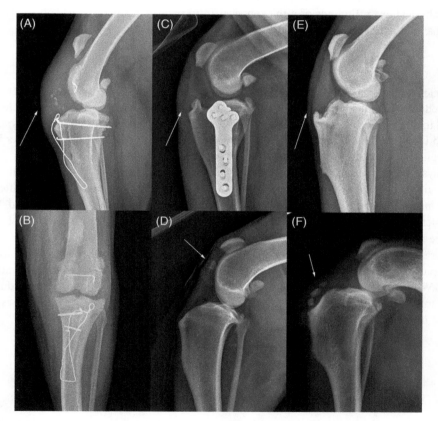

Figure 19.19   Examples of patellar desmopathies in five patients. *Patient I* (A, B) adult patient that sustained patellar ligament rupture after surgical correction of patellar luxation. Note the (white arrow) calcified and thickened patellar ligament. *Patient II* (C) typical (white arrow) patellar ligament thickening after TPLO surgery. *Patient III* (D) traumatic fracture of the distal patella resulting in disruption of the extensor mechanism. *Patient IV* (E) nontraumatic patellar desmopathy without a history of surgery. Note the (white arrow) thickening and enthesopathy. *Patient V* (F) nontraumatic patellar desmopathy without a history of surgery. Note the (white arrow) thickening and calcification of the patellar ligament.

STIFLE REGION

19.9.1   Nontraumatic Patellar (Ligament) Desmopathy

Patellar ligament thickening and desmopathy has been described following tibial tuberosity advancement (TTA) and TPLO in up to 80% of the cases (Dan et al. 2019). This is thought to occur due to increased stress placed on the ligament. In most cases, it does not result in clinical lameness and appears to be self-limiting.

A similar condition may be observed in patients that have not undergone surgical treatment. As with people (Dan et al. 2019), it may be caused by chronic overuse and intense athletic activities. The authors have observed it in large-breed, athletic dogs. Lameness is typically progressive and intermittent, with worsening of pain during exercise and jumping.

Physical exam may reveal varying but typically mild degrees of pelvic limb lameness. Tenderness or pain may be elicited with direct palpation of the ligament and flexion of the stifle. Some cases have visually evident or palpable patellar ligament thickening.

Thickening of the patellar ligament (or surrounding region) is easily recognized radiographically but it may be difficult to differentiate patellar ligament from abnormal peritendinous soft tissues. To assess the structural integrity of the ligament, ultrasound or MRI can be used. Using a combination of physical exam findings of a thickened, painful patellar ligament, plus soft tissue specific imaging allows the best assessments for therapeutic intervention.

19.9.2   Patellar Ligament Laceration/Rupture

Traumatic patellar ligament desmopathy is an uncommon injury in dogs (Das et al. 2014) and is associated with high leaps and falls, bites, lacerations, and other traumas. Any breed of dog is susceptible to sharp trauma. However, puppies are more likely to avulse the tibial apophysis rather than rupture the tendon from falls and other trauma. Iatrogenic laceration has been described as a complication of stifle surgery (Das et al. 2014).

On physical exam, rupture of the patellar ligament prevents active stifle extension and causes involuntary stifle collapse during the stance phase. If sharp trauma is suspected, the stifle should be examined for lacerations or wounds. A chronically ruptured tendon may be thickened. In cases of complete tears, the patella will be displaced proximally throughout flexion and extension ROM. The stifle may be painful especially if other tissue trauma is present.

A lateral radiograph in the flexed and extended position can document a proximally displaced patella, particularly in stifle flexion, as well as thickened tendon and any avulsion fragments when present. With complete rupture, the patella is located proximal to the trochlear groove due to the contraction of the quadriceps. Imaging of the tendon itself with ultrasound or MRI allows visualization of integrity of the remaining tendinous soft tissue.

19.10   Other Diseases Affecting the Stifle Region

19.10.1   Angular Limb Deformity

The most common types of stifle joint ALD are an excessive TPA (i.e. a TPA of 35° or greater) and frontal and transverse plane deformities of the femur. The latter is a common cause of patellar luxation in dogs. The former generally presents in combination with (and because of symptoms associated with) CCLD and has been reported to be associated with early neutering in large-breed dogs (Duerr et al. 2007). It can also be the result of undetected or untreated proximal tibial physeal injury/fracture. As sagittal plane deformity is generally well tolerated in dogs, observation of this deformity is difficult on physical exam, although some patients may show a compensatory gait of stifle flexion to keep the tibial joint surface parallel with the ground.

ALD due to trauma, nutritional deficiencies, hypertrophic osteodystrophy, retained cartilaginous cores, and other genetic/congenital skeletal dysplasias can result in various complex deformities. These deformities may result in secondary patellar luxation or hip pathology. Pure, isolated frontal plane deformity of the proximal tibia is rare, but spontaneous proximal tibial valgus deformity has been described in large- or giant-breed dogs (Olsen et al. 2016).

19.10.2 Gastrocnemius Injury

Injury to the origin of the Gastrocnemius muscle is a rare injury in dogs that may be caused by acute trauma or chronic overuse. Gastrocnemius myotendinopathy has been described in both pet or athletic, medium- to large-breed dogs and presents most commonly as none to mild, chronic pelvic limb lameness (Kaiser et al. 2016). The lateral head of the muscle is typically affected. Physical exam findings include pain upon palpation of the muscle origin at the medial supracondylar tuberosity, stifle pain, and effusion, but with no stifle instability. Since the gastrocnemius muscle is a stifle flexor and tarsal extensor, simultaneous stifle extension and tarsal flexion while palpating the origin of the muscle may exacerbate pain. Radiographs may reveal chronic changes (enthesopathy and mineralization) at the origin of the muscle and fabella (Figure 19.14) and mild joint effusion. However, advanced imaging (MRI or ultrasound) is necessary to establish the diagnosis if radiographs are normal.

Acute, traumatic, and atraumatic avulsion of the muscle has also been reported. Likely this condition describes the precursor of the above-described chronic myotendinopathy. However, clinical symptoms can be more severe and result in non-weight-bearing lameness and a slightly dropped hock, or even mild plantigrade stance. Radiographs may show distal displacement of one (Figure 19.20) or both fabellae, fracture or fragmentation of the fabellae.

19.10.3 Long Digital Extensor Tendon Injury

LDE tendon injuries include rupture, luxation, and chronic tendinopathies. The LDE tendon can be *traumatically* injured in dogs of any age, although avulsion fractures of the origin of the tendon typically happen in juvenile animals (Fitch et al. 1997). Dogs with traumatic luxation, tears, or avulsion fracture will have stifle joint effusion, pain with flexion of the stifle, and crepitus if the injury is chronic. Iatrogenic laceration during the lateral approach to the stifle joint can also occur. *Luxation* is a rare cause of lameness in dogs and can either be nontraumatic or traumatic. This condition should be considered a differential diagnosis for "popping" sounds originating from the stifle. The diagnosis can be made by placing a finger over the tubercle of Gerdy (located on the lateral, proximal tibia) while placing the stifle joint through ROM. Clinical signs vary but may include intermittent lameness or skipping gait making it a differential diagnosis for patellar luxation. Luxation of the LDE has also been reported as a complication after TPLO (Haaland and Sjöström 2007). *Calcification* of the LDE tendon (Figure 19.20) has been reported in a dog that also suffered from CCLD (Kennedy et al. 2014).

Radiographs may be normal or show cranial displacement of the fat pad with joint effusion. In dogs with an avulsion fracture, a bony fragment may be seen in the craniolateral aspect of the joint. The LDE itself can be imaged via MRI, CT, ultrasound, and arthroscopy. On ultrasound, the LDE can be seen as a hypoechogenic linear structure just cranial to the lateral meniscus (Soler et al. 2007).

STIFLE REGION

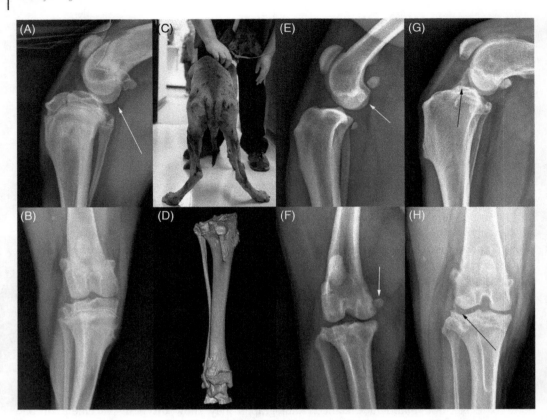

Figure 19.20 Other diseases affecting the stifle region: (A–D) patient with proximal tibial valgus resulting in visible (C) angular limb deformity – note that the (A) lateral view shows (white arrow) both condyles (rather than the condyles being superimposed) indicating the deformity. The extent of the deformity can further be classified based on the (B) craniocaudal view and (D) CT; (E, F) patient with traumatic avulsion of the medial head of the gastrocnemius muscle – note the (white arrow) distally displaced medial fabella. The stifle is otherwise normal indicating that this is an isolated injury; (G, H) patient with (black arrows) calcification of the LDE tendon and changes indicative of CCLD (which was confirmed at the time of surgery).

19.10.4 Stifle Region Neoplasia

Neoplasia of the stifle region is a common differential diagnosis because of the predilection site for osteosarcoma (Figure 22.1). Histiocytic sarcoma, villonodular synovitis, and lymphoma have all been reported in the stifle. Radiography as a first-line diagnostic and additional imaging and/or diagnostics should be considered if neoplasia is suspected. Further details about neoplastic conditions affecting the region are provided in Chapters 11 and 22.

19.10.5 Miscellaneous Other Conditions

Although *Panosteitis* more commonly affects the long bones of the thoracic limb, it can also affect the femur and tibia and should therefore be considered a differential diagnosis in juvenile patients with shifting limb lameness and pain on long bone palpation (Chapter 14).

Septic arthritis is an important differential diagnosis particularly if the patient has a history of recent stifle surgery. However, hematogenous or local spread as well as spontaneous septic arthritis (Chapter 14) have all been described in the stifle.

Quadriceps contracture can result secondary to femoral fractures (i.e. quadriceps "tie down" or "fracture disease") or because of infectious disease (i.e. "parasitic" quadriceps contracture). Please refer to Chapter 20 for further details.

Happy Jack Skip (also referred to as "Jack Russell Tick") is a condition that has not been described in the peer-reviewed veterinary literature but anecdotally is described as intermittent, non-weight-bearing lameness without an identifiable cause. The condition presents similarly to a Grade 2 MPL (i.e. a "skipping" pelvic limb lameness); however, the patella is stable during palpation. It is seen in Jack Russell Terriers but the authors have observed it in other terriers and small-breed dogs. Proposed reasons for the skipping include dynamic patellar luxation (e.g. the luxation only occurs during certain maneuvers/muscle contractures), neurologic disorders (e.g. nerve impingement that may be dynamic), hip pathology, or a behavioral condition.

Other rare causes of lameness associated with pathology in the stifle region include epiphyseal dysplasia (Chapter 20 and Figure 20.16), ganglion and synovial cysts (Franklin et al. 2011; Murata et al. 2014), osteochondromatosis (Smith et al. 2012), synovial hemangioma (Arias et al. 2009), and avulsion of the popliteal muscle (Tanno et al. 1996).

References

Arias, J.I., Torres, C., and Saez, D. (2009). Synovial hemangioma in a dog. *Vet Surg* 38 (4): 463–466.

Baker, L.A. and Muir, P. (2018). Epidemiology of cruciate ligament rupture. In: *Advances in the Canine Cranial Cruciate Ligament* (ed. P. Muir), 109–114. Hoboken: Wiley-Blackwell.

Beer, P., Bockstahler, B., and Schnabl-Feichter, E. (2018). Tibial plateau leveling osteotomy and tibial tuberosity advancement: a systematic review. *Tierarztl Prax Ausg K Kleintiere Heimtiere* 46 (4): 223–235.

Bergh, M.S., Sullivan, C., Ferrell, C.L. et al. (2014). Systematic review of surgical treatments for cranial cruciate ligament disease in dogs. *J Am Anim Hosp Assoc* 50 (5): 315–321.

Bosio, F., Bufalari, A., Peirone, B. et al. (2017). Prevalence, treatment and outcome of patellar luxation in dogs in Italy. *Vet Comp Orthop Traumatol* 30 (5): 364–370.

Cabassu, J.P., Ivanoff, S., Haroutunian, G., and Besse, J. (2001). Rupture bilatérale des ligaments patellaires chez un chien pendant un traitement à l'enrofloxacine. *Traitement Revue Méd Vét* 152 (7): 523–530.

Campbell, C.A., Horstman, C.L., Mason, D.R., and Evans, R.B. (2010). Severity of patellar luxation and frequency of concomitant cranial cruciate ligament rupture in dogs: 162 cases (2004–2007). *J Am Vet Med Assoc* 236 (8): 887–891.

Comerford, E.J., Smith, K., and Hayashi, K. (2011). Update on the aetiopathogenesis of canine cranial cruciate ligament disease. *Vet Comp Orthop Traumatol* 24 (2): 91–98.

Dan, M.J., Crowley, J., Broe, D. et al. (2019). Patella tendinopathy zoobiquity: What can we learn from dogs? *Knee* 26 (1): 115–123.

Das, S., Thorne, R., Lorenz, N.D. et al. (2014). Patellar ligament rupture in the dog: repair methods and patient outcomes in 43 cases. *Vet Rec* 175 (15): 370.

De Rooster, H. and Van Bree, H. (1999a). Popliteal sesamoid displacement associated with cruciate rupture in the dog. *J Small Anim Pract* 40 (7): 316–318.

De Rooster, H. and Van Bree, H. (1999b). Radiographic measurement of craniocaudal instability in stifle joints of clinically normal dogs and dogs with injury of a cranial cruciate ligament. *Am J Vet Res* 60 (12): 1567–1570.

De Rooster, H. and Van Bree, H. (1999c). Use of compression stress radiography for the detection of partial tears of the canine cranial cruciate ligament. *J Small Anim Pract* 40 (12): 573–576.

Denny, H.-R. and Gibbs, C. (1980). Osteochondritis dissecans of the canine stifle joint. *J Small Anim Pract* 21 (6): 317–322.

Di Dona, F., Della Valle, G., and Fatone, G. (2018). Patellar luxation in dogs. *Vet Med (Auckl)* 9: 23–32.

Dillon, D.E., Gordon-Evans, W.J., Griffon, D.J. et al. (2014). Risk factors and diagnostic accuracy of clinical findings for meniscal disease in dogs with cranial cruciate ligament disease. *Vet Surg* 43 (4): 446–450.

Dudley, R.M., Kowaleski, M.P., Drost, W.T., and Dyce, J. (2006). Radiographic and computed tomographic determination of femoral varus and torsion in the dog. *Vet Radiol Ultrasound* 47 (6): 546–552.

Duerr, F.M., Duncan, C.G., Savicky, R.S. et al. (2007). Risk factors for excessive tibial plateau angle in large-breed dogs with cranial cruciate ligament disease. *J Am Vet Med Assoc* 231 (11): 1688–1691.

Duval, J.M., Budsberg, S.C., Flo, G.L., and Sammarco, J.L. (1999). Breed, sex, and body weight as risk factors for rupture of the cranial cruciate ligament in young dogs. *J Am Vet Med Assoc* 215 (6): 811–814.

Fitch, R.B., Wilson, E.R., Hathcock, J.T., and Montgomery, R.D. (1997). Radiographic, computed tomographic and magnetic resonance imaging evaluation of a chronic long digital extensor tendon avulsion in a dog. *Vet Radiol Ultrasound* 38 (3): 177–181.

Fithian, D.C., Kelly, M.A., and Mow, V.C. (1990). Material properties and structure-function relationships in the menisci. *Clin Orthop Relat Res* (252): 19–31.

Fitzpatrick, N., Yeadon, R., Van Terheijden, C., and Smith, T.J. (2012). Osteochondral autograft transfer for the treatment of osteochondritis dissecans of the medial femoral condyle in dogs. *Vet Comp Orthop Traumatol* 25 (2): 135–143.

Franklin, A.D., Havlicek, M., and Krockenberger, M.B. (2011). Stifle synovial cyst in a Labrador Retriever with concurrent cranial cruciate ligament deficiency. *Vet Comp Orthop Traumatol* 24 (2): 157–160.

Franklin, S.P., Cook, J.L., Cook, C.R. et al. (2017). Comparison of ultrasonography and magnetic resonance imaging to arthroscopy for diagnosing medial meniscal lesions in dogs with cranial cruciate ligament deficiency. *J Am Vet Med Assoc* 251 (1): 71–79.

Fujita, Y., Sawa, S., and Muto, M. (2017). Radiographic measurement of the angle of the tibial translation in the Beagle dog. *Vet Rec* 180 (10): 252–252.

Gatineau, M., Dupuis, J., Plante, J., and Moreau, M. (2011). Retrospective study of 476 tibial plateau levelling osteotomy procedures. *Vet Comp Orthop Traumatol* 24 (5): 333–341.

Gilbert, S., Langenbach, A., Marcellin-Little, D.J. et al. (2019). Stifle joint osteoarthritis at the time of diagnosis of cranial cruciate ligament injury is higher in Boxers and in dogs weighing more than 35 kilograms. *Vet Radiol Ultrasound* 60 (3): 280–288.

Griffith, C.J., Laprade, R.F., Coobs, B.R., and Olson, E.J. (2007). Anatomy and biomechanics of the posterolateral aspect of the canine knee. *J Orthop Res* 25 (9): 1231–1242.

Griffon, D.J. (2010). A review of the pathogenesis of canine cranial cruciate ligament disease as a basis for future preventive strategies. *Vet Surg* 39 (4): 399–409.

Haaland, P.J. and Sjöström, L. (2007). Luxation of the long digital extensor tendon as a complication to tibial plateau levelling osteotomy. *Vet Comp Orthop Traumatol* 20 (3): 224–226.

Hayes, G.M., Granger, N., Langley-Hobbs, S.J., and Jeffery, N.D. (2013). Abnormal reflex activation of hamstring muscles in dogs with cranial cruciate ligament rupture. *Vet J* 196 (3): 345–350.

Jackson, G.M. and Wendelburg, K.L. (2012). Evaluation of the effect of distal femoral elevation on radiographic measurement of the anatomic lateral distal femoral angle. *Vet Surg* 41 (8): 994–1001.

Johnson, A.L. and Olmstead, M.L. (1987). Caudal cruciate ligament rupture a retrospective analysis of 14 dogs. *Vet Surg* 16 (3): 202–206.

Kaiser, S.M., Harms, O., Konar, M. et al. (2016). Clinical, radiographic, and magnetic resonance imaging findings of gastrocnemius musculotendinopathy in various dog breeds. *Vet Comp Orthop Traumatol* 29 (6): 515–521.

Kalff, S., Butterworth, S.J., Miller, A. et al. (2014). Lateral patellar luxation in dogs: a retrospective study of 65 dogs. *Vet Comp Orthop Traumatol* 27 (2): 130–134.

Kennedy, K.C., Perry, J.A., Duncan, C.G., and Duerr, F.M. (2014). Long digital extensor tendon mineralization and cranial cruciate ligament rupture in a dog. *Vet Surg* 43 (5): 593–597.

Knight, R.C., Thomson, D.G., and Danielski, A. (2017). Surgical management of pivot-shift phenomenon in a dog. *J Am Vet Med Assoc* 250 (6): 676–680.

Korvick, D.L., Pijanowski, G.J., and Schaeffer, D.J. (1994). Three-dimensional kinematics of the intact and cranial cruciate ligament-deficient stifle of dogs. *J Biomech* 27 (1): 77–87.

Kowaleski, M., Boudrieau, R.J., and Pozzi, A. (2018). Stifle joint. In: *Veterinary Surgery: Small Animal*, 2e (eds. S.A. Johnston and K.M. Tobias), 1071–1168. St. Louis: Elsevier.

Marino, D.J. and Loughin, C.A. (2010). Diagnostic imaging of the canine stifle: a review. *Vet Surg* 39 (3): 284–295.

McCready, D.J. and Ness, M.G. (2016). Systematic review of the prevalence, risk factors, diagnosis and management of meniscal injury in dogs: part 2. *J Small Anim Pract* 57 (4): 194–204.

Might, K.R., Bachelez, A., Martinez, S.A., and Gay, J.M. (2013). Evaluation of the drawer test and the tibial compression test for differentiating between cranial and caudal stifle subluxation associated with cruciate ligament instability. *Vet Surg* 42 (4): 392–397.

Miles, J.E., Mortensen, M., Svalastoga, E.L., and Eriksen, T. (2015). A comparison of anatomical lateral distal femoral angles obtained with four femoral axis methods in canine femora. *Vet Comp Orthop Traumatol* 28 (3): 193–198.

Mostafa, A.A., Griffon, D.J., Thomas, M.W., and Constable, P.D. (2008). Proximodistal alignment of the canine patella: radiographic evaluation and association with medial and lateral patellar luxation. *Vet Surg* 37 (3): 201–211.

Murata, D., Sogawa, T., Tokunaga, S. et al. (2014). Ganglion cysts arising from a canine stifle joint. *J Vet Med Sci* 76 (3): 457–459.

Neal, B.A., Ting, D., Bonczynski, J.J., and Yasuda, K. (2015). Evaluation of meniscal click for detecting meniscal tears in stifles with cranial cruciate ligament disease. *Vet Surg* 44 (2): 191–194.

O'Connor, B.L. and Mcconnaughey, J.S. (1978). The structure and innervation of cat knee menisci, and their relation to a "sensory hypothesis" of meniscal function. *Am J Anat* 153 (3): 431–442.

Olsen, A.M., Vezzoni, L., Ferretti, A. et al. (2016). Hemiepiphysiodesis for the correction of proximal tibial valgus in growing dogs. *Vet Comp Orthop Traumatol* 29 (4): 330–337.

O'Neill, D.G., Meeson, R.L., Sheridan, A. et al. (2016). The epidemiology of patellar luxation in dogs attending primary-care veterinary practices in England. *Canine Genet Epidemiol* 3 (1): 4.

Pagnani, M.J., Cooper, D.E., and Warren, R.F. (1991). Extrusion of the medial meniscus. *Arthroscopy* 7 (3): 297–300.

Park, B.H., Banks, S.A., and Pozzi, A. (2018). Quantifying meniscal kinematics in dogs. *J Orthop Res* 36 (6): 1710–1716.

Petazzoni, M., De Giacinto, E., Troiano, D. et al. (2018). Computed tomographic trochlear depth measurement in normal dogs. *Vet Comp Orthop Traumatol* 31 (06): 431–437.

Plesman, R., Sharma, A., Gilbert, P. et al. (2012). Radiographic landmarks for measurement of cranial tibial subluxation in the canine cruciate ligament deficient stifle. *Vet Comp Orthop Traumatol* 25 (6): 478–487.

STIFLE REGION

Rey, J., Fischer, M.S., and Bottcher, P. (2014). Sagittal joint instability in the cranial cruciate ligament insufficient canine stifle. Caudal slippage of the femur and not cranial tibial subluxation. *Tierarztl Prax Ausg K Kleintiere Heimtiere* 42 (3): 151–156.

Rutherford, S., Bell, J.C., and Ness, M.G. (2012). Fracture of the patella after TPLO in 6 dogs. *Vet Surg* 41 (7): 869–875.

Sample, S.J., Racette, M.A., Hans, E.C. et al. (2017). Radiographic and magnetic resonance imaging predicts severity of cruciate ligament fiber damage and synovitis in dogs with cranial cruciate ligament rupture. *PLoS One* 12 (6): e0178086.

Smith, M.E.H., De Haan, J.J., Peck, J., and Madden, S.N. (2000). Augmented primary repair of patellar ligament rupture in three dogs. *Vet Comp Orthop Traumatol* 13 (3): 154–157.

Smith, T.J., Baltzer, W.I., Lohr, C., and Stieger-Vanegas, S.M. (2012). Primary synovial osteochondromatosis of the stifle in an English Mastiff. *Vet Comp Orthop Traumatol* 25 (2): 160–166.

Soler, M., Murciano, J., Latorre, R. et al. (2007). Ultrasonographic, computed tomographic and magnetic resonance imaging anatomy of the normal canine stifle joint. *Vet J* 174 (2): 351–361.

Sumner, J.P., Markel, M.D., and Muir, P. (2010). Caudal cruciate ligament damage in dogs with cranial cruciate ligament rupture. *Vet Surg* 39 (8): 936–941.

Tanno, F., Weber, U., Lang, J., and Simpson, D. (1996). Avulsion of the popliteus muscle in a Malinois dog. *J Small Anim Pract* 37 (9): 448–451.

Valen, S., Mccabe, C., Maddock, E. et al. (2017). A modified tibial compression test for the detection of meniscal injury in dogs. *J Small Anim Pract* 58 (2): 109–114.

Van Der Vekens, E., De Bakker, E., Bogaerts, E. et al. (2019). High-frequency ultrasound, computed tomography and computed tomography arthrography of the cranial cruciate ligament, menisci and cranial meniscotibial ligaments in 10 radiographically normal canine cadaver stifles. *BMC Vet Res* 15 (1): 146.

Vasseur, P.B. and Arnoczky, S.P. (1981). Collateral ligaments of the canine stifle joint: anatomic and functional analysis. *Am J Vet Res* 42 (7): 1133–1137.

Vezzoni, A., Bohorquez Vanelli, A., Modenato, M. et al. (2008). Proximal tibial epiphysiodesis to reduce tibial plateau slope in young dogs with cranial cruciate ligament deficient stifle. *Vet Comp Orthop Traumatol* 21 (4): 343–348.

von Pfeil, D.J., Decamp, C.E., Diegel, K.L. et al. (2009). Does Osgood-Schlatter disease exist in the dog? *Vet Comp Orthop Traumatol* 22 (4): 257–263.

von Pfeil, D.J., Decamp, C.E., Ritter, M. et al. (2012). Minimally displaced tibial tuberosity avulsion fracture in nine skeletally immature large breed dogs. *Vet Comp Orthop Traumatol* 25 (6): 524–531.

Witsberger, T.H., Villamil, J.A., Schultz, L.G. et al. (2008). Prevalence of and risk factors for hip dysplasia and cranial cruciate ligament deficiency in dogs. *J Am Vet Med Assoc* 232 (12): 1818–1824.

Wucherer, K.L., Conzemius, M.G., Evans, R., and Wilke, V.L. (2013). Short-term and long-term outcomes for overweight dogs with cranial cruciate ligament rupture treated surgically or nonsurgically. *J Am Vet Med Assoc* 242 (10): 1364–1372.

STIFLE REGION

20

Hip Region

Nina R. Kieves

Department of Veterinary Clinical Sciences, The Ohio State University, Columbus, OH, USA

20.1 Introduction and Common Differential Diagnoses

Lameness of the pelvic limb in the canine is often attributable to pathology associated with the coxofemoral joint and surrounding structures. These can include osseous conditions affecting the surrounding skeletal structures (pelvis and proximal femur) or the joint itself including, luxation, developmental disease (hip dysplasia [HD]), and avascular necrosis of the femoral head. Muscle conditions should also be included as differential diagnoses when investigating discomfort of the hip region, including quadriceps contracture, gracilis and semitendinosus/semimembranosus myopathy, and iliopsoas tendinopathy. The most commonly utilized tests include radiographs and ultrasound. Figure 20.1 and Table 20.1 outline common differential diagnoses and diagnostic steps for the hip region.

20.2 Normal Anatomy

The femoral head and acetabulum form the hip joint (Figure 20.2). Like the shoulder joint, its ball and socket configuration allow it to function with a large range of motion – with the ability for significant flexion, extension, as well as abduction and adduction. The primary joint stabilizers are comprised of the ligament of the head of the femur and the joint capsule. Secondary stabilizers include the acetabular labrum, a fibrocartilaginous band that extends laterally from the dorsal acetabular rim (DAR) and ventrally across the acetabular notch (i.e. the transverse acetabular ligament). Finally, hydrostatic pressure is created by joint fluid and the periarticular muscles of the joint.

Periarticular muscles of the hip include the gluteal muscles (deep, middle, and superficial), iliopsoas, quadratus femoris, gemelli, and the internal and external obturator muscles. The gluteal muscles function to extend the hip joint, as well as internally rotate and abduct the femur. The deep gluteal originates on the body of the ilium and the ischiatic spine extending caudally to insert on the cranial aspect of the greater trochanter. It functions to extend, and abduct the hip, while also medially rotating the femur. The largest of the gluteals, the middle, originates on the ilium and inserts on the dorsal greater trochanter. The piriformis also contributes to hip extension with its origin on the lateral surface of S3 and Cd1, inserting on the dorsal aspect of the greater trochanter

Table 20.1 Key features for diseases affecting the hip region.

Disease	Common signalment	Diagnostic test of choice	Exam findings	Treatment	Clinical pearls	Terminology
Fractures	Any breed or age	Radiographs (orthogonal views), may need additional views or fluoroscopy to diagnose slipped capital femoral physis	Pain, crepitus, non-weight-bearing lameness	Depends on location	Acetabular and severely displaced fractures of the ilium are generally treated surgically	
Coxofemoral luxation	Any breed or age; intact, male dogs predisposed (higher risk of trauma)	Radiographs (orthogonal views)	Pain, crepitus, non-weight-bearing; craniodorsal luxation: appearance of shorter limb, held with the thigh adducted rotating the stifle outward; ventral luxation: appearance of longer limb longer, abducted position with internal rotation	Closed or open reduction	Anesthetize for closed reduction attempts to relax muscles	Hip Luxation
Juvenile hip dysplasia	Any breed but more common in large- and giant-breeds (German Shepherd Dogs, Newfoundland, Retriever breeds, and Rottweilers), 5–12 months of age	Radiographs (orthogonal views) and PennHIP; Ortolani maneuver	Pain with range of motion, positive Ortolani, muscle atrophy	JPS if diagnosed before 5 months of age; Medical management for osteoarthritis and pain; total hip arthroplasty or femoral head and neck ostectomy	Normal Radiographs do not r/o disease	
Adult hip dysplasia	Same breeds as juvenile, mature age	Radiographs (orthogonal views)	Pain, crepitus, decreased ROM, and muscle atrophy	Medical management for OA; total hip arthroplasty or femoral head and neck ostectomy	Most cases respond well to medications and rehabilitation; if medical management fails, surgery should be considered	

Condition	Signalment	Diagnosis	Clinical signs	Treatment	Comments	Synonyms
Avascular necrosis of the femoral head	Small-breed dogs, 4–11 months of age; genetic in Miniature Poodle and West Highland White Terrier	Radiographs (orthogonal views), CT for early presentation	Pain, crepitus, variable lameness, can be non-weight-bearing	Surgical: total hip arthroplasty or femoral head and neck ostectomy	Can be bilateral and frequently patients also have patellar luxation	Legg-Perthes, Calve-Perthes, Legg-Calve-Perthes, aseptic necrosis of the femoral head, osteochondritis juvenilis, and coxa plana
Gracilis contracture	German Shepherd Dog, males 3–7 years of age	Palpation of muscle; biopsy for definitive diagnosis	Distinctive gait: shortened stride with reduced stifle extension jerking motion of the limb	Medical management; surgery unrewarding	Can be bilateral; dogs non-painful	
Quadriceps contracture	Young, often after femur fracture	Physical exam; muscle biopsy	Unable to flex stifle	If secondary to trauma – prevention is the best treatment; if secondary to Neospora and caught early medical management may avoid progression	Differentiate etiopathogenesis (d/t fracture orparasitic) based on history. Perform titers for Neospora and toxoplasmosis if bilateral and no history of trauma	Fracture disease; quadriceps "tie down," parasitic quadriceps contracture
Iliopsoas myotendinopathy	Any breed or age; however, working dogs may be more prone	Ultrasound, MRI	Variable lameness; pain with hip extension and internal rotation	Rest, pain relief; rarely surgery	Ultrasound is operator dependent modality; Diagnosis based on palpation may result in overdiagnosis	
Neoplasia	Any breed or age	Radiographs, CT; biopsy for definitive diagnosis	Pain, crepitus, variable lameness	Based upon tumor type: surgery, radiation, ±chemotherapy	Can be difficult to differentiate neoplasia from severe osteoarthritis and sepsis	

r/o = rule out and dt/ = due to.

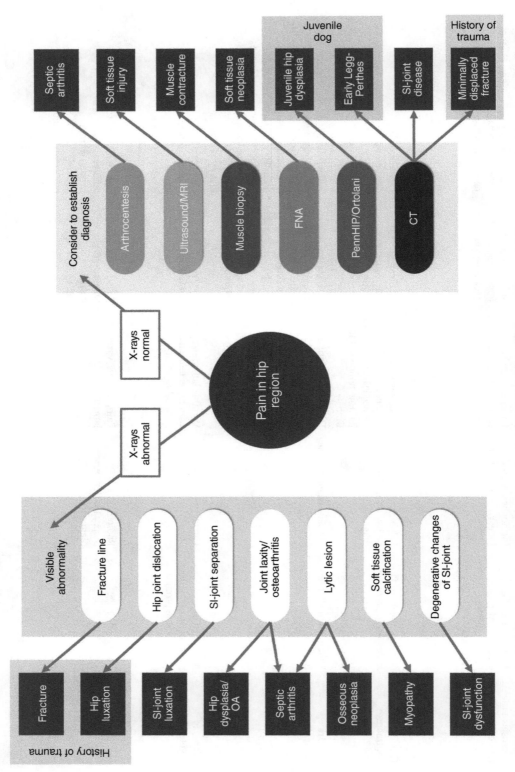

Figure 20.1   Schematic of common diseases affecting the hip region and the steps necessary to establish a diagnosis.

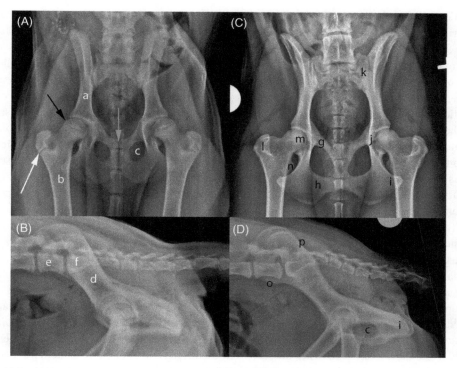

Figure 20.2 Normal anatomy of the hip region: (A) ventrodorsal and (B) lateral radiographic views of a normal immature dog; (C) ventrodorsal and (D) lateral radiographic views of a normal adult dog. The arrows indicate the (white arrow) physis of greater trochanter; (black arrow) capital physis; (red arrow) pubic symphysis; (a) pelvis; (b) femur; (c) obturator foramen; (d) ilial body; (e) L7; (f) sacrum; (g) pubis; (h) ischium; (i) ischiatic tuberosity; (j) acetabulum; (k) sacroiliac joint; (l) greater trochanter; (m) femoral head; (n) lesser trochanter; (o) tuber coxae; and (p) tuber sacrale.

with the middle gluteal tendon. The superficial gluteal extends the pelvic limb as well as contributing to abduction; its origin is the lateral border of the sacrum and Cd1 and the sacrotuberous ligament extending distal to insert on the third trochanter. The sacrotuberous ligament runs from the transverse process of S3 and Cd1 to the lateral angle of the ischiatic tuberosity. As a group, the gluteal muscles are innervated by the cranial and caudal branches of the gluteal nerve.

The quadratus femoris, gemelli, and the internal and external obturator muscles make up the caudal hip muscles. This group of muscles is innervated by the sciatic nerve and primarily allows rotation of the femur as the stifle turns outward (creating a supination-like effect). They also antagonize the middle gluteal muscle, which tends to pronate the femur (i.e. moves the stifle inward).

The adductor muscle is the primary adductor of the pelvic limb originating on the entire pelvic symphysis, ischiatic arch, and ventral pubis and ischium. It also has a large insertion area covering the entire lateral lip of the caudal surface of the femur. Also originating from the pubis at the iliopubic eminence of the pubic tubercle is the pectineus, inserting on the distal end of the medial lip of the caudal face of the femur. Along with the adductor, the pectineus contributes to hip adduction. They are both innervated by the obturator nerve.

The iliopsoas muscle is comprised of the psoas major and iliacus muscle and is innervated by the femoral nerve. The psoas major originates from the transverse processes of L2 and L3 and the bodies of L4 through L7. The iliacus originates on the ventral surface of the ilium. They combine to have a common insertion on the lesser trochanter of the femur. The function of the iliopsoas is primarily hip flexion, but it also contributes to external rotation of the femur as well as lumbar flexion.

Hip extension, thigh adduction, stifle flexion, and tarsal extension are controlled by the following group of muscles found superficially on the caudal portion of the medial thigh: the semitendinosus, semimembranosus, and gracilis muscles. The semitendinosus muscle originates on the ischiatic tuberosity and inserts at the cranial border of the tibia. It has an aponeurosis that spreads onto the crural fascia. A well-developed fibrous band extends from its caudal border and joins the calcanean tendon, inserting on the tuber calcaneus giving it the ability to extend the tarsus in addition to flexing the stifle and extending the hip. The semimembranosus originates on the ischiatic tuberosity and inserts on the distal mid-femur, as well as on the proximal end of the tibia. Its primary function is hip extension, with the ability to flex or extend the stifle depending upon the position of the limb. Extension of the hip is also aided by the gracilis that originates on the pubic symphysis and inserts on the cranial border of the tibia with the semitendinosus. In addition to hip extension, it contributes to adduction of the pelvic limb as well as flexion of the stifle. The semitendinosus and semimembranosus muscles are innervated by the sciatic nerve, while the gracilis is innervated by the obturator nerve.

The sartorius is made up of a cranial and caudal head, with the cranial head originating on the medial crest of the ilium and inserting on the patella with the quadriceps, and the caudal head originating on the cranial ventral iliac spine, inserting on the cranial medial border of the tibia with the gracilis muscle. While both heads contribute to flexion of the hip joint, the cranial belly extends the stifle, and the caudal head flexes the stifle. The sartorius is innervated by the femoral nerve.

The last muscle to contribute to hip extension is the large biceps femoris. It originates on the sacrotuberous ligament and ischiatic tuberosity, and inserts via the fascia lata to the patella, patellar tendon, and cranial border of the tibia, and via the crural fascia to the tuber calcanei. In this respect, it can contribute to stifle extension, and tarsal extension. Uniquely, the caudal portion of the muscle will flex the stifle. The biceps femoris is innervated by the sciatic nerve.

The sacroiliac (SI) joint is both a synovial and cartilaginous joint. Biomechanically, the SI joint functions to support the weight of the caudal portion of the body and to transfer propulsion forces from the pelvic limbs to the spine. The apposed crescent-shaped surfaces of the medial wing of the ilium and sacrum are covered by cartilage, with a thin joint capsule uniting their margins. This allows for some rotation and translational movement of the ilium relative to the sacrum. Dorsal to the auricular surfaces, the wing of the sacrum and the wing of the ilium are rough and possess irregular projections and depressions that tend to interlock. Fibrocartilage fills this space between the bony projections of both bones that unites the two wings. Through the medium of this fibrocartilage, the ilium and sacrum are firmly united in adulthood, forming the SI synchondrosis (synchondrosis sacroiliaca). The SI synchondrosis is located craniodorsal to the synovial portion of the joint.

The SI joint does have a small amount of normal motion, though it is very slight (Gregory et al. 1986). How much motion is not fully known, one study estimated ~7 degrees of rotation and likely a small amount of craniocaudal and dorsoventral motion, while an in vivo CT imaging study found only ~2 degrees of motion (Saunders et al. 2013). The SI joint is primarily stabilized by the dorsal and ventral SI ligaments and the sacrotuberous ligament, and is innervated by S1–S3/4 with sensory input from L1–S3.

The SI joint is connected to the wings of the ilium and sacrum via four soft tissue structures: a craniodorsal synchondrosis component, a caudoventral synovial component, the dorsal SI ligaments, and the ventral SI ligaments. The dorsal SI ligaments are divided into a short and a long part and are more extensive than the ventral SI ligaments, which are composed of many short, fibrous fascicles that are arranged in two groups. Those of the cranial ventral group run medially and caudally from the ilium to the sacrum. Those of the shorter caudal ventral group run medially and cranially. The thin joint capsule appears between them.

20.3 Fractures of the Hip Region

Fractures of the pelvis occur commonly with motor vehicle trauma or other high energy traumas such as falling from a height. Fractures can occur to the pelvic bones, SI joint, or the coxofemoral joint itself – fractures of the femoral head, femoral neck, and acetabulum.

Dogs will typically present non-weight-bearing on the affected limb, or possibly laterally recumbent depending upon concurrent injuries. Patient stabilization is the primary objective before any orthopedic issues are addressed, as many dogs with such trauma will have concurrent injuries (e.g. pneumothorax, pulmonary contusions, and urogenital injury).

Orthogonal radiographs should be obtained under heavy sedation or general anesthesia to confirm the presence of fracture(s) and to assess the fracture anatomy. The pelvis can be considered a rigid box-like structure, with fractures commonly occurring in specific locations and patterns. Because of this box-like structure, for there to be displacement the pelvis must fracture in at least three places. However, because SI luxation may also act like a fracture, displacement can occur under that scenario (e.g. pubic and ischial fracture in combination with SI luxation would also allow for displacement; Figure 20.3). CT may be indicated in cases of acetabular factures or more complex cases and may be combined to assess for comorbidities.

20.3.1 SI Joint Luxation and Sacral fractures

Sacroiliac luxation-fracture (SIL/F) denotes traumatic separation of the ilial wing from the sacrum (Figure 20.4). As with fractures of the pelvis, for displacement to occur several other fractures or luxations must be present, unless bilateral luxation is present with an intact pelvis. The iliac wing will typically displace cranially and dorsal to the sacrum due to the pull of attached musculature. While SIL/F can involve a small portion of the sacral wing fracturing, this should be differentiated from a true sacral fracture (Figure 20.5), where the sacral bone is significantly involved. Cases of sacral fracture are typically more painful than SIL/F, and dogs will commonly have neurologic deficits unlike those with simple SIL/F. If such signs are noted on physical exam, sacral fracture should be considered. CT imaging elucidates the extent of damage more readily than survey radiographs. SIL/F can be treated surgically or nonsurgically (Fauron and Déjardin 2018). Considerations to include in selection of treatment include patient level of pain, degree of instability of the pelvis, and amount of narrowing of the pelvic canal.

20.3.2 Fractures of the Ilium

Fractures of the ilium are most commonly long oblique fractures oriented from cranioventral to caudodorsal (Figure 20.3). While most are midbody, they can also extend cranially involving a portion of the SI joint, or caudally over the dorsal aspect of the acetabulum (not involving the joint). Ilial fractures are generally accompanied by fractures of the ischium and pubis, which are generally not treated surgically. Treatment can be surgical or nonsurgical and usually depends on displacement.

HIP REGION

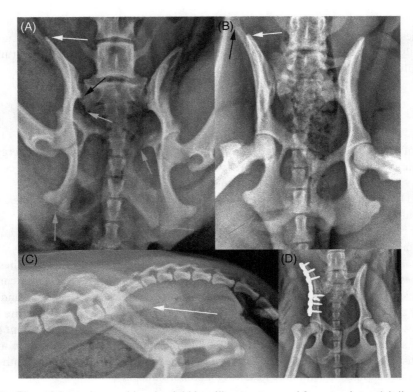

Figure 20.3 The pelvis can be considered a rigid box-like structure and for any substantial displacement to occur, at least three fractures have to be present (unless an SI luxation is also present). (A) Typical appearance of a dog with multiple fractures of (red arrows) pubis and ischium and an (black arrow) SI luxation; the green arrow illustrates the distal aspect of the sacrum, the location where the articular surface of the ilium should be located. This allows for (white arrow) displacement of the ilium (i.e. it is located further cranial than the tip of the ilium of the contralateral side). (B) Example of an iliac fracture illustrating the concept of the "pelvic box." Note that while the (white arrow) wing of the ilium itself is not displaced, the fractured (black arrow) body of the ilium can be seen cranial to the tip of the wing of the ilium. Also note the location of the obturator foramina indicating the displacement. (C) The fracture itself is best visualized on the lateral radiograph (white arrow); (D) note restoration of the structural integrity of the pelvis, including the symmetric location of the obturator foramina and tips of the ilial wings, after surgical repair of the fracture illustrated in (B, C).

20.3.3 Fractures of the Coxofemoral Joint

With fracture of the coxofemoral joint there will be pain and crepitus with range of motion of the joint. This can sometimes be difficult to assess given the patients generalized discomfort, or with fractures of the ilium near the coxofemoral joint. These are intra-articular fractures and surgical intervention is generally recommended to achieve the best outcome for the patient. Even with surgical intervention, such injury predisposes the patient to develop osteoarthritis (OA) in the joint over time.

20.3.3.1 Fractures of the Acetabulum

In cases of possible acetabular involvement, a CT scan can be useful to determine exact location and extent of the fracture. If CT is not available for imaging, oblique lateral views can be useful to remove some of the superimposition of the pelvis aiding in assessment for acetabular involvement and comminution. Caudal acetabular fractures may not necessarily require

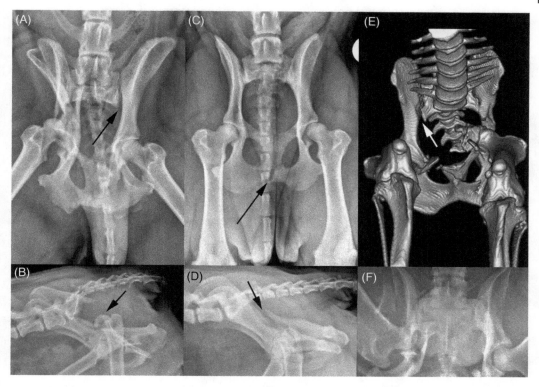

Figure 20.4 Pelvic fractures I: (A, B) multiple pelvic fractures including SI luxation (illustrated by black arrow in image (A) and the cranially located tip of the ilial wing) and comminuted ilial and acetabular fractures of the opposing side. The lack of bone dorsal to the femoral head, (illustrated by black arrow in image (B) clearly indicates that the fractures seen on the ventrodorsal view includes an acetabular fracture. (C, D) Minimally displaced, long-oblique acetabular fracture (black arrow, image (D) that cannot be identified on the ventrodorsal view; however, a fracture of the ischium (black arrow, image (C) can be visualized. (E, F) CT and ventrodorsal radiographs of a dog with multiple pelvic fractures. CT aided in establishing the diagnosis of SI luxation (white arrow) in this case, which was difficult to visualize radiographically.

surgical fixation; however, this has been disputed and some recommend fixation of all acetabular fractures (Boudrieau and Kleine 1988).

20.3.3.2 Slipped Capital Femoral Physis and Femoral Neck Fractures

In young dogs, Salter-Harris Type I or II fractures of the capital femoral physis most commonly occur secondary to trauma, with Type I being the most common (see Chapter 13 for review of the classification system). These fractures can be challenging to diagnose, as they are often reduced when a standard hip extended radiograph is evaluated. If there is pain on manipulation of the coxofemoral joint in a young dog and a capital physeal fracture is suspected, a frog leg view of the pelvis can help delineate such a fracture. Additionally, placing the hip through range of motion while taking fluoroscopic (or serial digital) images can help reveal such a fracture (Figure 20.5). In some cases, no trauma is noted, and the onset of lameness is gradual. Such atraumatic separation has been previously reported, but is rare (Moores et al. 2004) and is sometimes referred to as a slipped capital femoral physis based on a similar condition described in children (Dupuis et al. 1997). In children, it is broken down further into a pre-slip, acute, chronic, and acute-on-chronic stage.

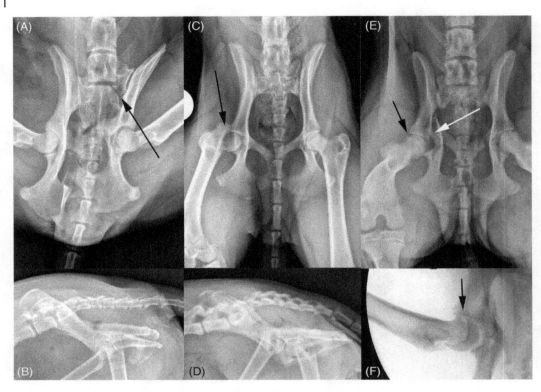

Figure 20.5   Pelvic fractures II: (A, B) sacral fracture (black arrow) and multiple fractures of the ischium and pubis in a dog; (C, D) severely displaced slipped capital physeal fracture that is easily identified on radiographs; (E, F) minimally displaced (black arrow) slipped capital physeal fracture and (white arrow) acetabular fracture. Note that the physeal fracture is difficult to identify on radiographs. (F) Fluoroscopy aided in establishing the diagnosis of (black arrow) mild displacement of the fracture.

Fractures of the femoral neck can occur in patients of any age and can be classified as intracapsular or extracapsular. These fractures can also be challenging to diagnose, particularly if they are minimally displaced, and may require additional imaging (e.g. CT or fluoroscopy) to accomplish a diagnosis. For both fractures (capital physeal and femoral neck fractures), surgical repair is generally recommended, or if not possible salvage with a femoral head and neck ostectomy or total hip arthroplasty.

20.4   Coxofemoral Luxation

Coxofemoral luxation (CFL) accounts for 90% of all luxations seen in dogs (Wardlaw and McLaughlin 2018). For the coxofemoral joint to luxate, two or more of the primary stabilizers must be disrupted. The amount of soft tissue injury that occurs allowing for CFL varies; however, at minimum a portion of the ligament of the head of femur and the joint capsule must be disrupted. In addition, surrounding musculature including the gluteal muscles may be disrupted, partially or fully. In some cases, avulsion of a portion of the head of the femur occurs with disruption to the ligament of the head of the femur. Damage to the acetabulum may also occur but is rare.

The most common type of CFLs is craniodorsal, comprising approximately 80% of all luxations. Typically, luxation occurs when a supraphysiologic force is applied to the femur. This causes the distal femur to be adducted, stretching/tearing the joint capsule and the ligament of the head of the femur. Then, the femoral head slides over the dorsal rim of the acetabulum completing the tearing of the ligament and the capsule. The gluteal and iliopsoas muscles act upon their insertion at the greater and lesser trochanters causing the head of the femur to move craniodorsally. Ventral luxation and caudodorsal luxation are rare. Ventral luxation most commonly occurs with a fall or slip where the stifle is abducted rapidly. The femoral head may luxate into the obturator foramen if the limb is rotated internally when it is luxating, or it may be adjacent to the pubis if the limb was undergoing simultaneous external rotation of the limb when the luxation occurs.

Nonsurgical (closed reduction) and numerous surgical techniques (open reduction) have been described for the treatment of CFL. Closed reduction is often attempted first in patients with normal anatomic configuration of the hip joint; however, this is associated with an approximately 50% failure rate for single attempts at reduction. Historically, after closed reduction, it is recommended that the limb be placed in an Ehmer sling for 10–14 days to prevent reluxation (McLaughlin 1995). When a closed reduction fails, or there are concurrent orthopedic injuries (HD, pelvic fractures, intra-articular fractures), open reduction with stabilization, total hip arthroplasty, or femoral head and neck ostectomy is warranted.

20.4.1   Signalment and History

The majority of CFLs in dogs are the result of external trauma, with vehicular trauma composing 59–83% of cases (Bone et al. 1984; Basher et al. 1986; McLaughlin 1995). Trauma may happen to any age or breed of dog; however, young intact male dogs are more likely to undergo vehicular trauma. Dogs with HD are predisposed to both craniodorsal and ventral hip luxation compared to dogs with normal hip coxofemoral joint conformation. Spontaneous luxations have been reported in a series of dogs with minimal to no evidence of HD and no trauma (Trostel et al. 2000).

20.4.2   Physical Exam

CFL is often suspected based upon physical examination of the patient. Dogs will often present non-weight-bearing on the affected limb, or non-ambulatory in the rear if they have sustained bilateral CFL, which occurs in approximately 6% of cases (Basher et al. 1986). If any trauma was associated with the injury, the entire patient should be assessed for stability prior to addressing any luxation. Dogs may be intermittently weight-bearing if the luxation occurred sometime ago. In all cases, severe discomfort and crepitus are present with range of motion of the hip.

With a craniodorsal luxation, the affected limb typically appears shorter than the contralateral limb and is held with the thigh adducted rotating the stifle outward (externally) and the hock inward (Video 20.1). On palpation of the hip region, the greater trochanter will be elevated compared to the normal limb and there will be increased space between the greater trochanter and the tuber ischii. In a normal non-luxated coxofemoral joint, palpation of the greater trochanter, the

---

Video 20.1:

Hip luxation gait.

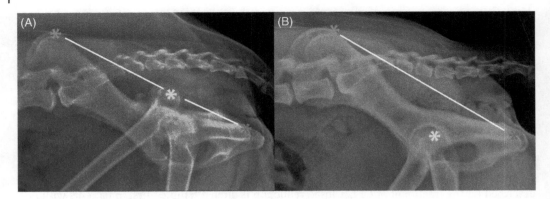

Figure 20.6   Coxofemoral luxation palpation: (A) lateral radiograph of a patient with craniodorsal coxofemoral luxation; the location of the greater trochanter (yellow star) is on a "line" between the cranial dorsal iliac spine (red star) and ischiatic tuberosity (blue star) while in a (B) normal dog it is located below this line.

cranial dorsal border of the wing of the ilium, and the ischiatic tuberosity will form a triangle with the greater trochanter positioned distal to a line between the cranial dorsal iliac spine and the ischiatic tuberosity. This normal triangle becomes a line when the coxofemoral joint is luxated in a craniodorsal direction with the greater trochanter being easily palpated between the two other landmarks (Figure 20.6). Additionally, the clinician's thumb may be placed between the greater trochanter and ischiatic tuberosity in the ischiatic notch and the femur externally rotated to palpate for a luxation. If the hip is luxated the clinician's thumb will be pinched with this motion, but if it is not luxated the thumb will be displaced with this motion.

Conversely, with ventral hip luxation the affected limb appears longer than the contralateral normal limb, and the limb is held in an abducted position with internal rotation. The greater trochanter will be in a more medial location than expected, and the femoral head may be entrapped within the obturator foramen, inhibiting internal rotation and adduction of the femur.

20.4.3   Diagnostics

Diagnosis of CFL is confirmed via orthogonal radiographs (standard ventrodorsal and lateral views; Figure 20.7). These should be thoroughly evaluated for concurrent trauma such as acetabular or pelvic fractures, slipped capital physeal fractures and fractures of the greater trochanter in young patients, femoral head or femoral neck fractures, and SI luxation. Evidence of HD should also be noted, as this affects treatment recommendations. At least, thoracic radiographs should be considered in all cases of known trauma.

20.5   Hip Dysplasia

HD is a developmental disease where there is joint laxity and inadequate coverage of the femoral head by the acetabulum. It is the most common orthopedic disease seen in dogs (King 2017). The exact etiology is unknown; however, several studies have shown it to be a genetic disease with a complex inheritance pattern (numerous genes), which is likely influenced by environmental factors that influence its expression (Ginja et al. 2015; King 2017). Initially, there is laxity of the

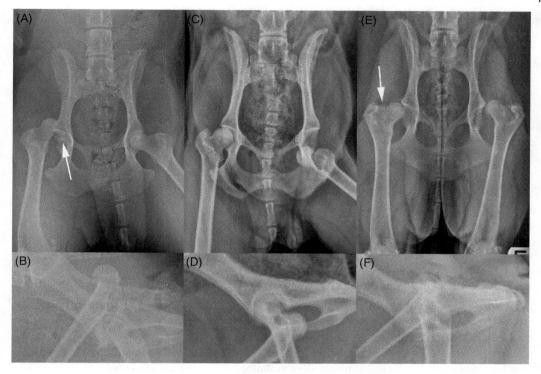

Figure 20.7 Coxofemoral luxation: (A, B) traumatic cranio-dorsal luxation; (C, D) traumatic caudo-ventral luxation; and (E, F) luxation secondary to hip dysplasia. (A) Note the avulsion fragment of the femoral head (white arrow) – a contraindication for closed reduction. (E) The bilateral nature in combination with the degenerative changes (the white arrow indicates femoral neck thickening) suggests that this dog is not suffering from traumatic coxofemoral luxation, but rather severe laxity due to hip dysplasia.

coxofemoral joint without evidence of OA. This laxity allows subluxation of the hip joint to occur, eventually giving rise to a shallow acetabulum, flattening of the femoral head from wear on the DAR, and eventually the development of OA of the joint. Treatment for HD most commonly consists of medical management; however, numerous surgical options are available. Early diagnosis of HD is key since some treatment options, such as juvenile pubic symphysiodesis (JPS), are only effective if performed before 5 months of age (Schachner and Lopez 2015).

20.5.1 Signalment and History

HD is most commonly seen in large-breed dogs, but can be seen in most breeds, with Sighthounds being a protected group of dogs. Some more commonly affected breeds include German Shepherd Dogs, Newfoundlands, Retriever breeds, and Rottweilers with a reported prevalence of up to 17% (Witsberger et al. 2008). Early gonadectomy (<5 months of age) has been associated with a higher risk of developing HD (Spain et al. 2004). One study found castrated male dogs to be significantly more likely to be affected by the disease (Witsberger et al. 2008).

A clinical bimodal presentation – dogs presenting as juveniles (juvenile form) or as middle-aged dogs (chronic form) – is seen in dogs affected by HD (Demko and McLaughlin 2005; Witsberger et al. 2008; Smith et al. 2018). However, radiographic progression has been reported to be linear (Smith et al. 2006). Dogs presenting at a young age generally are more severely affected and have pain associated with their coxofemoral laxity and resulting inflammatory changes (e.g. synovitis). These dogs will present with a history of exercise intolerance compared to other puppies, reluctance to climb stairs and jump onto things/into the car, generalized muscle atrophy of the pelvic limbs, a bunny hopping and short-strided gait (Video 20.2), narrow stance, and occasionally vocalization with petting of the hip region or manipulation of the hip joint. Later in life, presentation is associated with OA of the hip joint and a history of decrease in activity, stiffness when rising, worsening lameness with heavy activity, reluctance to jump, muscle atrophy of the pelvic limbs, and possible change in behavior associated with pain being reported by owners.

Video 20.2:

Hip dysplasia gait examples.

20.5.2 Physical Exam

Diagnosis is most commonly made based on physical exam findings and orthogonal radiographs. Dogs with HD experience pain particularly during hip extension. Differential diagnosis for pain on extension of the coxofemoral joint include any other coxofemoral joint disease (e.g. aseptic necrosis of the femoral head in young patients, femoral head and neck fracture, sepsis, and neoplasia), neurological disease affecting the lower back (e.g. lumbosacral disease), stifle pathology (most notably cranial cruciate ligament rupture), or pathology of any muscle stretched during hip extension (e.g. sartorius, iliopsoas muscle). Therefore, further manipulation of the hip joint (flexion and abduction) should be performed as the next diagnostic step. If pain is elicited during these latter two maneuvers, true pathology of the hip joint is more likely. If no pain is elicited, further evaluation of the differential diagnoses should be pursued (Figure 20.8 and Video 3.1).

In young dogs, examination will reveal generalized pelvic limb muscle atrophy, pain with manipulation of the coxofemoral joint, and joint laxity. Hip laxity can be assessed with specific tests such as the Ortolani maneuver (Figure 20.9 and Video 20.3), whereby the hip is subluxated and subsequently reduced (Syrcle 2017). The Ortolani test is typically performed with the dog in lateral recumbency, but can also be done with the dog in dorsal recumbency. The clinician places one hand on the dorsal aspect of the pelvis and spine to stabilize it, the second hand is placed on the stifle to maneuver the hip joint. Initially, the hip is subluxated by adducting the stifle and placing gentle pressure proximally to allow the femoral head to subluxate/luxate above the dorsal rim. This aspect of the Ortolani test is also known as the Barlow test. Next, gentle proximal pressure is maintained along the axis of the femur while the limb is abducted. A clunk or click may be heard, and palpated when the hip is reduced, this is considered a positive test. The Barden's test, which is less frequently used, also assesses for laxity of the hip joint. This is done by placing a lateral force on the femur with one had while the dog is in lateral recumbency without abducting the limb. The other hand is placed on the greater trochanter to assess for motion. If there is more than ½″ of

---

Video 20.3:

How to perform the Ortolani maneuver.

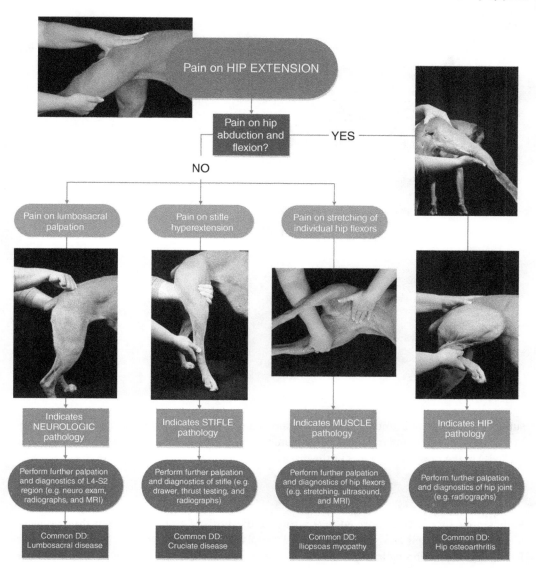

Figure 20.8 Algorithm to differentiate the four differential diagnoses for pain on hip extension: hip, stifle, neurologic, or muscular pathology.

motion, it is suggestive of laxity of the joint. The Ortolani test may be inaccurate in dogs <4 months of age; however, Gatineau et al. (2012) found that dogs with evidence of hip OA at 2 years of age all had a positive Ortolani test at 6 months of age. On the other hand, only 50% of dogs with a positive Ortolani test at 6 months of age went on to develop radiographic hip OA at 2 years of age. Thus, a positive Ortolani test has a strong sensitivity, but poor specificity at 6 months of age for predicting the development of radiographic OA at 2 years of age (Gatineau et al. 2012).

In comparison to younger dogs suffering mainly from laxity, older dogs will present primarily with signs of OA including a weight-bearing lameness that is typically bilateral, though one limb may be worse. They will have generalized pelvic limb muscle atrophy, decreased range of motion (particularly in extension and abduction) possibly with palpable crepitus, and in cases with severe

(A)

(B)

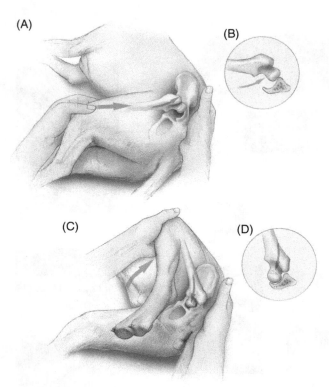

(C)

(D)

Figure 20.9 When performing the Ortolani maneuver (A) gentle dorsal pressure during adduction of the hip is applied. If laxity is present, this (B) results in subluxation of the hip joint. The (C) limb is then abducted, which (D) results in reduction of the joint, which can be palpated or heard as a "clunk," defined as a positive Ortolani sign.

subluxation the greater trochanter may be palpated more dorsally than expected due to subluxation of the hip joint (similarly to CFL). Ortolani testing is not indicated in these patients as there is no laxity in the progressive stages of the disease.

20.5.3 Diagnostics

Radiographs should be performed to confirm the diagnosis of HD and rule out the presence of other pathology such as septic arthritis and neoplasia, or fractures of the femoral head/neck. Radiographic positioning is imperative for accurate evaluation of laxity of the coxofemoral joint. Standard films include a lateral pelvis, and a ventrodorsal view with the hips extended. For the lateral view the ilial wings should be superimposed with one pelvic limb pulled in front of the other. The ventrodorsal view should be performed so that the pelvis is straight, and the limbs are extended and parallel to the imaging table. A straight pelvis will have symmetrical obturator foramens, and the width of the wings of the ilium will be equal. If one side is wider than the other, the patient is crooked (with the thinner side being elevated further from the table). Additionally, the vertebrae should be assessed for alignment; with straight alignment, symmetrical transverse processes and a spinous process centered on the body of the vertebrae will be observed. The femurs should be parallel to the table or they will appear foreshortened. A portion of the lesser trochanter should be visible and the patella should be within the trochlear groove with the fabellae bisecting the cortices (Figure 20.10).

In young dogs, minimal to no OA may be noted, although evidence of subluxation or full luxation may be present (which is generally assessed on the ventrodorsal leg extended view,

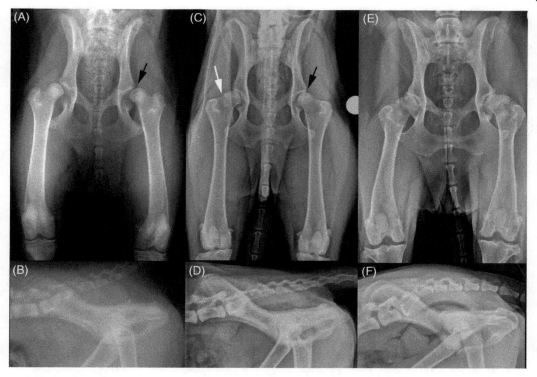

Figure 20.10 Radiographic views of three patients diagnosed with coxofemoral osteoarthritis secondary to hip dysplasia displaying the radiographic progression: (A, B) juvenile patient displaying (black arrow) severe subluxation without arthritic changes; (C, D) adult patient displaying (white arrow) arthritic changes namely a thickened femoral head and (black arrow) subluxation; (E, F) adult patient displaying severe osteoarthritic changes of the hip joint. Note that this patient is the only patient that displays obvious changes on the lateral view.

unless luxation is present). It is important to note that in some dogs with juvenile HD, conventional radiographs may not show any pathology, including a lack of subluxation/decreased coverage of the femoral head by the acetabulum on the ventrodorsal view. This is because maximum hip laxity occurs in a neutral position (similar to weight-bearing standing position) and when performing the standard leg extended radiographs, the joint capsule is twisted and forces the femoral head into the acetabulum (also called "windup mechanism"; Figure 20.11; Heyman et al. 1993). However, as the disease progresses with age, evidence of OA will develop including periarticular osteophyte formation on the femur (caudolateral curvilinear osteophyte), osteophytes on the cranial and caudal acetabular rim, joint remodeling including flattening of the femoral head and subchondral sclerosis of the craniodorsal aspect of the acetabulum. Often, the acetabulum will also be shallow compared to a normal coxofemoral joint. The lateral projection may show complete dorsal luxation of the hip joint, or loss of normal joint space, but these changes are only observed with more severe disease.

Numerous specific radiographic assessments have been developed for evaluating dogs for HD with two common methods including the Orthopedic Foundation for Animals (OFA) evaluation and PennHIP (the University of Pennsylvania Hip Improvement Program) to help try and determine which dogs may develop clinical HD over time. OFA radiographic evaluation consists of

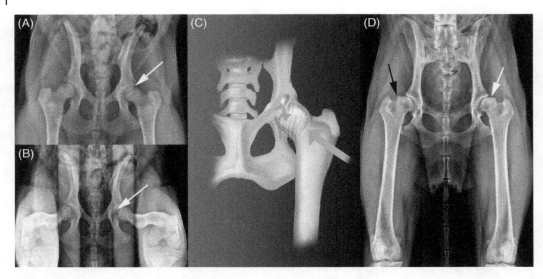

Figure 20.11 Windup mechanism: juvenile animals with mild-moderate hip laxity (i.e. hip dysplasia) may have (A) normal appearing standard radiographs with normal femoral head coverage (white arrow). (B) PennHIP radiographs can be used to demonstrate pathologic laxity (white arrow). (C) This is explained by the so-called "windup mechanism," when standard leg extended ventrodorsal hip radiographs are performed the joint capsule is twisted which forces the femoral head into the acetabulum artificially improving the radiographic appearance of the hip joint. While (D) degenerative changes (black arrow) and subluxation (white arrow) will become more obvious as the animal grows and the disease progresses, early intervention (e.g. juvenile pubic symphysiodesis) may prevent such progression. As such, early diagnosis (i.e. by 20 weeks of age) is crucial.

subjective evaluation of a ventrodorsal hip extended view for evaluation of hip conformation associated with joint subluxation, joint congruity, and evidence of OA. A grade of excellent, good, fair (all considered within normal limits), borderline, and mild, moderate, or severe (considered dysplastic) is assigned based on these secondary changes. Dogs must be 2 years of age or older to have an official score given.

If subluxation is not obvious, PennHIP (Figure 20.12) may be performed as soon as 16 weeks of age to more objectively evaluate laxity (Butler and Gambino 2017). PennHIP requires a certification process, mandatory submission of the radiographs to a for-profit company (that will also evaluate the radiographs and provide a report) and the use of a fulcrum device. The PennHIP report includes a reported distraction index (DI) that is given relative to other dogs of the same breed. The report also stratifies risk as low, mild, moderate, or high for developing OA based on the laxity of the individual. The DI measures the maximal femoral head displacement from the center of the acetabulum when a custom fulcrum device is used to place lateral stress to the proximal femur. It is calculated by dividing the distance between the geometric center of the femoral head and geometric center of the acetabulum by the radius of the femoral head. As the DI increases, so does the risk of developing OA with age; dogs with a DI≥0.3 are more at risk. PennHIP radiographs should always be performed prior to testing for a positive Ortolani to avoid cavitation (Figure 20.12).

While the PennHIP distraction method appears to be highly predictive for the development of OA, not all clinicians have access to the equipment and certified personnel required to perform this series of radiographs. One method for performing distraction-stress radiography without the use of a specific device was described by Flückiger et al. (1999). In dorsal recumbency femoral heads are displaced manually in a craniodorsal direction and a subluxation index is calculated by comparing

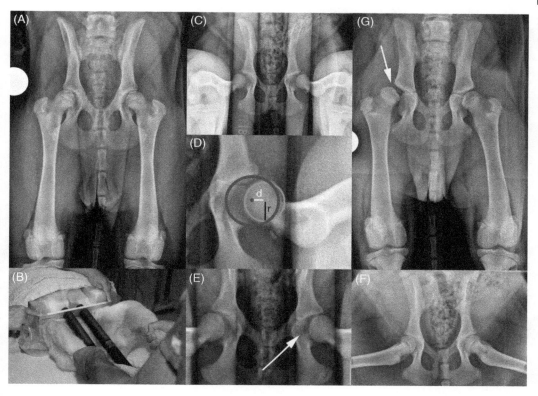

Figure 20.12 Coxofemoral osteoarthritis in patients with (A–F) mild and (G) severe juvenile hip dysplasia: images (A–F) are from the patient with juvenile hip dysplasia that did not show (A) evidence of pathology on routine ventrodorsal radiographic views. Based on clinical suspicion, the (B) PennHIP distraction technique was used to establish the diagnosis. Please note that the image is for the purpose of illustration of the distraction device and its position only; appropriate protective equipment should be worn when performing the procedure. PennHIP radiographs consist of a (C) distraction view that allows for measuring of the distraction index (DI). This is performed by (D) placing a circle over the acetabulum (indicated by blue circle) and the femoral head (indicated by red circle). The distance (d) between these two is then divided by the radius (r) of the femoral head circle. When performing PennHIP, it is important to avoid cavitation (see white arrow in image (E) indicating gas bubbles from excessive distraction) since this does not allow for accurate readings. As such, Ortolani testing should not be performed until after the procedure. Image (F) illustrates the frog leg view also requested by PennHIP that is used to evaluate acetabular filling. Image (G) is of a juvenile patient of the same age that is displaying obvious subluxation (white arrow). In this case, further evaluation with PennHIP is not necessarily due to the severity of the disease.

the distraction films to conventional hip extended pelvic radiographs (Flückiger et al. 1999). The dorsolateral subluxation test is another method that evaluates joint subluxation with dogs positioned in a weight-bearing position and can be performed between 4 and 8 months of age (Farese et al. 1998).

Other specific radiographic techniques to evaluate for evidence of HD include the DAR radiographic projection (Meomartino et al. 2002), and the Norberg angle (NA). The DAR projection is used to evaluate and measure the dorsal acetabular slope (DAS). In a normal dog, the DAR is sharply pointed; whereas, with the development of HD, the rim progresses from being slightly blunted and rounded to eroded. The DAS slope increases with worsening (more laxity) of HD.

Gatineau et al. (2012) found an increased DAS to be correlated to an increased risk of developing OA. Though it should be noted, the DAS was most predictive when the DI was >0.7.

Another measurement used to quantitatively evaluate HD is the NA. To make this measurement a hip extended ventrodorsal view is used. First, a line is drawn connecting the centers of the femoral heads, then a line is drawn from the center of the femoral head to the ipsilateral craniolateral acetabular rim. If the NA $\geq 105°$, it is considered normal. However, Gaspar et al. (2016) compared NA to DI and dorsolateral subluxation score and found that a cutoff of 105° was not highly predictive for HD suggesting that a much higher angle should be used, such as $\geq 112°$ in order to predict laxity in dogs with a DI of ≤ 0.3.

Distraction radiography appears to hold more promise to screen animals for HD compared to hip-extended radiographs (Verhoeven et al. 2012). Evidence of hip laxity remains the most predicative risk factor for the development of OA in dysplastic hips (Smith et al. 2001). In the future, blood sample testing may simplify screening for HD, though a DNA test that recently became available was found to be of low diagnostic value (Ginja et al. 2015; Manz et al. 2017).

In older dogs with OA who have sudden worsening of one side, or present with toe touching to non-weight-bearing lameness, cranial cruciate ligament rupture, sepsis, or neoplasia should be considered as a differential diagnosis. Radiographs of dogs with severe OA can be difficult to differentiate from infection and/or neoplasia (Figure 20.16). In these cases, arthrocentesis may assist in making a definitive diagnosis. Additional imaging with CT scan may also be useful. If warranted, arthroscopy, ultrasound or CT guided biopsy can be performed as well (Butler and Gambino 2017).

20.6 Avascular Necrosis of the Femoral Head

Avascular necrosis of the femoral head is known by many names: Legg-Perthes, Calve-Perthes, Legg-Calvé-Perthes, aseptic necrosis of the femoral head, osteochondritis juvenilis, and coxa plana (Demko and McLaughlin 2005). It is a disease affecting the vascularity of the femoral head and neck of small-breed dogs, causing a noninflammatory aseptic necrosis. The definitive etiology of the disease is not known; however, several theories have been proposed including anatomic conformation, deficiency in blood clotting factors, hereditary factors, hormonal imbalances, infection, infarction and obstruction of the venous drainage of the femoral head and neck, and trauma.

Regardless of the exact etiology, the progression of the disease is well delineated. Initially, the compromise to the blood supply leads to ischemia and necrosis of the femoral head. This is followed by an attempt at repair with fibrovascular tissue. Due to the underlying compromise to the bone, subsequent repeated forces on the bone cause fissures and clefts to develop in the articular cartilage of the femoral head, leading to collapse of the subchondral bone and flattening of the femoral head. The damage to the joint surface will eventually lead to the development of OA.

Conservative treatment with pain management is only reported to be adequate in 25% of cases, thus surgical intervention with femoral head and neck ostectomy or total hip arthroplasty is typically recommended.

20.6.1 Signalment and History

Numerous breeds have been reported as being afflicted with the disease, with toy breeds and terriers being predisposed to developing avascular necrosis of the femoral head. It has been determined to be an autosomal recessive trait in the miniature poodle and the West Highland white terrier (Robinson 1992; Demko and McLaughlin 2005). Males and females are equally affected, with most dogs presenting between 4 and 11 months of age. Approximately 12–16% of cases are affected bilaterally. Dogs will present with unilateral or bilateral pelvic limb lameness (Demko and McLaughlin 2005).

20.6.2 Physical Exam

Dogs will have pain and crepitus with range of motion of the affected hip joint(s). They may have accompanying atrophy of the limb from disuse. Given the prevalent signalment of toy-breed dogs, concurrent patella luxation may be present. This may confuse the veterinary exam; however, if both are present the hip pathology generally causes more pain than the stifle pathology in these cases.

20.6.3 Diagnostics

Diagnosis of avascular necrosis of the femoral head is suspected based on signalment, history, and physical exam findings. It is confirmed via orthogonal radiographs of the pelvis (Figure 20.13). In the early stages of the disease, there may be an increased joint space. Once vascular necrosis has occurred, radiographic changes will be seen within the femoral head and neck as areas of lucency. Ultimately, there may be flattening of the femoral head, collapse of the joint space, and progressive degeneration of the joint. CT scan may also be performed if radiographs are unequivocal (during early stages of the disease). Differential diagnosis include fracture (slipped capital physeal fracture, femoral neck fracture), infection, and neoplasia.

20.7 Muscle Contractures

Muscle contraction describes the normal, physiologic process of muscle shortening during activation. Muscle contracture, on the other hand, is a pathologic process that results in permanent shortening of the muscle leaving it unable to stretch. The normal muscle fibers are replaced by fibrous connecting tissue, which will shorten the affected muscle. Muscle contracture is also referred to as "fibrotic myopathy" or "fibrotic contracture" in the literature (Taylor and Tangner 2007; Adrega Da Silva et al. 2009; Cabon and Bolliger 2013). Muscle contractures are different from acute strain injuries because of their chronicity. However, it is possible that muscle strains trigger muscle contractures (Section 20.9.3; Nielsen and Pluhar 2005).

20.7.1 Gracilis Contracture

A syndrome known as gracilis contracture (also referred to as gracilis myopathy), can affect not only the gracilis muscle, but also the semitendinosus and semimembranosus, and rarely the biceps femoris muscles, individually, or concurrently (Lewis et al. 1997; Steiss 2002; Spadari et al. 2008).

The exact etiology of gracilis contracture is not known. It has been theorized to develop secondary to acute trauma, chronic repetitive trauma, infection, autoimmune disease, neurogenic disorders, vascular abnormalities and even drug reactions, though none have been proven (Taylor and Tangner 2007). Affected dogs frequently participate in tracking-obedience-protection work from a young age (Steiss 2002), giving some credence to repetitive stress/trauma as a cause

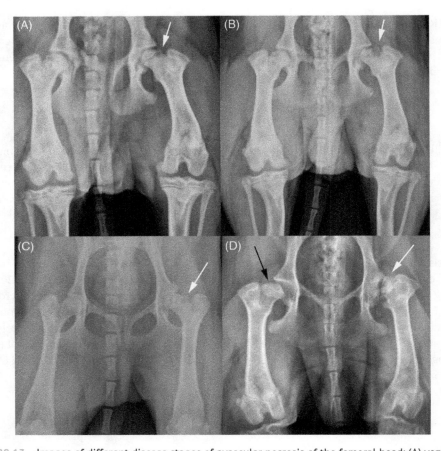

Figure 20.13 Images of different disease stages of avascular necrosis of the femoral head: (A) very early changes showing a mild irregularity of the femoral neck (white arrow); (B) progression of the same changes as noted in image A; (C) similar changes in a different patient affecting the femoral neck and head; (D) severe changes associated with chronic avascular necrosis of the femoral head (white arrow), note that the animal is also showing degenerative changes of the contralateral limb that are more consistent with coxofemoral osteoarthritis.

of the contracture. Histologic evaluation shows normal muscle being replaced by a dense network of collagenous connective tissue.

Unfortunately, to date no treatment for gracilis myopathy has been proven to be successful. Various surgical methods of treatment have been attempted, but none have been shown to be successful long term: Surgical resection of the muscle results in resolution of clinical signs for two to three months, when symptoms recur (Lewis et al. 1997). Although gracilis myopathy may affect a dog's overall performance and the pathognomonic gait abnormality remains for the life of the patient, it is not thought to be painful by their owners to the extent that patients can function well enough to have good daily quality of life.

20.7.1.1 Signalment and History

This disease most commonly affects male German Shepherd Dogs between the ages of 3–7 years but has been reported in Rottweilers and Doberman Pinchers as well (Steiss 2002). Dogs will present with a unique and consistent gait abnormality. The gait comprises a shortened stride in the affected limb with reduced stifle extension and a quick, almost elastic jerking motion of the limb with internal/medial rotation of the foot with external rotation of the calcaneus and concurrent internal rotation of the stifle during the mid and late swing phase (Video 20.4). In the early stages of the disease, these changes in gait can be subtle. However, the disease typically progresses until it becomes pathognomonic for gracilis contracture.

Video 20.4:

Gracilis contracture gait.

20.7.1.2 Physical Exam

Physical exam will reveal a taught fibrous band palpable along the caudomedial aspect of the thigh (Figure 20.14). If the gracilis and semitendinosus muscle complex is stretched, there may be some muscle spasming. This is done by concurrently flexing the hip, extending the stifle, and abducting the limb. In later stages of the disease, the stifle is often unable to be fully extended. Generally, the

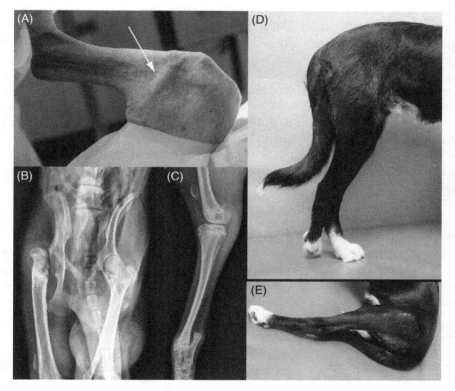

Figure 20.14   Muscle contractures: (A) gracilis contracture; (B–E) quadriceps contracture: (A) note the fibrotic gracilis muscle (white arrow); (B–E) two dogs suffering from quadriceps contracture due to (B, C) Neospora infection and (D, E) fracture disease. (B) ventrodorsal radiographs showing luxation of the hip joint due to (C) severe stifle and hock extension. (D, E) Note the classic straight limb and non-weight-bearing position with stifle and hock extension due to inability to flex these joints seen with quadriceps contracture.

HIP REGION

fibrosis affects the more distal myotendinous region and not the origin of the muscle. While the disease can be unilateral, it often progresses to affect the dog bilaterally.

20.7.1.3   Diagnostics

Definitive diagnosis is made via muscle biopsy; however, the characteristic gait and physical exam findings generally suffice to make a clinical diagnosis of the disease. Ultrasound may also be used to confirm muscle pathology. Differential diagnosis for gracilis myopathy includes acute injury to the gracilis muscle (Section 20.9.3).

20.7.2   Quadriceps Contracture

Quadriceps contracture, sometimes referred to in the literature as tie down, or stiff stifle disease, is significantly more common than gracilis myopathy. It most commonly occurs following femur fracture in puppies, or prolonged fixation of the stifle with external coaptation at a young age. Unlike gracilis contracture, it is a significantly debilitating process as it causes the dog to be unable to flex the femur or the hock (Bardet 1987).

In addition to contracture occurring following femoral fracture, quadriceps contracture can occur secondary to parasitic muscle diseases such as *Neospora caninum* and *toxoplasmosis*. These dogs are frequently puppies and are often affected bilaterally. They will initially have weakness and muscle atrophy in the rear limbs as inflammation secondary to the infection affects the muscles and nerve roots of the pelvic limb. With progression of the disease they lose their patellar reflex as lower motor neuron damage progresses, ultimately leading to further muscle atrophy and fibrosis leading to rigid hyperextension of the pelvic limbs (Crookshanks et al. 2007; Reichel et al. 2007).

Given the two different etiologies and treatment considerations it is important to differentiate between fracture disease (i.e. quadriceps "tie down" after femur fracture) and parasitic quadriceps contracture (i.e. due to infectious myositis). Prognosis is considered to be guarded once the disease has advanced; however, successful surgical management has been reported in cases with fracture disease (Moores and Sutton 2009). Therefore, early treatment with appropriate antibiotics (for parasitic quadriceps contracture) and/or rehabilitation is indicated to prevent development of irreversible changes.

20.7.2.1   Signalment and History

Quadriceps tie down most commonly occurs following femur fracture repair in puppies, but it can occur in adult animals as well. The risk for development of contracture increases if repair of the fracture is not appropriate, leading to poor limb use, or if there is a prolonged period of immobilization. Dogs with parasitic quadriceps contracture are also frequently puppies and may have a history of traveling from or being located in areas exposed to the known pathogens.

20.7.2.2   Physical Exam

On palpation, the quadriceps muscle will feel like a tight band, similar to gracilis contracture. With fracture disease, there are adhesions between the muscle and femur as well as periarticular fibrosis. Dogs may initially only show atrophy of the quadriceps with poor limb use. As the muscle fibrosis progresses, function will decrease significantly, and the dog will have difficulty ambulating. In severe cases, since dogs cannot flex their stifle or hock, they will walk with a straight limb, often scraping the dorsum of the foot leading to open wounds (Figure 20.14). The stifle and tarsocrural joints are unable to be flexed, even under heavy sedation. There may be pain associated with palpation of the muscle belly. In extreme cases, there may be genu recurvatum (i.e. stifle bent backwards) and secondary hip pathology (subluxation), patellar luxation, and eventually ankylosis of the stifle joint (Vaughan 1979).

20.7.2.3 Diagnostics

Young dogs with no known traumatic injury should have *N. caninum* and *toxoplasmosis* titer levels checked and/or muscle biopsy taken for histopathology which reveals multifocal lymphohistiocytic myositis (Crookshanks et al. 2007). Histologically, the muscle fibers are replaced by fibrous connective tissue in fracture disease.

Radiographs are used to evaluate fracture healing or to evaluate for secondary changes such as hip luxation and patellar luxation as well as genu recurvatum (Figure 20.16).

20.8 Iliopsoas Tendinopathy

The iliopsoas muscle is comprised of the psoas major and iliacus muscles, whose primary function is flexion of the coxofemoral joint along with adduction and external rotation of the femur. It also contributes to core stabilization and flexion of the lumbar spine.

Iliopsoas injuries can present as isolated, acute injuries or as chronic overuse injuries. It has also been suggested that iliopsoas injury may occur as a secondary, compensatory problem due to a primary disease (Cabon and Bolliger 2013; Cullen et al. 2017). Since pain upon palpation of the muscle is often found in conjunction with concurrent orthopedic or neurologic conditions, a thorough evaluation of the patient is essential to ensure a primary injury/pathology is not missed (Nielsen and Pluhar 2005).

Treatment most frequently is nonsurgical; however, tenotomy of the iliopsoas tendon can be performed in refractory or severe cases (Stepnik et al. 2006; Ragetly et al. 2009; Cabon and Bolliger 2013).

20.8.1 Signalment and History

In acute cases, strains most commonly occur when there is a sudden abduction of the limb (Breur and Blevins 1997). Common history includes slipping while walking, jumping out of a vehicle, or rough play. During such motions, eccentric contraction is occurring – the muscle is contracted while being stretched (Nielsen and Pluhar 2005). Chronic injury is thought to be secondary to microtrauma to the muscle fibers from repetitive use. Sporting and working dogs may be at increased risk for both forms (Cabon and Bolliger 2013; Cullen et al. 2017).

20.8.2 Physical Exam

Iliopsoas tendinopathy can cause varying degrees of pelvic limb lameness. Degree of lameness varies depending upon severity of the strain. If there is current inflammation of the muscle or there is significant fibrosis, the femoral nerve may be entrapped causing toe touching to non-weight-bearing lameness (Stepnik et al. 2006; Adrega Da Silva et al. 2009).

Dogs can present with unilateral or bilateral injury. On gait evaluation, dogs will often have a shortened stride as they do not fully extend their pelvic limbs. There may be pain with extension of the hip joint, exacerbated by internal rotation of the limb. Hip extension is often decreased due to pain or in some cases fibrosis of the muscle. This may occur with primary or secondary compensatory injury.

HIP REGION

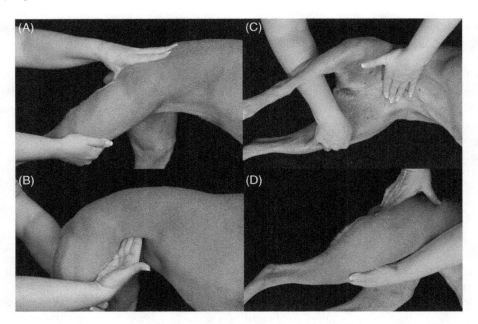

Figure 20.15 Iliopsoas palpation: the Iliopsoas muscle can be palpated (A, B) in standing or (C, D) recumbent position. Pain during (A) hip extension may be caused by the iliopsoas muscle or stifle, hip or neurologic pathology (Figure 20.8). As such, further palpation of the muscle is required to evaluate whether the source of pain is originating from the iliopsoas muscle: (B) palpation of the abdominal portion of the muscle below the vertebral column can be performed while the animal is standing or (C) while in lateral recumbency. Stretching of the muscle is performed by (D) hyperextending the spine, while simultaneously extending the hip joint and internally rotating the limb.

Direct palpation of the iliopsoas can cause pain, which is often most pronounced at the insertion near the lesser trochanter. Palpation is performed either in lateral recumbency or with the dog standing (Figure 20.15). Muscle strain can occur at any portion of the muscle. While generally muscle strains are thought to occur frequently at the myotendinous junction, the most frequent site of injury in a recent report was the tendon of insertion (Cullen et al. 2017). Both the insertion at the lesser trochanter and the more proximal muscle belly should be assessed. The muscle belly can be palpated by cupping the hands and gently placing dorsal and medial pressure along the body of the psoas muscle cranioventral to the wing of the ilium. When truly injured and sore, significant pressure is rarely required to elicit a pronounced reaction.

Because the groin region is generally a sensitive area even in normal dogs, caution in overinterpreting a response from the dog while palpating the area is needed. If there is pain on coxofemoral extension, but no exacerbation of discomfort with internal rotation of the femur, or direct palpation of the iliopsoas muscle, primary coxofemoral joint pathology is most likely. To help differentiate lumbosacral pain from primary coxofemoral pathology the author prefers to lay the dog in lateral recumbency and ensure the pelvis is stable when performing hip extension to avoid any flexion or hyperextension of the lumbosacral joint and lumbar spine while extending the hip (as often occurs when extending the hip from a standing position).

Other muscle groups near the iliopsoas should also be assessed for discomfort including the gracilis, semitendinosus, sartorius, and pectineus muscles. In a small case series of 22 dogs, the iliopsoas was the most common muscle strained in cases of pelvic limb muscle strains. However, isolated pectineus muscle strains occurred 23% of the time, and concurrent iliopsoas and pectineus muscle strain was found in 25% of cases (Nielsen and Pluhar 2005).

20.8.3   Diagnostics

As mentioned above, muscle palpation is a subjective assessment and therefore confirming a tentative diagnosis based upon palpation with objective imaging is ideal. Establishing a definitive diagnosis should include ruling out comorbidities or alternate diseases including lumbosacral pathology, pathology of the coxofemoral joint, and stifle pathology. Radiographs may show dystrophic mineralization or avulsion fractures (Vidoni et al. 2005), but in general they appear normal (unless comorbidities are detected) and cannot assess muscle fiber pattern for evidence of strain.

Imaging of the iliopsoas muscle typically consists of ultrasonography or MRI. Ultrasonographic features of the muscle have been described (Cannon and Puchalski 2008) and many dogs that showed pain upon palpation of the muscle had ultrasonographic changes in one study (Cullen et al. 2017). Several grading systems (stage/grade I–III with I = mild and III = severe) have been proposed (Cabon and Bolliger 2013; Cullen et al. 2017). However, these grading systems have been challenged recently (Mueller-Wohlfahrt et al. 2013).

20.9   Other Diseases Affecting the Hip Region

20.9.1   Sacroiliac Joint

Pain in or around the SI joint is commonly recognized in human medicine secondary to misalignment of the joint, abnormal movement, or insufficient stabilization of the joint. To date, it has received little attention in veterinary medicine. The SI joint serves to transmit the propulsive forces from the pelvic limbs to the vertebral column. It also supports the weight of the torso and may help buffer ground impact forces (Saunders et al. 2013). SI pain is recognized in horses (Jeffcott et al. 1985), but not well documented in dogs. However, given its innervation and similar anatomy, it can be postulated that disease at the SI joint could cause pain in dogs. A retrospective study evaluating canine survey radiographs found over 60% of radiographs to have calcification of the interosseous SI ligaments, and 44% to have calcification of the dorsal and/or ventral SI ligaments (Knaus et al. 2004). The clinical significance of such radiographic lesions has yet to be correlated with discomfort and performance issues.

As it is not a well-defined syndrome in dogs, a definitive diagnosis of SI joint pain is difficult to make. In humans, SI joint disease can cause sciatic pain secondary to compression from piriformis tension (piriformis syndrome) manifesting as buttock pain, without radiation of pain down the limb (Foster 2002). In dogs, it has been hypothesized that piriformis tension and muscle spasm may also occur with SI joint dysfunction and pain (Edge-Hughes 2007). Diagnosis of SI joint dysfunction has been proposed to be based upon movement, and stress testing, as well as evaluation of anatomic landmarks for asymmetry. Similar methods have been proposed for use in dogs as well. However, assessing pain of the SI joint specifically in dogs is difficult and subjective and while any of the below mentioned techniques have been proposed (Edge-Hughes 2007), they have not been validated and caution must be used when interpreting them.

Yet, evaluating symmetry of the ischial tuberosities, and the iliac crests can be useful. This is done by standing the dog in a square, equally balanced position, and palpating along the most caudal portion of the ischial tuberosities for ventral or dorsal rotation of the ilia. The iliac crests are also palpated for cranial or caudal slip by running the hands along the sides of the back until the wings of the ilia are found. Additional palpation may include strumming the piriformis muscle from caudal to cranial while assessing for pain, as well as evaluating the sacrotuberous ligament for asymmetry of its positioning and for pain on palpation. A pain provocation stress test based on a human thigh thrust technique has also been proposed: the dog is placed in lateral recumbency and slow, deliberate force is placed by holding the stifle and pushing the femur dorsally while the other hand stabilizes the sacrum. The hip is at neutral range of motion and held in slight abduction to differentiate hip pain from SI pain. Pain is thought to be elicited by stressing the dorsal SI ligaments. Movement testing is done in humans to evaluate amount and quality of movement of the SI joint with voluntary flexion of the limb and trunk. While not voluntary motion, a dog's hip can be flexed and extended and quality and amount of motion of the iliac spine can be assessed for symmetry (Edge-Hughes 2007). Muscles used for stabilization of the pelvis can be assessed for strength including the gluteals, latissimus dorsi, multifidus, abdominals, and epaxials. Caution must be used in making such assessments, however, as these can be weak with other orthopedic and neurologic disease such as HD, and lumbosacral or thoracolumbar disease. Along with muscle strength, flexibility testing can be performed, particularly of the hamstrings, piriformis, sartorius, iliopsoas, adductors, tensor fasciae, and latissimus dorsi. The abdominal obliques may show asymmetry. Finally, evaluating for hyper- and hypomobility of the SI joint via direct palpation while stressing the joint in a craniocaudal direction and dorsal-ventral direction can be performed.

As the diagnosis of SI joint dysfunction is in its infancy, no definitive treatment currently exists. Case reports of rehabilitation have been reported and a method of injecting the SI joint with ultrasound guidance was described in a cadaveric model (Jones et al. 2012), as this is commonly performed in humans and horses for pain non-responsive to physical therapy. Accuracy of injecting the SI synovial joint space was deemed fair to poor, although accuracy of injecting the synchondrosis and ventral and dorsal ligaments was deemed good. This modality needs further investigation to evaluate its potential for widespread clinical use.

20.9.2 Septic Arthritis

Septic arthritis (Figure 20.16) of the hip joint has been described and is generally seen in dogs with preexisting OA (Benzioni et al. 2008). Please refer to Chapter 14 for further information.

20.9.3 Muscle Strains and Tears

Muscle strains represent a common reason for pain and orthopedic dysfunction in people. Because these injuries are frequently self-limiting and diagnosis involves advanced imaging, only limited information exists in veterinary medicine. However, one study of canines reported that the adductor, pectineus, and iliopsoas may be prone to acute, stretch-induced injury (Nielsen and Pluhar 2005).

Acute gracilis muscle rupture, also termed "dropped back muscle," has been described in the racing greyhound (Eaton-Wells 1992). With such acute injury there is often significant soft tissue swelling and bruising, unlike with gracilis contracture. Repair of the muscle tear generally allows the dog to return to racing.

20.9.4 Hip Region Neoplasia

The most common neoplasia of the hip is proximal femoral osteosarcoma that may be difficult to differentiate radiographically from OA in some cases. OA and osteosarcoma may also occur simultaneously, making establishing a diagnosis even more challenging. Well positioned radiographs and additional views (e.g. frog leg) can help to detect subtle lucencies and pathologic fractures (Figure 20.16), but advanced imaging (e.g. CT/MRI) may be necessary. Further details about neoplastic conditions affecting the region are provided in Chapters 11 and 22.

20.9.5 Miscellaneous Other Conditions

Sorjonen et al. (1990) described *compression of the sciatic nerve* between the sacrotuberous ligament and secondary changes from severe hip OA.

Calcification of the gluteal muscles has been described and may indicate chronic trauma or overuse (Liu and Dorfman 1976).

MacInnes et al. reported a benign unicameral *bone cyst* of the hip joint causing mild lameness in an 11 year old dog (MacInnes et al. 2005).

Epiphyseal dysplasia, also known as multiple epiphyseal dysplasia, is a rare osteochondrodysplasia that causes a growth disturbance of bone and cartilage (Rorvik et al. 2008). It results in defects of ossification of the epiphyses and most commonly affects the shoulder, stifle and hip joint (Figure 20.16).

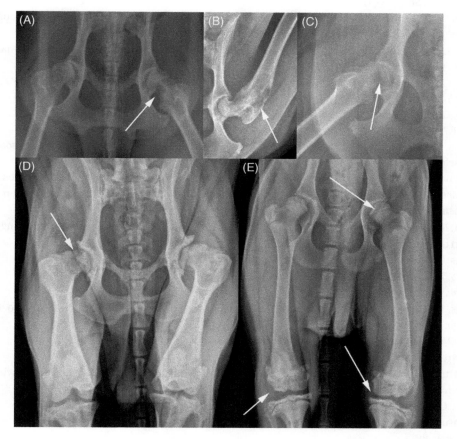

Figure 20.16   Other diseases of the hip region: (A–C) proximal femoral osteosarcoma; (D) septic arthritis; (E) epiphyseal dysplasia. (A, B) Images of a dog diagnosed with coxofemoral osteoarthritis and osteosarcoma; (A) note that the osteolytic changes are fairly subtle on the conventional X-ray; however, (B) they are more obvious on a frog leg, oblique view (white arrows). (C) This dog suffered from a pathologic fracture secondary due to osteosarcoma, note that the lytic changes are again very subtle and displacement of the fracture (white arrow) is minimal and therefore can easily be missed. (D) Septic arthritis in a dog previously diagnosed with coxofemoral osteoarthritis. Note that the osteoarthritic changes are very similar to the changes associated with sepsis (white arrow). (E) Epiphyseal dysplasia affecting the stifle and hip joint of a juvenile dog. Note failure of normal ossification (white arrows), which is more obvious in the stifles.

References

Adrega Da Silva, C., Bernard, F., Bardet, J.F. et al. (2009). Fibrotic myopathy of the iliopsoas muscle in a dog. *Vet. Comp. Orthop. Traumatol.* 22 (3): 238–242.

Bardet, J.F. (1987). Quadriceps contracture and fracture disease. *Vet. Clin. North Am. Small Anim. Pract.* 17 (4): 957–973.

Basher, A.W.P., Walter, M.C., and Newton, C.D. (1986). Coxofemoral Luxation in the Dog and Cat. *Vet. Surg.* 15 (5): 356–362.

Benzioni, H., Shahar, R., Yudelevitch, S., and Milgram, J. (2008). Bacterial infective arthritis of the coxofemoral joint in dogs with hip dysplasia. *Vet. Comp. Orthop. Traumatol.* 21 (3): 262–266.

Bone, D.L., Walker, M., and Cantwell, H.D. (1984). Traumatic coxofemoral luxation in dogs results of repair. *Vet. Surg.* 13 (4): 263–270.

Boudrieau, R.J. and Kleine, L.J. (1988). Nonsurgically managed caudal acetabular fractures in dogs: 15 cases (1979–1984). *J. Am. Vet. Med. Assoc.* 193 (6): 701–705.

Breur, G.J. and Blevins, W.E. (1997). Traumatic injury of the iliopsoas muscle in three dogs. *J. Am. Vet. Med. Assoc.* 210 (11): 1631–1634.

Butler, J.R. and Gambino, J. (2017). Canine hip dysplasia: diagnostic imaging. *Vet. Clin. North Am. Small Anim. Pract.* 47 (4): 777–793.

Cabon, Q. and Bolliger, C. (2013). Iliopsoas muscle injury in dogs. *Compend Contin. Educ. Vet.* 35 (5): E1–E7.

Cannon, M.S. and Puchalski, S.M. (2008). Ultrasonographic evaluation of normal canine iliopsoas muscle. *Vet. Radiol. Ultrasound* 49 (4): 378–382.

Crookshanks, J.L., Taylor, S.M., Haines, D.M., and Shelton, G.D. (2007). Treatment of canine pediatric *Neospora caninum* myositis following immunohistochemical identification of tachyzoites in muscle biopsies. *Can. Vet. J.* 48 (5): 506–508.

Cullen, R., Canapp, D., Dycus, D. et al. (2017). Clinical evaluation of iliopsoas strain with findings from diagnostic musculoskeletal ultrasound in agility performance canines: 73 cases. *Vet. Evid.* 2 (2) https://www.veterinaryevidence.org/index.php/ve/article/view/93.

Demko, J. and McLaughlin, R. (2005). Developmental orthopedic disease. *Vet. Clin. North Am. Small Anim. Pract.* 35 (5): 1111–1135.

Dupuis, J., Breton, L., and Drolet, R. (1997). Bilateral epiphysiolysis of the femoral heads in two dogs. *J. Am. Vet. Med. Assoc.* 210 (8): 1162–1165.

Eaton-Wells, R. (1992). Surgical repair of acute gracilis muscle rupture in the racing Greyhound. *Vet. Comp. Orthop. Traumatol.* 5 (1): 18–21.

Edge-Hughes, L. (2007). Hip and sacroiliac disease: selected disorders and their management with physical therapy. *Clin. Tech. Small Anim. Pract.* 22 (4): 183–194.

Farese, J.P., Todhunter, R.J., Lust, G. et al. (1998). Dorsolateral subluxation of hip joints in dogs measured in a weight-bearing position with radiography and computed tomography. *Vet. Surg.* 27 (5): 393–405.

Fauron, A.H. and Déjardin, L.M. (2018). Sacroiliac luxation in small animals: treatment options. *Companion Anim* 23 (6): 322–332.

Flückiger, M.A., Friedrich, G.A., and Binder, H. (1999). A radiographic stress technique for evaluation of coxofemoral joint laxity in dogs. *Vet. Surg.* 28 (1): 1–9.

Foster, M.R. (2002). Piriformis syndrome. *Orthopedics* 25 (8): 821–825.

Gaspar, A.R., Hayes, G., Ginja, C. et al. (2016). The Norberg angle is not an accurate predictor of canine hip conformation based on the distraction index and the dorsolateral subluxation score. *Prev. Vet. Med.* 135: 47–52.

HIP REGION

Gatineau, M., Dupuis, J., Beauregard, G. et al. (2012). Palpation and dorsal acetabular rim radiographic projection for early detection of canine hip dysplasia: a prospective study. *Vet. Surg.* 41 (1): 42–53.

Ginja, M., Gaspar, A.R., and Ginja, C. (2015). Emerging insights into the genetic basis of canine hip dysplasia. *Vet. Med. (Auckl)* 6: 193–202.

Gregory, C.R., Cullen, J.M., Pool, R., and Vasseur, P.B. (1986). The canine sacroiliac joint. Preliminary study of anatomy, histopathology, and biomechanics. *Spine* 11 (10): 1044–1048.

Heyman, S.J., Smith, G.K., and Cofone, M.A. (1993). Biomechanical study of the effect of coxofemoral positioning on passive hip joint laxity in dogs. *Am. J. Vet. Res.* 54 (2): 210–215.

Jeffcott, L.B., Dalin, G., Ekman, S., and Olsson, S.E. (1985). Sacroiliac lesions as a cause of chronic poor performance in competitive horses. *Equine Vet. J.* 17 (2): 111–118.

Jones, J.C., Gonzalez, L.M., Larson, M.M. et al. (2012). Feasibility and accuracy of ultrasound-guided sacroiliac joint injection in dogs. *Vet. Radiol. Ultrasound* 53 (4): 446–454.

King, M.D. (2017). Etiopathogenesis of canine hip dysplasia, prevalence, and genetics. *Vet. Clin. North Am. Small Anim. Pract.* 47 (4): 753–767.

Knaus, I., Breit, S., Kunzel, W., and Mayrhofer, E. (2004). Appearance and incidence of sacroiliac joint disease in ventrodorsal radiographs of the canine pelvis. *Vet. Radiol. Ultrasound* 45 (1): 1–9.

Lewis, D.D., Shelton, G.D., Piras, A. et al. (1997). Gracilis or semitendinosus myopathy in 18 dogs. *J. Am. Anim. Hosp. Assoc.* 33 (2): 177–188.

Liu, S.-K. and Dorfman, H.D. (1976). A condition resembling human localized myositis ossificans in two dogs. *J. Small Anim. Pract.* 17 (6): 371–377.

Macinnes, T.J., Thompson, M.S., and Lewis, D.D. (2005). What is your diagnosis? Benign bone cysts. *J. Am. Vet. Med. Assoc.* 227 (10): 1561–1562.

Manz, E., Tellhelm, B., and Krawczak, M. (2017). Prospective evaluation of a patented DNA test for canine hip dysplasia (CHD). *PLoS One* 12 (8): e0182093.

McLaughlin, R.M. (1995). Traumatic joint luxations in small animals. *Vet. Clin. Small Anim. Pract.* 25 (5): 1175–1196.

Meomartino, L., Fatone, G., Potena, A., and Brunetti, A. (2002). Morphometric assessment of the canine hip joint using the dorsal acetabular rim view and the centre-edge angle. *J. Small Anim. Pract.* 43 (1): 2–6.

Moores, A.P., Owen, M.R., Fews, D. et al. (2004). Slipped capital femoral epiphysis in dogs. *J. Small Anim. Pract.* 45 (12): 602–608.

Moores, A.P. and Sutton, A. (2009). Management of quadriceps contracture in a dog using a static flexion apparatus and physiotherapy. *J. Small Anim. Pract.* 50 (5): 251–254.

Mueller-Wohlfahrt, H.W., Haensel, L., Mithoefer, K. et al. (2013). Terminology and classification of muscle injuries in sport: the Munich consensus statement. *Br. J. Sports Med.* 47 (6): 342–350.

Nielsen, C. and Pluhar, G.E. (2005). Diagnosis and treatment of hind limb muscle strain injuries in 22 dogs. *Vet. Comp. Orthop. Traumatol.* 18 (4): 247–253.

Ragetly, G.R., Griffon, D.J., Johnson, A.L. et al. (2009). Bilateral iliopsoas muscle contracture and spinous process impingement in a German Shepherd Dog. *Vet. Surg.* 38 (8): 946–953.

Reichel, M.P., Ellis, J.T., and Dubey, J.P. (2007). Neosporosis and hammondiosis in dogs. *J. Small Anim. Pract.* 48 (6): 308–312.

Robinson, R. (1992). Legg-Calve-Perthes disease in dogs: genetic aetiology. *J. Small Anim. Pract.* 33 (6): 275–276.

Rorvik, A.M., Teige, J., Ottesen, N., and Lingaas, F. (2008). Clinical, radiographic, and pathologic abnormalities in dogs with multiple epiphyseal dysplasia: 19 cases (1991–2005). *J. Am. Vet. Med. Assoc.* 233 (4): 600–606.

Saunders, F.C., Cave, N.J., Hartman, K.M. et al. (2013). Computed tomographic method for measurement of inclination angles and motion of the sacroiliac joints in German Shepherd Dogs and Greyhounds. *Am. J. Vet. Res.* 74 (9): 1172–1182.

HIP REGION

Schachner, E.R. and Lopez, M.J. (2015). Diagnosis, prevention, and management of canine hip dysplasia: a review. *Vet. Med. (Auckl)* 6: 181–192.

Smith, G.K., Leighton, E.A., Karbe, G.T., and McDonald-Lynch, M.B. (2018). Pathogenesis, diagnosis, and control of canine hip dysplasia. In: Veterinary Surgery: Small Animal, 2e (eds. S.A. Johnston and K.M. Tobias), 964–991. St. Louis: Elsevier.

Smith, G.K., Mayhew, P.D., Kapatkin, A.S. et al. (2001). Evaluation of risk factors for degenerative joint disease associated with hip dysplasia in German Shepherd Dogs, Golden Retrievers, Labrador Retrievers, and Rottweilers. *J. Am. Vet. Med. Assoc.* 219 (12): 1719–1724.

Smith, G.K., Paster, E.R., Powers, M.Y. et al. (2006). Lifelong diet restriction and radiographic evidence of osteoarthritis of the hip joint in dogs. *J. Am. Vet. Med. Assoc.* 229 (5): 690–693.

Sorjonen, D.C., Milton, J.L., Steiss, J.E. et al. (1990). Hip dysplasia with bilateral ischiatic nerve entrapment in a dog. *J. Am. Vet. Med. Assoc.* 197 (4): 495–497.

Spadari, A., Spinella, G., Morini, M. et al. (2008). Sartorius muscle contracture in a German Shepherd Dog. *Vet. Surg.* 37 (2): 149–152.

Spain, C.V., Scarlett, J.M., and Houpt, K.A. (2004). Long-term risks and benefits of early-age gonadectomy in dogs. *J. Am. Vet. Med. Assoc.* 224 (3): 380–387.

Steiss, J.E. (2002). Muscle disorders and rehabilitation in canine athletes. *Vet. Clin. North Am. Small Anim. Pract.* 32 (1): 267–285.

Stepnik, M.W., Olby, N., Thompson, R.R., and Marcellin-Little, D.J. (2006). Femoral neuropathy in a dog with iliopsoas muscle injury. *Vet. Surg.* 35 (2): 186–190.

Syrcle, J. (2017). Hip dysplasia: clinical signs and physical examination findings. *Vet. Clin. North Am. Small Anim. Pract.* 47 (4): 769–775.

Taylor, J. and Tangner, C.H. (2007). Acquired muscle contractures in the dog and cat. A review of the literature and case report. *Vet. Comp. Orthop. Traumatol.* 20 (2): 79–85.

Trostel, C.D., Peck, J.N., and Dehaan, J.J. (2000). Spontaneous bilateral coxofemoral luxation in four dogs. *J. Am. Anim. Hosp. Assoc.* 36 (3): 268–276.

Vaughan, L.C. (1979). Muscle and tendon injuries in dogs. *J. Small Anim. Pract.* 20 (12): 711–736.

Verhoeven, G., Fortrie, R., Van Ryssen, B., and Coopman, F. (2012). Worldwide screening for canine hip dysplasia: Where are we now? *Vet. Surg.* 41 (1): 10–19.

Vidoni, B., Henninger, W., Lorinson, D., and Mayrhofer, E. (2005). Traumatic avulsion fracture of the lesser trochanter in a dog. *Vet. Comp. Orthop. Traumatol.* 18 (2): 105–109.

Wardlaw, J.L. and McLaughlin, R. (2018). Hip luxation. In: Veterinary Surgery: Small Animal, 2e (eds. S.A. Johnston and K.M. Tobias), 956–964. St. Louis: Elsevier.

Witsberger, T.H., Villamil, J.A., Schultz, L.G. et al. (2008). Prevalence of and risk factors for hip dysplasia and cranial cruciate ligament deficiency in dogs. *J. Am. Vet. Med. Assoc.* 232 (12): 1818–1824.

21

Neurological Disease of the Pelvic Limb

Lisa Bartner

Department of Clinical Sciences, College of Veterinary Medicine and Biomedical Sciences, Colorado State University, Fort Collins, CO, USA

21.1 Introduction

Dogs with monoparesis and/or neurogenic lameness are frequently presented to the veterinary practitioner, although less commonly so than those with spinal cord conditions. It is important to recognize and differentiate these neurologic deficits from orthopedic lameness since the causes, treatment, and prognosis often differ greatly. Clinical signs of neurologic gait abnormalities can be challenging to differentiate from lameness derived from orthopedic origin and therefore are the focus of this chapter. Table 21.1 outlines common differential diagnoses and diagnostic steps for neurological disease affecting the pelvic limb.

21.2 Relevant Anatomy

Similar to the thoracic limb, the anatomic structures of the nervous system that can be implemented in causing a pelvic limb lameness or monoparesis include the intumescence of the spinal cord and the efferent neuron (i.e. motor nerve) and all its constituents. The lumbosacral intumescence is located within the central nervous system (CNS) and is composed of spinal cord segments L4–S3, with small contributions from L3. The cell body of the efferent neurons is within the intumescence, while the remaining aspects are located in the peripheral nervous system (PNS).

There are seven pairs of lumbar nerves exiting the spinal cord bilaterally, through a similarly numbered intervertebral foramen and caudal to the same numbered vertebra. As the spinal cord courses caudally, each segment is shorter than the vertebral segment and as a result the spinal cord ends around the fifth or sixth vertebral bodies (Figure 4.2). In large dog breeds, this may be more cranially positioned (fifth lumbar vertebra) and in small dogs, this can be located more caudally (e.g. sixth lumbar vertebra). Thus, the entirety of the lumbosacral intumescence lies within the spinal canal between the third and fifth lumbar vertebral bodies (Figure 4.2). For this reason, the last several pairs of spinal nerves extend longer distances within the vertebral canal before exiting their respective intervertebral foramen.

The dorsal nerve root branches exit the foramina and innervate epaxial muscles while the last four or five ventral branches of the lumbar nerves and the ventral rootlets of all sacral nerves join

Table 21.1 Key features of select neurologic diseases causing monoparesis or neurogenic lameness of the pelvic limb.

Disease	Common signalment	Diagnostic test of choice	Clinical presentation and course	Distinguishing exam findings	Treatment	Clinical pearls
Intervertebral disc (IVD) extrusion (Hansen Type I)	Young- to middle-aged adults; chondrodystrophic	History and examination MRI	Acute, progressive, or wax/wane	Depends on severity and location; spinal hyperesthesia common	Depends on clinical signs; conservative or surgical	Common cause of lameness or monoparesis; frequently lateralized and acute
IVD protrusion (Hansen Type II)	Older dogs; non-chondrodystrophic	History and examination MRI	Chronic and usually progressive	Mild to no hyperesthesia	Depends on clinical signs; conservative or surgical	Often occurs in DLSS at L7–S1 and at this location commonly causes lameness or monoparesis; otherwise rarely causes unilateral signs
Fibrocartilaginous Embolism (FCE)	Young to middle-aged, large- and giant-breed	History and examination MRI	Peracute, non-progressive after 24 hours	Usually non-painful and asymmetric signs	Conservative	Common cause of lameness or monoparesis
Degenerative Lumbosacral Stenosis (DLSS)	Older, large-breed dogs (e.g. GSD); males	History and examination MRI CT Radiographs	Usually chronic	Can be vague; urinary/fecal incontinence	Depends on clinical signs, conservative, or surgical	Common cause of monoparesis or lameness especially at L7–S1; foraminal stenosis and Type II IVDH commonly present
Discospondylitis	Medium- to large-breed; male dogs overrepresented	History and examination Radiographs MRI CT	Acute, wax/ wane, or chronic, generally progressive	Hyperesthesia; generally, no or minimal neurologic deficits	Conservative (>12 months antibiotics); surgery only warranted with compression (IVDH, subluxation)	Lameness or monoparesis can be encountered, especially with foraminal stenosis
Neoplasia of the spinal nerve or spinal cord	Older but any age	History and examination Radiographs MRI, CT Electrodiagnostics	Acute or chronic and progressive	Sensory exam (cutaneous testing) and muscle atrophy	Conservative, surgical, and radiation therapy	Common cause of monoparesis or lameness

Peracute = several hours; acute = several days; chronic = weeks or longer.

and form the *lumbosacral plexus*. The lumbar portion of this plexus innervates the cranial and medial muscles and skin of the thigh while the sacral plexus supplies the caudal muscles and skin of the thigh, tarsus, and foot. Because the series of sacrocaudal nerve roots are forming the S1-caudal spinal cord segments and their respective nerves resemble a horse's tail, this portion of the spinal cord and spinal roots is called the *cauda equina*. Thus, the cauda equina is part of the PNS. Injury or disease affecting only the cauda equina will not cause paresis or lameness because of no contribution to the femoral and sciatic nerves.

The major spinal nerve contributions to the lumbosacral plexus are summarized in Table 21.2, though individual variations exist on the actual contributions to the named nerves. The two nerves that would result in a monoparesis are the femoral nerve and the sciatic nerve with its tibial and fibular branches. Clinically significant deficits in the obturator and genitofemoral nerves are rarely reported in dogs. Sensory loss to the skin innervated by the genitofemoral nerve may be appreciated during testing and can further aid in mapping of deficits.

The *femoral nerve* arises predominantly from the fifth lumbar spinal nerves, along with substantial portions from L4 and L6. It is formed within the psoas major muscle and continues caudally, protected within this muscle. Proximally it supplies the psoas major and iliopsoas muscles as well as sending the saphenous nerve before diving between the rectus femoris and vastus medialis. It supplies all four heads of the quadriceps (rectus femoris, vastus medialis, vastus intermedius, and vastus lateralis) and therefore plays the major role in extending the stifle. Consequently, injury to this nerve will result in inability to support body weight in the affected limb(s); when the dog attempts to bear weight on the limb, the stifle will passively flex. The saphenous branch of the femoral nerve innervates the skin on the medial surface of the foot, stifle, and thigh.

The *sciatic nerve* (also known as the ischiatic nerve) is a mixed sensory and motor nerve that arises from the spinal cord segments L6, L7, S1, and occasionally S2 and is the extrapelvic continuation of the lumbosacral trunk (the largest part of the lumbosacral plexus). As the nerve exits the plexus, it continues as the sciatic nerve and exits the pelvis caudomedial to the coxofemoral joint, deep to and in between the tuber ischii and the greater trochanter of the femur. It courses distally along the thigh between the semimembranosus and biceps femoris muscles. Branches of the sciatic nerve supply the muscles that extend the hip (biceps femoris, semimembranosus, and semitendinosus), flex the stifle (biceps femoris, semimembranosus, and semitendinosus), and extend the tarsus (biceps femoris). The sciatic nerve divides at the level of the distal femur into fibular (previously called peroneal) and tibial nerves. The *fibular nerve* innervates the muscles that flex the hock (cranial tibial and long digital extensor muscles) and extend the digits (long digital extensor muscle). Therefore, injury to this nerve will result in unopposed extension of the tarsus and knuckling of the digits. The *tibial nerve* supplies the tarsal extensors (gastrocnemius, semitendinosus, and superficial digital flexor muscles) and digital flexors (superficial digital flexor and deep digital flexor muscles). Therefore, injury to this nerve will result in hyperflexion of the hock and plantigrade posture.

21.3 Neurological Diseases Affecting the Pelvic Limb

21.3.1 Myelopathies and Radiculopathies

Unilateral spinal cord lesions caudal to the T2 spinal cord segment (i.e. T3–L3 or L4–S3) can cause pelvic limb monoparesis; however, the quality of paresis will depend on the location of the injury. A lesion at the lumbosacral intumescence affecting the L4–S3 spinal cord segments will result in a lower motor neuron (LMN) paresis and coinciding deficits, while a lesion in the T3–L3 spinal cord

Table 21.2 Summary of the major motor and sensory distribution of the lumbosacral plexus.

Nerve	Spinal cord segments	Muscle innervated	Motor function	Cutaneous sensory zone	Segmental spinal reflex	Signs of dysfunction
Sciatic	L6, L7, S1, S2	Biceps femoris, gastrocnemius, cranial tibial, semitendinosus, and semimembranosus	Extension of hip, extension and flexion of stifle (see tibial and peroneal branches)	Entire limb (via tibial and peroneal branch) except for medial aspect and first digit	Flexor withdrawal reflex (stifle flexion)	Severe gait dysfunction Paw is knuckled, but able to support weight Hip cannot be extended, hock cannot flex or extend (in more proximal lesions, hip is flexed and drawn toward the midline) Absent flexor reflex Loss of cutaneous sensation distal to stifle (except for areas supplied by saphenous nerve)
Fibular (peroneal) branch of the sciatic nerve	L6, L7, S1, S2	Tarsal flexors and digital extensors	Flexion of hock and extension of digits	Dorsal aspect of metatarsus and paw	Cranial tibial reflex and withdrawal reflex (hock flexion)	Hock is straightened, and foot tends to knuckle Poor hock flexion on flexor reflex Loss of sensation on cranial surface distal to stifle
Tibial branch of the sciatic nerve	L6, L7, S1, S2	Tarsal extensors and digital flexors	Extension of hock and flexion of digits	Plantar aspect of metatarsus and paw	Gastrocnemius reflex	Hock is dropped Loss of sensation on caudal surface of limb distal to stifle
Femoral	L3, L4, L5, L6	Quadriceps group and psoas group	Extension of stifle and flexion of hip	Medial aspect of thigh and paw, first digit	Patellar reflex	Severe gait dysfunction Non-weight-bearing Decreased or absent patellar reflex Anesthesia in medial limb and medial digit
Obturator	L4, L5, L6	Adductors	Adduction of pelvic limb	None	None	Little gait abnormality Abduction on slick surface
Genitofemoral	L3, L4	None	None	Proximal aspect of the medial thigh and pudendal region	None	Loss of sensation medial thigh

region will produce a bilateral upper motor neuron (UMN)-paresis (i.e. paraparesis) with general proprioceptive (GP) ataxia (Chapter 4). Sensory deficits usually accompany motor deficits. If the injury is at the level of the intumescence, multiple spinal cord segments are typically involved in most cases, causing a polyneuropathy.

21.3.1.1 Neoplasia

Tumors affecting the nervous system of the pelvic limb, either at the intumescence or the nerves, commonly cause pelvic limb monoparesis. For any lameness that does not quickly respond to empirical therapy, such as anti-inflammatory medications, neurologic conditions should be considered. Particularly in older animals, neoplasia is a common differential diagnosis (Chapter 11).

21.3.1.2 Spinal Cord Injury

Hansen Types I and II intervertebral disc herniation (IVDH), acute non-compressive nucleus pulposus extrusion (ANNPE), and fibrocartilaginous embolism (FCE) are also frequent causes of myelopathies and radiculopathies affecting the pelvic limbs. The clinical features of these diseases are discussed in Chapter 16. Vertebral fracture and luxation (VFL) in the lumbar spine constitute almost one-third of all VFL (Jeffery 2010). Multisite VFL also occurs with some frequency. In contrast to thoracolumbar IVDH, prognosis is grave if nociception is absent secondary to VFL.

Degenerative myelopathy (DM) can result in LMN paralysis but only with longer disease duration (Coates and Wininger 2010). The classic presentation of DM is a slow and progressive clinical course with asymmetric signs localizing to the T3–L3 spinal cord segments. Thus, it would not be a differential for monoparesis or lameness.

21.3.1.3 Degenerative Lumbosacral Stenosis and Foraminal Stenosis

In degenerative lumbosacral stenosis (DLSS; also called lumbosacral disease, lumbosacral instability, and cauda equina syndrome), stenosis results from chronic bony and/or soft tissue proliferation, especially Type II IVD protrusion, reducing the size of the spinal canal and/or intervertebral foramen, with resulting compression, inflammation, or entrapment of the cauda equina and/or seventh lumbar nerve as it exits, respectively (De Risio et al. 2000). This is a disease of older, large-breed, working dogs, especially the German Shepherd Dog, with a predilection for males. The L7–S1 intervertebral disc (IVD) is the most commonly affected site, but any site from L5 to S3 can be affected. Stenosis of the intervertebral foramen, called foraminal stenosis, can also occur anywhere in the lumbar spine but is most prevalent at the L7–S1 and is frequently a component of DLSS. The resulting nerve entrapment is a common cause of pelvic limb lameness or monoparesis. Clinical signs will be dependent on the specific nerves roots or spinal nerves affected. Dogs usually present for vague pelvic limb problems such as trouble rising, reluctance to jump, difficulty climbing stairs, lameness, and pain which can be ambiguous. Lameness is reported commonly and may be intermittent, shifting, unilateral, or bilateral. Regional pain, either occurring spontaneously or detected during physical examination, is common and, occasionally, may be the only historical problem. Care should be taken to differentiate discomfort on vertebral extension from hip extension. Applying digital pressure over the lumbosacral junction (Figure 20.8 and Video 3.1) and extending the lumbosacral junction by lifting the pelvis while pressing on the lumbar vertebrae (lordosis test) are two specific methods of assessing lumbosacral pain. Extension or traction of the tail and palpation of the lumbosacral joint on rectal examination are other methods. Careful assessment of pain responses during hip palpation and extension is required to identify coxofemoral disease (Chapter 20). If other neurologic deficits such as limb, tail, or anal sphincter paresis are apparent, a tentative diagnosis of DLSS can be based on these findings. Fecal and/or urinary incontinence may be historically reported.

Radiography is of some benefit, though, it rarely provides enough information to define or even diagnose DLSS. Many clinically normal older dogs will have degenerative abnormalities on radiographs, like spondylosis. However, conventional radiographs are indicated in patients having signs consistent with DLSS, as part of a complete workup. Special attention should be paid to the vertebrae (e.g. L7–S1 orientation, ventral spondylosis, erosive bony changes, facet changes, end plate sclerosis or osteophytes, and intervertebral foramen size and shape), hips (conformation and osteophyte presence), and intrapelvic structures (lymphadenopathy, prostate and colon/rectal abnormalities, and bladder or urethral stones).

Advanced imaging studies are necessary to define and diagnose DLSS, with MRI being preferred to CT for soft tissue detail and three-dimensional analysis of anatomy. Images may show impingement of the cauda equina and/or L7 nerve(s) from a central vertebral canal lesion (IVD protrusion), foraminal protrusion, or dorsal interarcurate ligamentous compression. However, this does not rule out the potential for disease elsewhere in the pelvic limbs, nor does it prove the compression is causing the clinical signs. Similar to radiographs, many older dogs that are apparently normal can have degenerative changes in the lumbosacral region. Furthermore, the apparent severity of cauda equina compression does not correlate with the severity of clinical signs. Electrodiagnostics can support diagnosis of a nerve disorder. Consequently, a final diagnosis of DLSS must be based on historical and clinical presentation combined with neuroimaging findings.

Conservative management is generally pursued for mild cases; surgical decompression may be warranted in more severe cases or those that fail medical management. Fecal and urinary incontinence should insight urgency in considering surgical decompression, as chronicity carries a poor prognosis in reversing these clinical signs.

21.3.1.4 Discospondylitis

Discospondylitis and associated osteomyelitis are typically bacterial (and less commonly fungal or algal) infections that begin either at the cartilaginous end plates of the vertebral bodies and spread to the IVD or remain confined to the vertebra, respectively (Thomas 2000). The L7–S1 disc space is most commonly affected, but other spaces including those affecting the thoracic limbs can be involved. Discospondylitis affects large, middle-aged dogs most commonly, especially those used for hunting, and male dogs outnumber females by about two to one.

Most patients affected with discospondylitis present with clinical symptoms associated with spinal pain (e.g. decreased activity and unwillingness to jump). Other nonspecific clinical signs include fever, weight loss, and anorexia. Presentation can be peracute or can wax and wane. Lameness can be part of the presenting signs and may be unilateral or bilateral but more commonly affects the pelvic limbs. Chronic discospondylitis can cause a myelopathy or radiculopathy if the infection extends into the surrounding soft tissues (e.g. muscles and ligaments). This can lead to IVDH or instability resulting in vertebral subluxation.

With vague clinical signs, discospondylitis is notoriously difficult to diagnose. Imaging is critical to establish the diagnosis of discospondylitis. Radiography (Figure 21.1A-C) is usually diagnostic (Ruoff et al. 2018). However, radiographic abnormalities may not appear until two to six weeks after onset of infection. Thus, normal spinal radiographs do not rule out a diagnosis of discospondylitis. Nevertheless, radiographs are warranted in a dog presenting with poorly localizable pain, paraspinal pain, and minimal to no neurologic deficits including lameness. Sedated radiographs of the entire vertebral column are recommended. In one study, 40% of dogs had multiple lesions at diagnosis and in almost 20% of cases, the number of affected disc spaces increased during the course of treatment (Burkert et al. 2005). The earliest radiographic signs of discospondylitis appear as subtle irregularity of the vertebral end plates. The IVD space may be narrowed due to destruction of the disc. As the infection progresses, lysis of the vertebral end plates and osteolysis of adjacent vertebral bodies becomes more pronounced. As bone regeneration occurs, there will be a variable amount of sclerosis adjacent to the lytic regions. Because radiographic abnormalities are often delayed, establishing a diagnosis may require advanced imaging (CT, MRI, or nuclear imaging). Alternatively, serial radiographs may be appropriate, particularly if positive culture results support the tentative diagnosis of discospondylitis.

Identification of the infectious agent is important to determine appropriate treatment. Prior to initiation of antibiotic therapy, urine and blood culture samples should be obtained. A thorough physical examination is also important to detect other sites of infection, such as bacterial endocarditis, prostatitis, skin, teeth, and ear canals. Combining bacterial cultures of urine and blood is thought to provide the greatest chance in isolating the causal organism and infection by multiple agents is reported. Testing for *Brucella canis* is critical from a zoonotic standpoint. More invasive techniques have been used such as fluoroscopically guided percutaneous needle aspiration of the IVD and surgical biopsies with variable success.

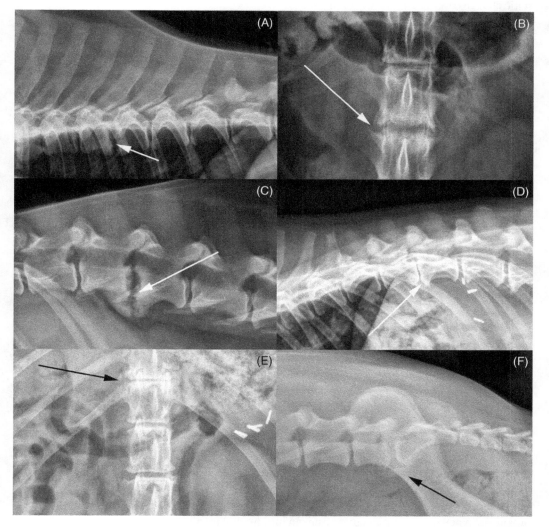

Figure 21.1 Survey spinal radiographic studies: (A–C) Lateral and ventrodorsal survey radiographic images of a dog with discospondylitis displaying vertebral end plate lysis of (A) thoracic and (B, C) lumbar vertebral bodies. (D, E) Lateral and ventrodorsal survey radiographic studies of a dog with a narrowed disc space secondary to IVDH. (F) Lateral radiograph demonstrating spondylosis deformans. Note that typically these degenerative changes alone do not indicate clinical relevance.

Treatment of discospondylitis most commonly involves pain management and long-term antibiotic therapy (typically 12–24 months). Since relapse is very common following cessation of antibiotics, follow-up diagnostic imaging is suggested prior to stopping therapy. There is no published data to guide the best method in decision-making for discontinuation of treatment. Serial radiographs performed until there is no evidence of disease has been recommended by some authors. Radiographic markers of quiescence used include absence of the lytic focus, smoothing and then loss of the lytic focus, and replacement by bridging of the involved vertebrae. However, it can be difficult to differentiate discospondylitis from normal healing processes, as well as degenerative end plate changes or new infection superimposed with degenerative spinal disease. Nuclear imaging, MRI, and CT have all been used for monitoring disease resolution and may be more reliable, but with limitations, including general anesthesia requirements, expense, and availability. The author typically performs radiographs at three- to six-week intervals until there is evidence of static changes over at least three serial studies.

21.3.2 Neuropathies (Nerves and Lumbosacral Plexus)

21.3.2.1 Sciatic Nerve Injury

The anatomic location of the sciatic nerve makes it particularly subject to injury from lumbosacral fractures and subluxations, lumbosacral stenosis, and pelvic or femoral fractures. The proximal portion of the nerve can be damaged by fractures of the ilium, acetabulum, and proximal femur. Iatrogenic injury can occur during surgical procedures (e.g. retrograde intramedullary pin placement in the femur, suture entrapment during hernia repair). More distal portions of the sciatic nerve (i.e. the fibular or tibial nerves along the caudal aspect of the femur) can incur injury from intramuscular injections given in the caudal thigh or distal femoral fractures. Less commonly, severe hip dysplasia can be associated with sciatic nerve damage (Sorjonen et al. 1990).

Clinical signs will depend on the location of the injury. Traumatic injuries to the lumbosacral region rarely result in a mononeuropathy since axons forming other nerves, such as pelvic, pudendal, and caudal nerves, are also injured. If there is damage to the nerve fibers in the spinal canal, at the level of the cord, then the injury and deficits will usually be bilateral. Lesions at, or proximal to, the lumbosacral trunk will result in complete loss of sciatic nerve function as well as signs of fibular and/or tibial nerve dysfunction where the patient will be unable to extend the hip, flex the stifle, or flex and extend the hock and digits. The animal will be able to extend the stifle and thus bear weight on the limb since femoral nerve function is intact but may stand or walk on the dorsum of the foot "knuckled over" or otherwise assume a plantigrade stance. Sensation will be compromised laterally (fibular nerve), caudally (tibial nerve), and dorsally (fibular nerve) but preserved medially from the intact saphenous branch of the femoral nerve. The withdrawal reflex is weak or absent with lack of flexion in the stifle, hock, and digits, especially with stimulation of the lateral digits. Stimulation of the medial digits might still elicit a conscious response and flexion of the hip due to femoral innervation. Severe pain may occur with nerve entrapment and self-mutilation may be an accompanying sign.

Treatment will vary with the cause and severity of the neuropathy but at minimum should include intense physiotherapy and adequate skin care. Nerve regeneration following iatrogenic injury is determined by the degree of injury (Chapter 16), with crushing injuries having a worse prognosis. When due to impingement from an intramedullary pin, removal of the pin usually leads to clinical improvement. Prognosis depends on the severity of injury making careful assessment of both sensory and motor function crucial to determine distribution and nerve involvement. Most injuries are neuropraxic and will often resolve in one to two months. Cutaneous sensation is typically preserved in these cases and supports a better prognosis. However, markedly decreased or absence of pain perception suggests severe injury. Similar to brachial plexus injuries, limb amputation may need to be considered if self-mutilation or injury from dragging the limb occurs.

21.3.2.2 Fibular (Peroneal) Nerve Injury

The fibular nerve is most susceptible to injury as it crosses the lateral aspect of the stifle joint. Injury to the fibular nerve can occur as a result from a damaging insult to the lateral aspect of the stifle; this can occur with trauma, surgery (such as lateral suture placement for cranial cruciate ligament rupture), or inadvertent intraneural injections.

Clinically affected animals will have weak hock flexion, the hock may be overextended, and the foot may also "knuckle over." There will be decreased cutaneous sensation on the dorsal surface of the paw and cranially overlying the hock and tibia; however, the dorsal surface of the foot does not tend to get as ulcerated as with more proximal sciatic nerve lesions. Most dogs learn to accommodate by greater flexion at the hip and extension at the stifle giving the impression of a "high-stepping gait" and the classic "sciatic gait" (Video 21.1). This must not be confused with hypermetria associated with cerebellar ataxia or the overreaching stride sometimes seen in GP ataxia (Chapter 4). Hock flexion will be severely decreased during testing of the withdrawal reflex and the conscious response will be diminished with stimulation to the dorsal aspect of the foot or digits; if the plantar surface of the digits is pinched (tibial nerve), then the animal will have a conscious response (afferent arm of the reflex) but the flexor reflex will be reduced (efferent arm of the reflex). Proprioceptive deficits are usually present.

Video 21.1:

Fibular nerve injury gait (sciatic gait).

Treatment and prognosis are variable depending on cause and severity as for other injuries. Removal of inappropriately placed sutures usually results in improvement and therefore should be performed immediately if severe pain is noted after stifle surgery (lateral suture).

21.3.2.3 Tibial Nerve Injury

Tibial nerve injury is less common than fibular nerve injury but can occur secondary to similar causes. In most animals, tibial nerve injuries occur together with fibular nerve lesions. Animals presenting with pure tibial nerve injury will display loss of hock extension, loss of sensation on the plantar surface of the paw, and proprioceptive deficits. The hock is dropped when the dog walks or when weight is supported on the limb. Trophic ulceration on the plantar surface can occur. The flexor withdrawal reflex is decreased when the plantar surface of the paw is stimulated but may be present when the dorsal surface is pinched. Dogs with tibial nerve dysfunction alone can usually accommodate well, and therefore treatment is conservative in most cases. Pantarsal arthrodesis and/or the use of orthotic devices may be helpful in those animals who do not improve. If sensory function remains intact, then the animal has a fairly good prognosis and conservative treatment is recommended. The presence of sensory deficits (decreased or absent nociception) carries a more guarded to poor prognosis.

21.3.2.4 Femoral Nerve Injury

Femoral nerve injuries are less common than those of the sciatic nerve, largely because of better protection afforded by the sublumbar and quadriceps musculature. Unilateral lesions restricted to the ventral gray matter of the L4–L6 segments can result in femoral neuropathy. Injury can be associated with trauma, iliopsoas myopathies (Stepnik et al. 2006), retroperitoneal abscess, hematoma, neoplasia, and positioning in ventral recumbency during surgery (i.e. extreme extension of the hips).

Clinical features with femoral nerve injury are distinct. They include severe monoparesis, with a loss of the ability to extend the stifle to allow for weight-bearing. The limb may be carried or may collapse when weight is placed on it and the patellar reflex will be reduced or absent. However, the flexor withdrawal reflex is almost normal, except there may be decreased flexion of the hip. With complete support, proprioceptive placement will be normal, although the hopping postural reaction will be greatly diminished because the dog will be unable to support weight on the affected limb. Rapid neurogenic atrophy becomes apparent in the quadriceps muscles and cutaneous sensation may be lost to the medical aspect of the limb and medial digits, regions of sensory innervation by the saphenous branch of the femoral nerve.

Generally speaking, lesions closer to the muscle innervated carry a more favorable prognosis than those more proximal. Treatment recommendations and prognosis are as described in Section 21.3.2.1. If there is no improvement seen in three months, recovery is unlikely; amputation may need to be considered.

21.3.3 Myopathies and Junctionopathies

Myopathies and junctionopathies can begin as shifting leg lameness or stiff gait, sometimes affecting the pelvic limbs before the thoracic. Idiopathic polymyositis is the most common example; others include endocrine and infectious myopathies. Junctionopathies refer to conditions altering the neuromuscular junction, with myasthenia gravis being the most reported and investigated. In most cases, these conditions are characterized by pain, generalized weakness/paresis, exercise intolerance, and/or stiff and stilted gait. Clinical signs are typically bilaterally symmetric but can occasionally demonstrate a shifting or unilateral leg lameness, particularly in the early stages. Many times, spinal reflexes are normal, discerning these from spinal cord diseases. Distinguishing features that point towards these PNS disorders rather than orthopedic disease include gait abnormalities that worsen with activity, neurogenic muscle atrophy, and elevated muscle enzyme levels, and electrodiagnostic abnormalities.

Serum muscle enzyme levels, including creatine kinase (CK), lactate dehydrogenase, and aspartate aminotransferase, may be significantly elevated in inflammatory conditions like myositis. Myoglobinuria may be detected with inflammatory myopathies (e.g. idiopathic polymyositis). In cases of endocrine myopathies, such as hyperadrenocorticoid (Cushing's) myopathy, for example, other supportive evidence is usually seen on serum chemistry analysis (e.g. elevated alkaline phosphatase). Total serum protein can be elevated in infectious myositis due to the presence of increased β- and γ-globulins. Electrodiagnostic tests can be used to confirm that PNS disease is present, but they will usually not diagnose the specific condition. However, in most cases, muscle and nerve biopsy samples are required to establish a final diagnosis; these techniques are described in detail elsewhere (Dickinson and Lecouteur 2002; Lecouteur and Williams 2012). Definitive diagnosis of myasthenia gravis relies on detecting serum antibodies to the acetylcholine receptors. If signs of megaesophagus are present, thoracic radiographs are also warranted. Some clinical features aid in deriving a list of differentials. For example, neurogenic, generalized muscle atrophy is a classic characteristic of polymyositis, especially when CK levels are elevated; whereas, dogs affected with myasthenia gravis rarely develop neurogenic muscle atrophy.

Ischemic neuromyopathy in dogs, most commonly caused by aortic thromboembolism (ATE), can have subacute or chronic onset with milder neurologic deficits that can be intermittent, in contrast to cats. Clinical signs usually involve the pelvic limbs and generally present as lameness, knuckling, paresis, or paralysis. Pelvic limb reflexes may be abnormal, and the extremities can be cool and/or painful. Serum CK levels are markedly elevated. Underlying conditions associated with ATE include cardiac disease, neoplasia, renal disease, immune-mediated hemolytic anemia, sepsis, and endocrine disorders (e.g. hypothyroidism and hyperadrenocorticism).

While not a neurologic condition, *fibrotic myopathies* such as quadriceps, gracilis, and/or semitendinosus contracture may be confused with a neurologic condition. They cause classic gait deficits without neurologic deficits (Chapter 20).

21.3.4 Other Neurologic and Spinal Diseases Affecting the Pelvic Limb

Rarely, other inflammatory diseases such as myelitis or meningomyelitis and protozoal neuritis cause acute progressive monoparesis; more typically these are generalized conditions. Some dogs with immune-mediated polyarthritis (IMPA) first present with shifting leg lameness and spinal hyperesthesia (Chapter 16).

Spondylosis deformans, diffuse idiopathic skeletal hyperostosis (DISH), multiple cartilaginous exostosis (MCE), and spinal dural ossification may all affect the pelvic limb. These conditions have been described in Chapter 16.

References

Burkert, B.A., Kerwin, S.C., Hosgood, G.L. et al. (2005). Signalment and clinical features of diskospondylitis in dogs: 513 cases (1980–2001). *J. Am. Vet. Med. Assoc.* 227 (2): 268–275.

Coates, J.R. and Wininger, F.A. (2010). Canine degenerative myelopathy. *Vet. Clin. North Am. Small Anim. Pract.* 40 (5): 929–950.

De Risio, L., Thomas, W.B., and Sharp, N.J.H. (2000). Degenerative lumbosacral stenosis. *Vet. Clin. North Am. Small Anim. Pract.* 30 (1): 111–132.

Dickinson, P.J. and Lecouteur, R.A. (2002). Muscle and nerve biopsy. *Vet. Clin. North Am. Small Anim. Pract.* 32 (1): 63–102.

Jeffery, N.D. (2010). Vertebral fracture and luxation in small animals. *Vet. Clin. North Am. Small Anim. Pract.* 40 (5): 809–828.

Lecouteur, R.A. and Williams, D.C. (2012). Neurodiagnostics. In: *Veterinary Surgery: Small Animal* (eds. K.M. Tobias and S.A. Johnston), 340–356. St. Louis: Elsevier/Saunders.

Ruoff, C.M., Kerwin, S.C., and Taylor, A.R. (2018). Diagnostic imaging of discospondylitis. *Vet. Clin. North Am. Small Anim. Pract.* 48 (1): 85–94.

Sorjonen, D.C., Milton, J.L., Steiss, J.E. et al. (1990). Hip dysplasia with bilateral ischiatic nerve entrapment in a dog. *J. Am. Vet. Med. Assoc.* 197 (4): 495–497.

Stepnik, M.W., Olby, N., Thompson, R.R., and Marcellin-Little, D.J. (2006). Femoral neuropathy in a dog with iliopsoas muscle injury. *Vet. Surg.* 35 (2): 186–190.

Thomas, W.B. (2000). Diskospondylitis and other vertebral infections. *Vet. Clin. North Am. Small Anim. Pract.* 30 (1): 169–182.

22

Neoplastic Conditions of the Pelvic Limb

Bernard Séguin

Department of Clinical Sciences, College of Veterinary Medicine and Biomedical Sciences, Flint Animal Cancer Center, Colorado State University, Fort Collins, CO, USA

22.1   Introduction

Neoplastic conditions of the pelvic limb are similar to those of the thoracic limb though osteosarcoma is less prevalent, and neoplasia of the peripheral nervous system is also less frequently seen. On the other hand, the lumbar area is the most common site for spinal metastasis. Please refer to Chapter 11 for details regarding the diagnostic workup of neoplasia.

22.2   Neoplasia of Specific Regions

22.2.1   Distal Limb Region

Digital and non-digital tumors should be considered as differential diagnoses and the diagnosis and treatment options are the same as for the thoracic limb (Section 17.2.1). Digital squamous cell carcinoma affects the pelvic limb less frequently than the thoracic limb.

22.2.2   Tarsal Region

Similar to the carpus region of the thoracic limb, the lack of soft tissue coverage surrounding the tarsus frequently results in earlier diagnosis of neoplasia of the region since owners may observe a swelling, particularly in short-haired dogs.

In contrast to the thoracic limb, osteosarcoma occurs in the metaphyseal areas of the proximal and distal femur and tibia at a similar rate (Brodey et al. 1963). Therefore, the maxim "osteosarcoma stays close to the stifle," meaning osteosarcoma is more common in the distal femur and proximal tibia and rare in the distal tibia and proximal femur, is not true. In fact, if a bone tumor of the distal tibia is diagnosed, it is most likely an osteosarcoma. The diagnostic approach and treatment is similar to primary bone tumors of the distal radius. Limb-sparing techniques for primary bone tumors are not well developed for the pelvic limb, and full limb amputation is most frequently performed as a treatment.

22.2.3   Stifle Region

Osteosarcoma is frequently diagnosed in the distal femur and proximal tibia (Figure 22.1). While osteosarcoma may occur independently, there is an ongoing discussion about a possible association with Tibial Plateau Leveling Osteotomy (TPLO) surgery. Explanations for this possible association include corrosion of the bone plate or local infection leading to an altered local cellular activity (Selmic et al. 2018). Implants that are not meeting the current regulatory standards (such as cast TPLO plates which are not sold anymore) are associated with an increased metal ion release when

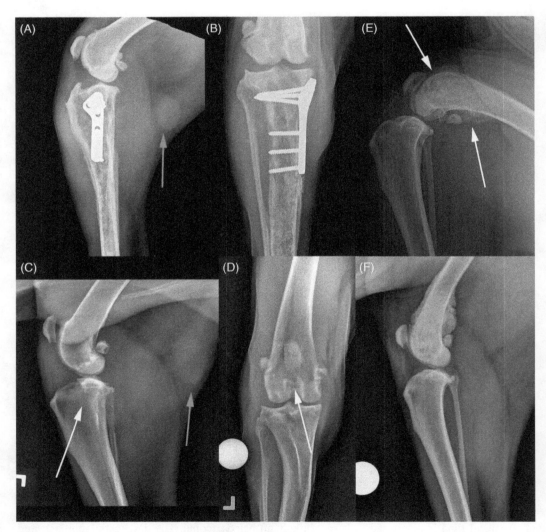

Figure 22.1   Radiographs of stifle joint neoplasia associated with (A, B) proximal tibial osteosarcoma, (C, D) histocytic sarcoma, and (E, F) distal femoral osteosarcoma: (A) lateral and (B) craniocaudal radiographs of a dog that developed osteosarcoma of the proximal tibia after Tibial Plateau Leveling Osteotomy (TPLO). Note the enlarged popliteal lymph node (red arrow); (C) lateral and (D) craniocaudal radiographs of the stifle joint with histiocytic sarcoma and an enlarged popliteal lymph node (red arrow). Note the severe soft tissue opacity in the stifle joint and subtle lysis of the proximal tibia, fibula, and intercondylar fossa of the femur (white arrows); (E) lateral radiograph at time of initial presentation and at (F) follow-up showing progression of the osteolytic and proliferative changes classic for distal femoral osteosarcoma.

compared to forged plates (i.e. currently used TPLO plates). This corrosion-related increased ion release may place patients at risk of tumor development (Sprecher et al. 2018). The risk of developing osteosarcoma after TPLO has been described to be very low. Sartor et al. (2014) retrospectively evaluated 2464 dogs with at least one-year follow-up after TPLO. In that study, 11 dogs developed osteosarcoma at the TPLO site (0.4% incidence) and 29 dogs developed osteosarcoma at a different site (1.2%). The authors calculated incidence density rates of OSA at the TPLO site to be between 10.2 and 30.4 per 10 000 dog-years at risk. Interestingly, all dogs that developed osteosarcoma at the TPLO site had cast TPLO plates implanted (Sartor et al. 2014). In a more recent matched case-control study, dogs that had received a TPLO in the last year were 40 times as likely to develop proximal tibial osteosarcoma as were dogs with no history of TPLO (Selmic et al. 2018). Unfortunately, the type of implant was not disclosed in that study. Regardless, proximal tibial osteosarcoma should be considered as a differential after TPLO which can easily be diagnosed with radiographs.

Presence of the classic findings of cranial cruciate ligament rupture, such as joint effusion and cranial drawer, do not rule out the possibility of neoplasia (Lahmers et al. 2002). While extremely rare, it is possible that stifle instability is secondary to neoplasia rather than due to degeneration. Several tumors of the stifle joint have been described. Specifically, the stifle is one of the three most common joints to develop periarticular histiocytic sarcoma. Villonodular synovitis has also been described in the stifle region of two dogs, one of which was bilateral (Marti 1997). Lymphoma of the synovium of the stifle joint has been reported in one dog (Lahmers et al. 2002).

Unfortunately, joint fluid analysis cannot be used to reliably diagnose stifle neoplasia and even in the case of synovial lymphoma, it failed to provide the diagnosis (Lahmers et al. 2002). Additionally, because radiographic abnormalities may be subtle, a biopsy is required to establish a diagnosis.

22.2.4 Hip Region

Osteosarcoma is the most common bone tumor of the proximal femur. Osseous tumors of the pelvis or soft tissue tumors of the pelvic canal can also cause a lameness. Lipomas in the inguinal area rarely cause a lameness unless they become large enough to interfere with normal range of motion. Another type of lipoma rarely associated with lameness is the intermuscular lipoma, which is typically encountered in the thigh region. This lipoma grows between the muscle bellies of the thigh, particularly those of the caudal thigh, and unlike the infiltrative lipoma does not invade the muscle bellies. Villonodular synovitis has also been described in the hip region of one dog (Kusba et al. 1983).

The rectal exam is an essential part to detect neoplasia of the hip region since it can reveal tumors of the pelvic canal or the pelvis (mostly caudal aspect, depending on the size of the dog and length of the finger of the examiner). Because of the large muscles surrounding the hip area, subtle lesions of the bones can be more easily missed on radiographs. Therefore, computed tomography is frequently used since it is more sensitive to show both soft tissue and bone pathology. Fine-needle aspirates and biopsies in this area frequently require imaging guidance. When tumors of the femoral neck or head are treated by amputation, an acetabulectomy en bloc is recommended.

22.2.5 Nervous System

Neoplastic diseases affecting the nervous system of the pelvic limb are similar to those of the thoracic limb (Chapter 17). Peripheral nerve sheath tumors can affect any component of the peripheral nervous system, but they are less commonly observed in the lumbosacral area compared to the

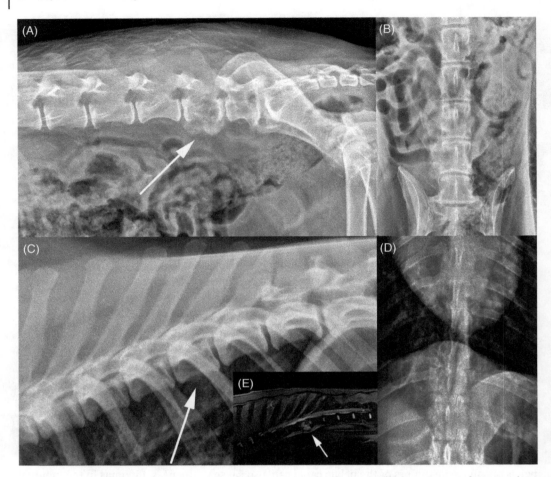

Figure 22.2 Vertebral tumors: (A) lateral and (B) ventrodorsal radiographs illustrate a case of metastatic anal gland adenocarcinoma affecting the sixth lumbar vertebrae (white arrow) that is easily visible on the lateral radiographs; (C) lateral and (D) ventrodorsal radiographs of a vertebral body mass that is easily missed on radiographs (white arrow indicates faint periosteal reaction), but clearly visible on (E) MRI.

cervicothoracic area (Brehm et al. 1995). On the other hand, the lumbar area is the most common site for spinal metastasis of tumors from other anatomic locations and therefore any diagnosis of neoplasia should trigger thorough staging of the patient (Figure 22.2).

Specific to the pelvic limbs, spinal cord blastoma (also called ependymoma, medulloepithelioma, neuroepithelioma, and nephroblastoma) has been described in young, large-breed dogs, especially German Shepherds and Retrievers. Liebel et al. (2011) located the tumor consistently between T9 and L2 and found that cytoreductive surgery improved survival time.

References

Brehm, D., Vite, C., Steinberg, H. et al. (1995). A retrospective evaluation of 51 cases of peripheral nerve sheath tumors in the dog. *J Am Anim Hosp Assoc* 31 (4): 349–359.

Brodey, R.S., Sauer, R.M., and Medway, W. (1963). Canine bone neoplasms. *J Am Vet Med Assoc* 143: 471–495.

Kusba, J.K., Lipowitz, A.J., Wise, M., and Stevens, J.B. (1983). Suspected villonodular synovitis in a dog. *J Am Vet Med Assoc* 182 (4): 390–392.

Lahmers, S.M., Mealey, K.L., Martinez, S.A. et al. (2002). Synovial T-cell lymphoma of the stifle in a dog. *J Am Anim Hosp Assoc* 38 (2): 165–168.

Liebel, F.-X., Rossmeisl, J.H., Lanz, O.I., and Robertson, J.L. (2011). Canine spinal nephroblastoma: long-term outcomes associated with treatment of 10 cases (1996–2009). *Vet Surg* 40 (2): 244–252.

Marti, J.M. (1997). Bilateral pigmented villonodular synovitis in a dog. *J Small Anim Pract* 38 (6): 256–260.

Sartor, A.J., Ryan, S.D., Sellmeyer, T. et al. (2014). Bi-institutional retrospective cohort study evaluating the incidence of osteosarcoma following tibial plateau levelling osteotomy (2000–2009). *Vet Comp Orthop Traumatol* 27 (5): 339–345.

Selmic, L.E., Ryan, S.D., Ruple, A. et al. (2018). Association of tibial plateau leveling osteotomy with proximal tibial osteosarcoma in dogs. *J Am Vet Med Assoc* 253 (6): 752–756.

Sprecher, C.M., Milz, S., Suter, T. et al. (2018). Retrospective analysis of corrosion and ion release from retrieved cast stainless steel tibia plateau leveling osteotomy plates in dogs with and without peri-implant osteosarcoma. *Am J Vet Res* 79 (9): 970–979.

Glossary

Name	Definition
Amble	Accelerated walk, maintaining the four-beat gait pattern
Apophysis	The site of a tendon or ligament attachment, such as the tibial tuberosity, that does not contribute to a joint; compare to epiphysis
Arthrokinematics	Joint surface movement, i.e. small amplitude movements of the bones at the joint surface such as roll, glide, spin; compare to osteokinematics
Ataxia	Failure of coordinated muscle movement; arises from disease affecting the spinal cord, cerebellum, or vestibular system
Axon	An elongated extension of the nerve cell that carries nerve impulses; a nerve fiber
Cauda Equina	Sacral and caudal spinal nerve roots
Central nervous system	The part of the nervous system comprising the brain and spinal cord
Concentric contraction	Shortening of a muscle during contraction – this happens when the force generated by the muscle is large enough to overcome the resistance, e.g. flexion of the elbow joint during biceps contraction (such as when lifting a glass of water from the table); compare to eccentric/isometric contraction
Crepitus	Grinding or grating sensation or sound that is caused by severe degeneration of the joint or intra-articular fractures
Diaphysis	Main (central or long part) of the bone; compare to metaphysis
Dimelia	Duplication of the whole or part of limb
Dysostoses	Constitutional bone diseases characterized by abnormal development of individual bones or parts of bones (such as ectrodactyly)
Eccentric contraction	Lengthening of a muscle during contraction – this happens when the force generated by the muscle is less than the resistance, e.g. extension of the elbow joint during biceps contraction (such as when lowering a glass of water to the table); compare to concentric/isometric contraction
Ectrodactyly	Congenital split formation (separation) between metacarpal bones
Encephalopathy	Brain disease/pathology
End-feel	Subjective description of the sensation that the observer experiences at the end of joint range of motion
Epiphysis	The end of a bone that contributes to a joint

(Continued)

Canine Lameness, First Edition. Edited by Felix Michael Duerr.
© 2020 John Wiley & Sons, Inc. Published 2020 by John Wiley & Sons, Inc.
Companion website: www.wiley.com/go/duerr/lameness

(Continued)

Name	Definition
Flaccid paresis	Paresis with decreased muscle tone (i.e. loss of muscle "power"). Flaccid paresis is indicative of an LMN lesion; compare to spastic paresis
Flexibility	Evaluation of muscle extensibility, i.e. the ability of the muscle to stretch or passively elongate when an external manual force is applied
Ganglion	Collection of nerve cell bodies in the PNS (i.e. the spinal ganglia is in the dorsal nerve root of spinal nerves; previously called dorsal root ganglia)
General proprioception	The sense of the relative position of parts of the body; muscle and joint position and movement, tactile input from the body, limbs, and head
Goniometry	Measurement of (joint) angles
Hamstrings	Caudal thigh muscles originating from the ischial tuberosity, i.e. the biceps femoris, semitendinosus, and semimembranosus (and abductor cruris caudalis) muscles
Hemimelia	Congenital absence of a part or all of one or more bones
Horner syndrome	Combination of clinical signs related to deficits in sympathetic innervation to the eye: enophthalmos, pupillary constriction (miosis), narrowing of the palpebral fissure (ptosis), and protrusion of the third eyelid. Partial Horner syndrome manifests as ipsilateral miosis due to ipsilateral sympathetic dysfunction
Intumescence	Normal spinal cord enlargement (cervical and lumbar)
Isometric contraction	Unchanged length of a muscle during contraction – this happens when the force generated by the muscle matches the resistance, e.g. maintaining the joint angle of the elbow joint during biceps contraction (such as when holding a glass of water); compare to concentric/eccentric contraction
Junctionopathies	Pathology of the neuromuscular junction
Kinematic gait analysis	The evaluation of motion throughout the complete gait cycle, frequently focused on joint angle evaluation
Kinetic gait analysis	Evaluates the forces produced when an animal's foot is in contact with the ground
Lameness	In orthopedics defined as a gait abnormality; compare to neurogenic lameness
Lower Motor Neuron	The neurons related to motor function that have their cell bodies in the grey matter of the CNS (brainstem and spinal cord) and axons that exit the CNS as nerves; in the spinal cord, this is via the ventral nerve roots to innervate skeletal muscles of the limb, head, or trunk
Metaphysis	Portion of the bone in between the epiphysis and diaphysis that contains the physis
Mononeuropathy	Disease or injury affecting a single nerve
Multiple mononeuropathies	Dysfunction of multiple (peripheral) nerves in the same limb (e.g. brachial plexus injury)
Myelopathy	Spinal cord disease
Myofascial pain syndrome	Muscle, sensory, motor, and autonomic nervous system symptoms caused by stimulation of myofascial trigger points (MTPs), i.e. myalgia that is characterized by the presence of MTPs
Myofascial trigger point	Discrete, focal, hyperirritable spots located in a taut band of skeletal muscle
Myopathy	Pathology of the muscles
Nerve	A collection of axons in the PNS that is usually grossly visible; Note: since a "nerve" by definition is part of the PNS, it is redundant to say "peripheral nerve"

(Continued)

Name	Definition
Nerve fiber	See axon
Nerve root signature (lameness)	See neurogenic lameness
Neurogenic lameness	Discomfort caused by pathology affecting the nerve roots and/or surrounding meninges (e.g. from a lateralized disc herniation), also frequently referred to as "nerve root signature (lameness)"
Neuron	Nerve cell (i.e. composed of a cell body and the nerve fibers)
Neuropathy	Pathology of the (peripheral) nerves
Osteokinematics	Gross movements of bones at joint (e.g. flexion/extension; abduction/adduction; and supination/pronation); compare to arthrokinematics
Pace	Two-beat, lateral gait in which ipsilateral limb pairs move in synchrony
Paralysis	Complete loss of voluntary motor function resulting in an inability to support weight (i.e. the most severe degree of paresis)
Paraparesis	Paresis of the pelvic limbs; Note: It is redundant to say, *pelvic limb paraparesis*
Paresis	Partial loss of voluntary movement that is due to disruption of the signal transmission from either the level of the upper motor neuron (UMN) or lower motor neuron (LMN). Note that in clinical neurology the term is sometimes used as synonym for weakness
Paronychia	Nonspecific inflammation of the nail/claw fold
Peripheral nervous system	Comprising cell bodies, bilateral spinal nerves arising as dorsal (sensory) and ventral (motor) nerve roots, nerves, neuromuscular junction, and muscle; the nerve cell bodies of the efferent (motor) axons are located in the ventral gray matter and the cell bodies of the afferent (sensory) axons are located in the spinal ganglia
Plegia	Paralysis
Polydactyly	Occurrence of one or more extra digits
Polyneuropathy	Disease or injury of multiple nerves (e.g. polyradiculoneuritis)
Radiculopathy	Nerve root disease
Somatic	Relating to, innervating or involving the voluntary (striated) muscle as opposed to the visceral (involuntary) muscle and its (autonomic innervation)
Spastic paresis	Paresis with increased muscle tone (i.e. inability to initiate gait voluntarily) which is caused by a disruption of signal transmission from the UMN to the LMN. Spastic paresis is indicative of a UMN lesion; compare to flaccid paresis
Spinal nerve	Spinal nerves arise after the fusion of the dorsal and ventral nerve roots at the level of the intervertebral foramen
Stretching	See flexibility
Synapse	Gap connection between one axon terminal and a neuron, muscle, or gland
Syndactyly	Partial or complete lack of separation between adjacent digits
Trigger point	See myofascial trigger point
Upper Motor Neuron	The neurons related to motor function that have their cell bodies in the grey matter of the CNS (cerebrum and brainstem) and axons that synapse on a LMN or interneuron
Weakness	Difficulty initiating gait due to LMN disease; Note: in clinical neurology sometimes used as synonym for paresis; however, weakness can be caused by other diseases

List of Abbreviations

ALD	Angular Limb Deformity
ANNPE	Acute Non-Compressive Nucleus Pulposus Extrusion
CCLD	Cranial Cruciate Ligament Disease
CNS	Central Nervous System
CSM	Cervical Spondylomyelopathy
CT	Computed Tomography
DISH	Diffuse Idiopathic Skeletal Hyperostosis
DJA	Diagnostic Joint Anesthesia
DM	Degenerative Myelopathy
ED	Elbow Dysplasia
FCE	Fibrocartilaginous Embolism
FCU	Flexor Carpi Ulnaris
FVA	Femoral Varus Angle
GP	General Proprioception
HD	Hip Dysplasia
HOD	Hypertrophic Osteodystrophy
IMPA	Immune-Mediated Polyarthritis
IOHC	Incomplete Ossification of The Humeral Condyle
LDE	Long Digital Extensor
LMN	Lower Motor Neuron
MCD	Medial Compartment Disease
MCE	Multiple Cartilaginous Exostoses
MPL	Medial Patellar Luxation
MPS	Myofascial Pain Syndrome
MRI/MR	Magnetic Resonance Imaging
MSI	Medial Shoulder Instability
MTP	Myofascial Trigger Point
OCD	Osteochondrosis/Osteochondritis Dissecans
OGA	Objective Gait Analysis
PNS	Peripheral Nervous System
PROM	Passive Range of Motion
RUIN	Radioulnar Ischemic Necrosis
SH	Salter-Harris

Canine Lameness, First Edition. Edited by Felix Michael Duerr.
© 2020 John Wiley & Sons, Inc. Published 2020 by John Wiley & Sons, Inc.
Companion website: www.wiley.com/go/duerr/lameness

SI	Sacroiliac
TNCC	Total Nucleated Cell Count
TPLO	Tibial Plateau Leveling Osteotomy
TP	Total Protein
UAP	Ununited Anconeal Process
UMN	Upper Motor Neuron

Index

Note: Page numbers in *italics* refer to figures, those in **bold** to tables and inset boxes.